Vitamins
unnecessary
P 376-78

Aids diet to
includes proteins P16

Chocolate 62%
saturated fats
P41

Eggs not
responsible for high
cholesterol which is
due to saturated fats

additives useful in
preserving food &
providing wider range
of foods available P10
in safe quantities

Ageing — men vs woman
P15

Galactose is
inability to convert
to glucose —
avoid meat,
brussel,
carrots
avoid e...

Fibre foods helps
to eliminate
cholesterol P 7B-72

Sugar has
calming effect
o not Hypertension

Liver risky...

D1469695

Rosemary Stanton's
Complete Book of

FOOD AND NUTRITION

For those I love, who have put up with my absence
while this book was being written.

Rosemary Stanton's Complete Book of

FOOD AND NUTRITION

ROSEMARY STANTON

BSc, C. Nut/Diet., Grad. Dip. Admin.

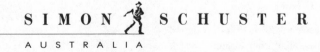

SIMON SCHUSTER

AUSTRALIA

ROSEMARY STANTON'S COMPLETE BOOK OF FOOD
AND NUTRITION

First published in Australasia in 1989 by
Simon & Schuster Australia
7 Grosvenor Place, Brookvale NSW 2100

Reprinted 1989
A division of Paramount Communications Inc.

National Library of Australia
Cataloguing in Publication data
    Stanton, Rosemary.
        Rosemary Stanton's complete book of food and nutrition.

        Includes index.
        ISBN 0 7318 0100 8.
        ISBN 0 7318 0033 8 (pbk.).

        1. Food — Handbooks, manuals, etc. 2. Nutrition. I.
        Title.

    641.1

Designed by Warren Penny
Cover photograph by Jonathan Chester
Illustrations by Fiona Lumsden
Photographs by Jonathan Chester

Typeset in Hong Kong by Setrite Typesetters Limited
Printed in Australia by Australian Print Group

INTRODUCTION

As a nutritionist, I am fascinated by the the interactions of food and health. As a lover of fine food, I am delighted that the food which nourishes and sustains the body can give such joy to the senses.

It is good that many people are beginning to realise that the body needs loving care and attention — including more attention to the foods we feed it — if it is going to give peak performance.

A lot of people are also becoming much more adventurous with the delights of food. Travel, migration and an expanding range of products are providing us with a thirst for more information about the foods we are currently eating or might introduce into our daily fare.

Nutrition is a young science and our knowledge about it has expanded rapidly over the past few years. Yet, until very recently, there has been little or no teaching about this vitally important area of human health. And the questions have been pouring in. Where can you find information about food and nutrition? What's found in various foods? Are they good for you? What are substances such as folacin or omega 3 fatty acids? Where do you find the important nutrients? What are the facts about cholesterol, calcium and carbohydrates? How many calories are there in a croissant? What is a wax jambu? How can you eat to maximise your body's performance?

There are thousands of questions about food and nutrition. This book aims to answer them as far as present knowledge allows. Some entries will be of interest to most people; others will have more limited appeal. I have no doubt that future editions of the book will be necessary as the exciting field of nutrition continues to grow.

The entries in the book have been designed to provide interest and information. No one book could contain information about every dish we eat. The foods which have been included range from raw foods to cooked dishes to menu terms. They have been chosen as items about which someone might want information.

Many topics of popular interest, such as cholesterol, fats, fibre, carbohydrates, protein, vegetarian diets, iron, calcium and vitamins have been given larger entries.

In the sections on major food groups such as fruits, vegetables, nuts, seeds, legumes or seafood, I have tried to include the varieties most likely to be encountered. I hope that you will consult some of these sections to find out about foods which may be new to you.

We do not yet have all the answers on nutrition. We do know that the greater the variety of foods eaten, the more likely it is that the diet will satisfy the body's nutritional needs. Those who try many different foods also know the pleasure to be derived from their eating adventures.

This book provides information which you might not easily find elsewhere. The extensive cross-referencing should make it easy to discover a great deal about both food and nutrition. My hope is that more information will lead to better nutrition as well as greater enjoyment of eating health-giving foods.

Rosemary Stanton

THE AUSTRALIAN NUTRITION FOUNDATION
Weight For Height Chart
(For Men and Women from 18 years onward)
Based on Body Mass Index (BMI) in Range of 18, 20, 25, 30.

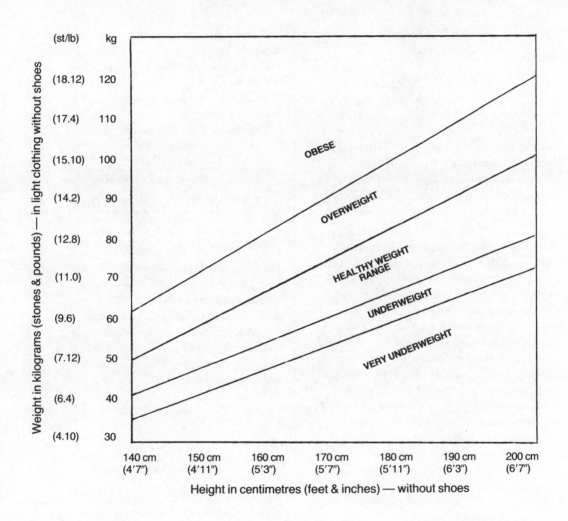

Height in centimetres (feet & inches) — without shoes

A

ABALONE
see Seafood.

ABERDEEN SAUSAGE

A Scottish sausage made by combining minced bacon, minced beef, breadcrumbs and seasoning, tying the mixture into a cloth and cooking in a boiling water bath. When cooked, the sausage is unwrapped, rolled in dried breadcrumbs and heated for a short time in a moderate oven. 100 g have 1145 kJ (275 Cals).

ABORIGINAL DIET

Australian Aborigines once had a rich and varied diet; the popular belief that they lived on a sparse and barely adequate diet is untrue. Most foods were eaten as they were collected and the Aborigines' harmony with their environment ensured a good supply of food. Fruits included bush apples, plums, passionfruit, bananas, tomatoes, gooseberries and quandongs. They also ate roots, tubers, seeds, nuts and the young shoots of plants. From the animal life they ate the well-known witchetty grubs, lizards, goannas, snakes, kangaroos, wallabies, echidnas, fruit bats, emus, many native birds and their eggs as well as freshwater fish, crustaceans and tortoises. Those in coastal areas added turtles, various molluscs and saltwater fish and crocodiles. Bush honey was a prized addition.

Nutritionally, the diet was high in protein and very low in fat. Food is much more than just nourishment to Aborigines. It is something to be shared and this involves complex interactions with relatives and other members of their tribe.

Some Australian Aborigines still eat bush foods. Many of those living in outlying areas are being encouraged to eat the highly nutritious foods they once enjoyed before being introduced to the poorer quality foods of Western civilisation.

See also Bush foods; Insects, Edible.

ABSINTHE
see Drinks, Alcoholic.

ABSORPTION OF NUTRIENTS
see Digestion.

ACACIA

Known as wattles in Australia, acacia trees have some edible parts. The seeds of some varieties can be ground into a flour and used to make bread or pancakes. A gum from acacia is used as gum arabic in confectionery and pharmaceuticals (it dissolves slowly so that drugs combined with it can thus be slowly released into the body).

ACEROLA
see Fruit.

ACESULFAME K
see Artificial sweeteners.

ACETALDEHYDE

A compound which forms when alcohol is oxidised. Has a slightly nutty flavour and a fruity odour and occurs in some sherries, especially fino sherry. Also used to make acetic acid.

ACETIC ACID

An acid produced by the fermentation of

carbohydrates and diluted to form vinegar. Also formed during chemical reactions to produce energy in the body and formed in the large intestine during the fermentation of dietary fibre.

ACETOACETIC ACID

A ketone (see page 197) which results when fats are not being completely burned in the body.

ACETONE

Normally a minor constituent in blood and urine but larger quantities may be produced in untreated diabetes, creating a health hazard. During starvation or fasting, acetone forms from the incomplete burning of fat and can be detected by its odour (rather like nail-polish remover) on the breath. Chemically, acetone is a ketone (see page 197).

ACETYLCHOLINE

A chemical substance needed for the transmission of impulses along nerves. Most acetylcholine is made in the body from choline (see page 73). Contrary to popular belief, taking extra choline, or lecithin (see page 203), which contains choline, will not improve nerve function in normal people.

ACETYLSALICYCLIC ACID

see Aspirin.

ACHLORHYDRIA

A condition where insufficient hydrochloric acid is produced in the stomach. Sometimes occurs with a deficiency of vitamin B_{12} or with cancer of the stomach. Some natural therapists attribute digestive upsets to a lack of acid in the stomach, although there is no evidence that this is the case.

ACIDOPHILUS

A bacterial culture which can be added to milk or yoghurt in the form of *lactobacillus acidophilus*. The culture may be used because it

happens to be available, or in the belief that it will cure intestinal problems and the vaginal yeast infection, candida. The truth of such claims has not been established with properly controlled trials.

ACIDOSIS

A condition in which the normal balance between acid and alkali in the blood is disturbed. May occur in untreated diabetes, in those with some kidney problems, and in starvation. Acidosis does not arise from eating lemons, tomatoes or other acid foods.

ACIDS

A class of chemical compounds with a pH content below 7 (see page 265). Acids generally taste sour. Many of the foods we eat are slightly acid, but there is little need to be concerned about this as the acidity levels in most foods are usually less than the acidity of the stomach (pH of 1.3—3.0). Lemons are fairly acid with a pH of 2; orange juice is pH 3.0 and coffee has a pH of 5.0. After digestion, most foods have an acid residue, the exceptions being plums, prunes and cranberries.

Weak acids are often used to preserve foods: for example vinegar or benzoic acid, sorbic acid or propionic acid are added to vegetables, fruits, dried fruits and breads to stop the growth of micro-organisms, such as bacteria, which would spoil the food.

Acids can also mimic cooking by causing proteins in foods to bond together into a solid mass (that is, to coagulate). For example, fish is often left in lemon juice or vinegar until its protein assumes almost the texture of cooked fish. It can then be eaten without cooking.

ACNE

A condition of pimply eruptions on the skin, commonly accompanying the hormonal changes of adolescence. There is no clear-cut relationship between diet and acne. Some people develop pimples after eating foods such as chocolate; others do not. A substance related to vitamin A is sometimes used to treat acne but vitamin A itself in large doses is too toxic to use. General dietary principles for healthy skin are to drink plenty of water, have a wide variety of fresh fruits and vegetables and avoid fatty foods. Exercise to improve blood flow to the skin is also important.

See also Adolescents and diet; Skin.

ACORNS

see Nuts.

ACTOMYOSIN

Complex filaments which make up muscle fibres of animals (including humans) and are important in muscle contractions. If the muscle fibres in animals are contracted when the animal is killed, the meat will have more actomyosin and will be tougher for eating.

ADAM'S APPLE

As well as being the common term for the epiglottis in the throat, Adam's apple is another name for a lime (see page 148).

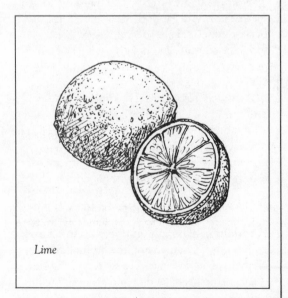

Lime

ADDITIVES, FOOD

The earliest food additives were salt and various chemical substances from smoke. These were followed by honey, spices and vinegar. In the good old days, food additives were also used to dilute and adulterate foods. For example, chalk was once added to flour to make white bread, cheaper chicory went into coffee, and many substances were added to alcoholic drinks. The idea that foods used to be more natural is something of a myth. It is also incorrect to think food additives today are more harmful than ever. With the benefit of scientific research and legislation covering food additives, many of those in use today are much safer than earlier products.

The preservation of foods is the major and legitimate use of food additives. The inclusion of colourings, artificial flavourings and various texture modifiers, has extended the uses which many food manufacturers claim to be 'essential'. It is the use of some of these additives that concerns nutritionists and many consumers.

In general, food additives can be beneficial in providing a wider range of foods to a greater number of people. It is not always food additives themselves which we need fear but more the overconsumption of certain food items containing them.

Many people fear food additives because they are chemicals, a word which often provokes apprehension. This fear is irrational since our bodies and all the natural foods we eat are made up of chemicals.

There is no such thing as a safe food additive; as with everything else we take into our bodies, there are only safe quantities. The use of food additives is controlled in some way in most countries, although many of the controls were imposed years ago when only a fraction of the food supply contained these substances. Tests for the safety of food additives are essential since some used in the past have been found to increase the risk of cancer or other diseases. Most, however, are harmless and more likely hazards exist with well-known food ingredients such as salt, sugar and fats.

Food additives generally fall into the following categories:

Anti-caking agents — stop powdered products from clumping together

Antioxidants — preserve food by controlling spoilage from oxygen reacting with fats or enzymes in foods

Artificial sweeteners — provide sweetness with fewer kilojoules than sugar

Bleaching agents — whiten products such as flour

Colourings — add to or alter colour

Emulsifiers — assist in the mixing of ingredients (usually fats) in foods so that they do not separate

Enzymes — accelerate the conversion of one substance into another

Flavours — enhance or provide particular flavours

Flour treatment agents — stimulate the growth of yeast and also hasten the natural ageing of flour to make it more suitable for breadmaking

Food acids — counteract the extreme sweetness of sugar in products such as soft drinks, control browning in fruits and vegetables, assist jam to gel and enhance the action of other preservatives used

Gums — thicken foods

Humectants — control moisture levels so that foods do not dry out

Minerals — replace those lost during processing

Mineral salts — modify foods by aerating, prevent unpleasant flavours which may come from the natural minerals, such as iron and manganese, present in foods, or increase the amount of water held in a food

Preservatives — control yeasts, moulds and bacteria which would otherwise make foods go bad

Propellants — used in pressurised foods

Thickeners — alter the consistency of foods

Vitamins — replace those lost during processing or add extra quantities

See also individual listings for details on some additives; E numbers; Labels, Food.

See pages 12 and 13 for a list of Australian Approved Additive Numbers.

ADENOSINE TRIPHOSPHATE (ATP)

A compound which carries chemical energy, is stored in every cell in the body and provides the energy for almost every function in the body. When energy is released from the combustion of foods eaten, ATP carries the chemical energy to the cells where it is used for the cell to stay alive. When substances are carried across the membranes of the body cells, or when any muscular work occurs, including the functioning of the heart muscle, ATP supplies the energy.

See also Energy.

ADIPOSE FAT

The correct term for body fat or the body's stored energy depots. Body fat has about 10 per cent water and 85 per cent fat and every kilogram represents an energy store of 30,000 kJ. Typical body fat level in men is around 15 per cent of the body weight; in women a normal level is around 25 per cent.

ADOLESCENTS AND DIET

In Western countries, the adolescent diet tends to be high in fat, sugar, salt and food additives, and lacks complex carbohydrates, dietary fibre and some minerals such as calcium, iron and zinc. Many of the fast foods which teenagers love to eat exacerbate these problems.

(*continued page 14*)

Approved Additive Numbers

The list below shows all the numbers approved by the National Health and Medical Research Council for approved food additives in Australia.

No.	Food Additive
100	Curcumin
101	Riboflavin
102	Tartrazine
107	Yellow 2G
110	Sunset yellow FCF
120	Cochineal, carminic acid
122	Carmoisine
123	Amaranth
124	Brilliant scarlet 4R
127	Erythrosine
132	Indigo carmine
133	Brilliant blue FCF
140	Chlorophylls
142	Green S
150	Caramel
151	Brilliant black BN
153	Carbo medicinalis vegetalis (charcoal)
155	Chocolate brown HT
160	Carotenoids
160(a)	Carotene, alpha-, beta-, gamma-
160(b)	Annatto (bixin, norbixin)
160(e)	Beta-apo-8' carotenal
160(f)	Ethyl ester of beta-apo-8' carotenoic acid
161	Xanthophylls
161(g)	Canthaxanthine
162	Beetroot red, betanin
163	Anthocyanins
170	Calcium carbonate
171	Titanium dioxide
172	Iron oxides and hydroxides
200	Sorbic acid
201	Sodium sorbate
202	Potassium sorbate
203	Calcium sorbate
210	Benzoic acid
211	Sodium benzoate
212	Potassium benzoate
213	Calcium benzoate
220	Sulphur dioxide
221	Sodium sulphite
222	Sodium bisulphite
223	Sodium metabisulphite
224	Potassium metabisulphite
234	Nisin
249	Potassium nitrite
250	Sodium nitrite
251	Sodium nitrate
252	Potassium nitrate
260	Acetic acid
261	Potassium acetate
262	Sodium acetates
263	Calcium acetate
270	Lactic acid
280	Propionic acid
281	Sodium propionate
282	Calcium propionate
283	Potassium propionate
290	Carbon dioxide
296	Malic acid
297	Fumaric acid
300	Ascorbic acid
301	Sodium ascorbate
306	Tocopherol-rich extracts of natural origin
307	Synthetic alpha-tocopherol
308	Synthetic gamma-tocopherol
309	Synthetic delta-tocopherol
310	Propyl gallate
311	Octyl gallate
312	Dodecyl gallate
320	Butylated hydroxy-anisole (BHA)
321	Butylated hydroxy-toluene (BHT)
322	Lecithins
325	Sodium lactate
326	Potassium lactate
327	Calcium lactate
330	Citric acid
331	Sodium citrates
332	Potassium citrates
333	Calcium citrates
334	Tartaric acid
335	Sodium tartrates

336	Potassium tartrates		464	Hydroxypropylmethylcellulose
337	Sodium potassium tartrate		465	Ethylmethylcellulose
339	Sodium orthophosphates		466	Sodium carboxymethylcellulose
340	Potassium orthophosphates		471	Mono- and diglycerides of fatty acids
341	Calcium orthophosphates		472(e)	Mono- and diacetyltartaric acid esters of mono- and diglycerides of fatty acids
350	Sodium malates			
351	Potassium malates		473	Sucrose esters of fatty acids
352	Calcium malates		475	Polyglycerol esters of fatty acids
353	Metatartaric acid		476	Polyglycerol polyricinoleate
354	Calcium tartrate		481	Sodium stearoyl-2-lactylate
355	Adipic acid		482	Calcium stearoyl-2-lactylate
363	Succinic acid		491	Sorbitan mono-stearate
380	Tri-ammonium citrate		500	Sodium carbonates
400	Alginic acid		501	Potassium carbonates
401	Sodium alginate		503	Ammonium carbonates
402	Potassium alginate		504	Magnesium carbonate
403	Ammonium alginate		508	Potassium chloride
404	Calcium alginate		529	Calcium oxide
405	Propylene glycol alginate		536	Potassium ferrocyanide
406	Agar		541	Sodium aluminium phosphate
407	Carrageenan		551	Silicon dioxide
410	Locust bean gum		553(b)	Talc
412	Guar gum		554	Sodium aluminium silicate
413	Tragacanth		558	Bentonite
414	Acacia		559	Kaolins
415	Xanthan gum		570	Stearic acid
416	Karaya gum		572	Magnesium stearate
420	Sorbitol		575	Glucono delta-lactone
421	Mannitol		621	Monosodium glutamate
422	Glycerol		627	Sodium guanylate
433	Polyoxyethylene (20) sorbitan mono-oleate		631	Sodium inosinate
			637	Ethyl maltol
435	Polyoxyethylene (20) sorbitan mono-stearate		900	Dimethylpolysiloxane
			901	Beeswaxes
436	Polyoxyethylene (20) sorbitan tristearate		903	Carnauba wax
			904	Shellac
440(a)	Pectin		905	Paraffins
442	Ammonium phosphatides		920	L-Cysteine and its hydrochlorides
450	Sodium and potassium polyphosphates		924	Potassium bromate
460	Microcrystalline cellulose, powdered cellulose		925	Chlorine
			926	Chlorine dioxide
461	Methylcellulose			

13

During adolescence, the growth spurt increases the need for protein, minerals and most vitamins. Kilojoule needs also increase, although this is usually much greater for boys than for girls. Most girls experience their growth spurt between 11 and 15, while for boys it occurs between 13 and 17. Some boys continue to grow until age 18 or 19. Appetite increases dramatically during periods of rapid growth.

Few teenagers will find their appetites satisfied with only 3 meals a day so snacking is common. Since the body's need for most nutrients increases with kilojoule requirements, snacks should consist of healthy foods such as breads, cereals, fruits, grain-based products, low-fat dairy products, nuts and seeds.

The kind of strict dieting often practised by overweight girls (and many who are not overweight), is not recommended. It can lead to anorexia nervosa (see page 24) or bulimia nervosa (see page 47). Hormone levels can easily be upset when body fat levels drop too low and the extreme thinness which is fashionable among some teenagers often stops menstruation.

Obesity in teenagers is also undesirable. Contrary to popular belief, it is not just puppy fat. More exercise and a concentration on healthy foods which are low in fat and sugar will solve the problem better than a strict diet.

See also Acne.

ADRENAL CORTEX

A part of the kidney which secretes hormones, including the hormone to control the amounts of sodium, potassium and water retained by the body.

ADRENALIN

The chemical which raises blood pressure, stimulates the conversion of liver glycogen and tissue protein to glucose to restore a flagging blood sugar level and increases the breakdown of body fat as an energy source.

ADUKI BEANS
see Legumes.

ADVERTISING AND FOOD

With thousands of foods available, advertising plays an important role in influencing food choice. Unfortunately, only foods with a high-profit margin tend to be advertised, and many of these foods have a high content of added sugars and fats. Fresh foods are advertised to a lesser extent. As a result of advertising, people are being influenced to choose more highly-processed foods with greater quantities of fat, salt, sugar and food additives. Children's eating habits, in particular, are being influenced adversely by the advertising of only a limited range of foods. When did you last see an advertisement for a carrot?

ADVOCAAT
see Drinks, Alcoholic.

AEROBIC ACTIVITY

Activity which requires oxygen. Examples include walking, swimming, running and various sports which depend on continuous activity rather than short sharp bursts. For example, playing hockey is aerobic activity; a single flick stroke from rest is not.

See also Anaerobic activity.

AFLATOXINS

A group of mycotoxins (see page 239) first isolated in 1961 following an outbreak of a disease called turkey X disease which occurred in poultry in the United Kingdom. They commonly occur in peanuts and are a major factor in the development of liver cancer in many developing countries. Awareness of the problem now ensures that peanut crops undergo stringent testing before being sold. Part of this testing involves looking for discolouration on peanuts — a possible sign of the toxins.

See also Aspergillus, Moulds.

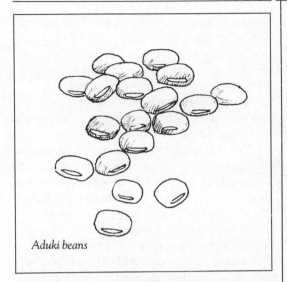

Aduki beans

AGAR-AGAR

A gelatine-like type of dietary fibre made from several varieties of red seaweed. Acts as a clarifying agent in brewing and wine-making and as a thickener in cream, salad dressings, marshmallows, some jellies and desserts. Main production areas include Australia, Japan, New Zealand, the United States and the Soviet Union. Agar is sold in strands or as a powder. It dissolves easily in hot water but will not dissolve in cold solutions.

AGARICUS BISPORUS

see Vegetables, Mushrooms.

AGEING AND DIET

Very little is known about the causes of ageing but various theories are put forward which claim to have the secret to stop the normal ravages of time.

Medical researchers view ageing as the process whereby the arteries become clogged, the bones lose some of their density and the chances of disease increase. The popular view of ageing, however, often ignores the biochemical aspects and concentrates on the avoidance of wrinkles and grey hair.

The length of life for any individual depends on genetic and environmental factors. From the moment of conception, a tiny fertilised egg weighing about one-thousandth of a gram grows and increases about 70 thousand million times into a complex, fully-developed individual.

Once the period of growth ceases, the body begins to go downhill. Little by little the active mass of every body cell is reduced and all body systems are progressively impaired. The loss of body cells occurs faster in men than in women, at least until the menopause. It has been estimated that between the ages of 25 and 65, men lose just over 16 per cent of their active cell mass, while women lose only about 8.5 per cent. These losses affect the heart, lungs and kidneys and increase their vulnerability to other environmental stresses.

Many of the biochemical aspects of ageing can be reduced by following a low-fat diet which still contains enough of the nutrients needed for health and includes plenty of physical activity. As well as reducing fats, older people need less alcohol, sugar and salt while dietary fibre and complex carbohydrate may need to be increased.

Free Radicals and Antioxidants

The ageing and degeneration of cells throughout the body occurs because substances called free radicals attack various parts of the cell. The accumulation of these free radicals can be prevented by certain enzymes (see page 113) which depend on a balanced supply of minerals such as manganese, copper, zinc and selenium. Without the appropriate enzymes, the free radicals multiply and damage the cells.

One of the major targets of free radicals is the membranes which surround every body cell. These membranes contain polyunsaturated fats — compounds which are very dependent on antioxidants to prevent oxidation and destruction.

Antioxidants help prevent the tissue-damaging effects of oxidation (see page 257). Some antioxidants occur naturally in foods, while others are synthetic. Both types are added to some processed foods so that they will keep longer.

Some people maintain that taking antioxidants, such as vitamins C and E, or the mineral selenium, or the preservatives BHA or BHT, will prevent the attack on the polyunsaturated fats in the cell membrane and the consequent damage to the cells caused by free radicals. Without this deterioration in the cells, they claim cells will be preserved and ageing will be prevented. Properly controlled tests have not yet established the truth of such claims. However, free radicals formed from cigarette smoke are now thought to initiate the cancer process. Research into free radicals continues.

In the meantime, there is probably not sufficient evidence to justify taking extra quantities of antioxidants apart from those present in a good diet. Vitamin C, one of the most useful antioxidants, is obtained from fruits and vegetables, while vitamin E occurs in seeds, wheatgerm, wholegrain products, nuts and vegetables. Selenium is widely distributed in vegetables, cereals and milk — providing the local soil contains adequate levels. See also page 24.

The idea that massive doses of vitamins will prevent wrinkles or grey hair has no scientific backing. Staying out of harsh sunlight helps prevent wrinkles and there is no dietary basis for greying of hair.

AIDS AND DIET

The Acquired Immune Deficiency Syndrome has no known cure at this stage. There are some who claim that a particular diet can help. Insofar as a healthy diet is useful for any body to combat infection, it is important that the diet of the AIDS sufferer be nutritionally as good as possible. However, there is no known 'magic' diet which will boost the immune system.

Taking extra zinc, massive doses of vitamins or following the candida diet (see page 54), have not been shown to be useful in controlled tests. However, because of the nature of the condition, it is possible that a natural regression may coincide with some dietary practice. This leads some people to ascribe curing properties to some foods.

As AIDS progresses, rapid and severe weight loss and muscle wasting occur. It is important to eat plenty of protein foods at this time. Fresh fruits and vegetables and wholegrain products should also be included to provide as much nourishment as possible. If the AIDS sufferer wants to try some new and unproved dietary combination, it is important that the diet does not restrict foods to the extent that weight loss becomes worse.

AIOLI

A sauce made from garlic, olive oil, lemon juice and egg yolk.

AKEE
see Fruit.

ALANINE

One of the amino acids which make up protein molecules. Alanine is released from muscle tissue during exercise, taken to the liver and converted into glucose which is then available to the muscle for energy. During brief periods of fasting, muscle protein is also broken down to provide alanine which can then be converted into glucose.

See also Amino acids.

ALBACORE
see Fish.

ALBILLO
see Wine, Varieties.

ALBUMEN

Strictly speaking albumen is called ovalbumin, and makes up the white of egg. It consists largely of protein and water and has small quantities of vitamins and minerals. An average-sized egg white has 60 kJ (14 Cals).

ALBUMIN

The main protein found in blood. One of its major functions is to regulate the level of water in the body.

ALCOHOL

Alcohols are organic compounds produced by yeasts (see page 405) when they ferment sugars. Suitable sugars include sucrose (from cane sugar), maltose (from malted cereals such as barley) or fructose (from fruits). During the fermentation process, the living yeasts synthesise proteins and vitamins of the B group, making the alcoholic liquid cloudy in the process. When beverages such as wines or beer are filtered to remove the yeast cells, most of the beneficial nutrients and dietary fibre are lost.

The most common form of alcohol, ethyl alcohol (or ethanol), is both a food and a drug. Alcohol is absorbed from the stomach, and this proceeds much more rapidly if there is no food in the stomach at the time. Alcoholic drinks containing carbon dioxide (such as champagne or whisky and soda) are absorbed even more quickly.

Once alcohol passes into the bloodstream, it is rapidly distributed throughout the body and produces a range of effects. A small concentration of alcohol in the blood produces a feeling of relaxation as some of the usual inhibitions are released.

As the concentration of alcohol in the brain increases, we begin to have lapses in concentration levels, in our ability to reason and make judgments. Memory loss may occur and muscular co-ordination also becomes difficult. These effects occur as alcohol affects the brain, beginning at the frontal lobe and moving into the areas which control speech, vision and the body's muscles.

Alcohol is processed by the liver at a rate of about 7 g of alcohol per hour (a standard drink has about 14 g of alcohol). Large quantities of alcohol will damage liver and brain cells. Some forms of cancer, such as cancer of the oesophagus or larynx, are much more likely in heavy drinkers. Because of its high kilojoule value (29 kJ/g or 7 Cals/g), alcoholic drinks can also increase weight. (See also page 112.)

Alcohol also causes the body to make less of its normal clotting proteins. This may be a reason why alcohol gives some protection against the formation of blood clots.

The rate at which alcohol is metabolised by the liver is not increased by exercise, coffee, vitamins or any other commonly available substance. Large quantities of fructose may hasten the removal of alcohol, but usually produce nausea. The only way to remove alcohol from the body is to allow the appropriate length of time for the liver to process the quantity consumed.

The old idea that alcohol is warming is incorrect; it causes flushing of the skin which is followed by a loss of body heat to the air. It is therefore foolish to give alcohol to anyone who is suffering from exposure or any type of stress.

Alcohol also interferes with some of the hormones which normally control the level of water in the body. Dehydration occurs, providing an unpleasantly dry mouth the next morning. Those who believe a few beers will replace the water they lose during sweating are wrong; alcoholic drinks cause more fluid to be lost from the body than they provide.

Other effects of alcohol include some irritation of the stomach lining, dilation of blood vessels (resulting in redness of the skin and also in headaches), gout (see page 168) and increased blood pressure. Pregnant women should avoid alcohol to reduce the risk of abnormalities in their babies.

Alcohol indirectly causes many deaths from motor vehicle accidents. Its effects on the brain can also increase violence. If the concentration of alcohol in the body becomes high enough, coma and death can result.

For all its faults, it is difficult to demonstrate that small quantities of alcohol (1—2 drinks a day) have any harmful effects. There is no doubt that large quantities should be avoided.

See also Drinks, Alcoholic; Cirrhosis.

ALDEHYDES

A class of chemical compounds which can be formed when alcohol reacts with oxygen. Some aldehydes are responsible for the toxic reactions which occur with heavy drinking. Other aldehydes are normal substances formed in the chemical reactions of the body, including vision and the production of some hormones.

ALE

see Drinks, Alcoholic, Beer.

ALEURONE

The layer just underneath the seed coat on grains containing a high concentration of the essential fatty acids, protein, vitamins and minerals. The aleurone layer is usually removed during the milling of cereal grains and is found in the bran portion. The dietary fibre in the aleurone layer consists of both soluble and insoluble fibre. In ordinary wheat bran, the soluble fibre binds the insoluble fibre which is not available to the body. A new process to split the aleurone layer from wheat bran will make this fibre available.

ALFALFA

see Vegetables.

ALGAE

Micro-organisms which use sunlight for energy, making them 10—50 times as efficient as conventional crops. They are so rich in protein that it has been estimated that the entire protein needs of the world could be produced in a volume of 10^{13} litres of algae. This would, of course, mean incorporating the algae into some

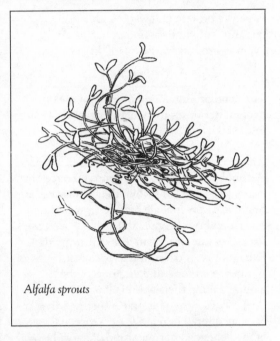

Alfalfa sprouts

palatable form, but this is not beyond the imagination of food scientists who can turn it into a powder or solid form to be cooked in with vegetables or other foods. Unfortunately, some algae also contain large quantities of substances which have the potential to increase uric acid levels in the body and thus cause gout. These would need to be removed before the algae would be useful.

ALGINATES

Gum-like derivatives of seaweed which are added to foods such as icecream to produce a slower melting product without large ice crystals. Also used in soups, sauces and some jellied foods. Alginates are good sources of soluble dietary fibre.

ALIMENTARY TRACT

The intestine or digestive tract, commencing at the mouth and ending at the anus. Carnivorous animals have a short alimentary tract while herbivores have a much longer tract.

See also Digestion.

ALKALINITY

A condition in which the pH is greater than 7 (see page 265). The only alkaline substances commonly found in the kitchen are egg white and bicarbonate of soda. Vegetables cooked with bicarb soda turn a bright green but also lose much of their vitamin content and soon go mushy. In parts of America, it has always been common practice to treat corn with alkali in the form of ashes and lime. This improves the balance of amino acids in corn and also releases the corn's niacin (vitamin B_3) so that it can be absorbed by the body.

In the body, the small intestine is alkaline and this counteracts the acidity of the stomach. The level of acidity/alkalinity in the blood is automatically controlled by the kidneys.

ALKALOIDS

A group of organic, nitrogen-containing compounds found in many plants and moulds. The group includes substances such as nicotine, morphine, strychnine and quinine. Most are toxic in large doses. Alkaloids in the skin of potatoes exposed to light are responsible for the nausea and vomiting which follows their consumption. Dangerous alkaloids in plants such as comfrey are also known to cause liver cancer. Caffeine is one of the most commonly consumed alkaloids; it stimulates the nervous system in small doses but is quite toxic in large amounts.

See also Caffeine.

ALKALOSIS

A condition in which the blood becomes excessively alkaline. Can arise from severe vomiting or taking diuretics.

ALLERGEN

A substance which is foreign to the human body and causes an allergic reaction. An allergen is a particular type of antigen.

ALLERGIES

A true allergy is a hypersensitive reaction involving the body's immune system, causing the formation of antibodies in the body's white blood cells. Food sensitivities or intolerances may cause symptoms but do not provoke a true allergic response by the body's immune system. Allergic reactions may be quite severe and usually occur in young children, whereas food sensitivity may arise (and disappear) at any stage of life.

Symptoms of food allergy include swelling of the throat, diarrhoea and vomiting, asthma, or eczema. The reaction usually occurs because a foreign substance (in this case, usually a protein or polysaccharide molecule in the offending food) causes the body to produce an antibody. When the foreign substance (properly known as an antigen) is again eaten, more antibodies are formed to fight the invading substance. Usually such a response is beneficial. For example, it prevents us catching a disease such as measles more than once. In the case of food allergy, the defence mechanism results in unpleasant and often dangerous symptoms.

Many young children grow out of their allergies as their digestive system matures, so that the original foreign substances are altered by their more mature digestive tract.

Foods which commonly cause allergic responses include milk, eggs (especially the white), fish, shellfish, wheat or other cereals, nuts, seeds, chocolate, tomatoes, some fruits and some meats.

It is important to distinguish between true food allergies which involve the immune system and food sensitivities. The latter may produce the same symptoms but are dose-related in that there is some critical quantity of a food or food additive which must be consumed before symptoms become apparent.

Skin and cytotoxic blood tests are not reliable in diagnosing food allergies or sensitivities since they do not always produce reliable positive or negative results. Food sensitivity is best diagnosed using an elimination diet in which all foods known to produce sensitive reactions are removed and then reintroduced in a specific way. Since many people have multiple sensitivities to foods, merely omitting a few foods will not always pinpoint all the culprits.

In young children, parents can keep a diary of foods eaten and timing of symptoms to provide some basis for possible reactions to particular foods. See also Hyperactivity.

The services of a qualified dietitian are required whenever a food allergy or sensitivity is suspected or found. There have been many instances where people omit certain foods and then find their diet is deficient in some essential nutrient.

See also Dermatitis; Eczema; Elimination diet.

ALLICIN

A sulphur-containing ingredient in garlic, thought to be responsible for its cholesterol-lowering properties. Much of the allicin in garlic is destroyed in most so-called 'odourless' garlic preparations.

ALLIGATOR PEAR

Another name for the avocado (see page 140).

ALLSPICE
see Spices.

ALMOND
see Nuts.

ALMOND OIL
see Oils.

ALOE VERA

This product comes from pulping the fleshy leaves of the cactus plant aloe vera. In large doses it has a rather violent laxative action. In the small quantities which find their way into everything from shampoos to face creams to slimming drinks, it is unlikely to have any effect at all except to expand the bank balances of those who charge high prices for it. Some products which claim to contain aloe vera do not. Claims that 'it is useful for' stretch marks, burns, vaginal infections, diabetes, arthritis, multiple sclerosis, cancer and various other diseases, have no scientific backing. Analyses of the juice from aloe vera have been unable to find any substance which could conceivably be beneficial.

ALOPECIA

The correct name for baldness. Can occur from large doses of vitamin A, but is mostly due to an effect of male hormones rather than any dietary factor.

ALPHA LINOLENIC ACID
see Linolenic acid.

ALPHA-TOCOPHEROL
see Vitamin E.

ALUMINIUM

An element which may be needed in minute quantities by humans but currently has no known function. Excessive amounts of aluminium (usually from antacids), can prevent the absorption of phosphorus and cause muscle weakness and bone problems. Using aluminium saucepans may allow aluminium to be absorbed, but the quantities are too small to present a health hazard. Some foods which release acids, alkalis or hydrogen sulphide (for example, boiled eggs), will make aluminium cooking vessels turn grey or black.

Excessive amounts of aluminium may make it easier for undesirable substances to enter the brain and contribute to Alzheimer's disease.

ALZHEIMER'S DISEASE

A condition in which some nerve cells in the brain degenerate causing severe memory impairment. The cause is not yet understood but may involve a deficiency of acetylcholine. There are also abnormally high levels of aluminium in the brain and some claim that aluminium cooking vessels are responsible for the condition.

AMARANTH
see Vegetables, Chinese spinach.

AMARANTH
see Colourings.

AMARETTO
see Drinks, Alcoholic.

AMBROSIA
see Cheese.

AMENORRHOEA

Cessation of menstrual periods which may occur when body fat levels drop too low. The exact level of body fat at which oestrogen levels function will vary from woman to woman. Some women will develop amenorrhoea if their body fat level drops below 20 per cent; others continue to menstruate normally at body fat levels as low as 16 per cent. (Normal body fat levels in women range from 20−25 per cent.) Amenorrhoea also develops in some female athletes who train for many hours each day. Once periods stop, oestrogen levels drop and much less calcium is retained by bones. This loss of calcium can lead to stress fractures in very thin women and elite athletes.

See also Menstruation and nutrition; Oestrogen.

AMINES

Nitrogen-containing chemical substances which occur in foods and in the blood from the breakdown of amino acids. They are found in bananas, avocados, cheese, yeast extracts, red wines (especially those made from Shiraz grapes), broad beans, pickled herrings and in any food which has been 'aged' (for example, some cheeses and fermented foods). Amines have the potential to constrict blood vessels and raise blood pressure. Some people are sensitive to amines and develop migraines or other symptoms if they consume too many foods containing them. Most people have no problems with amines, as an enzyme called monoamine oxidase (see page 232) causes them to break down. Some anti-depressant drugs prevent the action of this enzyme and anyone taking these drugs must avoid foods which contain amines.

AMINO ACIDS

There are 23 amino acids which make up proteins. 8 of these amino acids are called 'essential', as they cannot be made in the body and must be supplied from the diet. The remaining amino acids can be made from each other. Animal products such as eggs, fish, meat and milk contain all 8 essential amino acids; vegetable protein foods usually lack sufficient quantities of one or more. However, by eating a variety of vegetable foods such as grains, seeds, nuts, fruits and vegetables, all the essential amino acids can easily be supplied.

The 8 essential amino acids are isoleucine, leucine, lysine, methionine, phenylalanine, threonine, tryptophan and valine.

Histidine is also essential for children since their bodies seem to be unable to make this amino acid fast enough for their rapidly growing bodies. The other amino acids include alanine, arginine, aspartic acid, citrulline, cystine, cysteine, glutamic acid, glycine, histidine (for adults), hydroxylysine, hydroxyproline, ornithine, proline, serine, tyrosine. Citrulline, cystine and hydroxylysine do not occur in nature but are formed during chemical reactions within the body.

Athletes often take extra quantities of amino acids in an attempt to stimulate growth hormone and increase muscle mass. There is no evidence that this is effective.

See also Carnitine; Digestion.

AMMONIA

see Urea.

AMONTILLADO

see Drinks, Alcoholic.

AMYGDALIN

Extracted from apricot kernels, amygdalin is sometimes called vitamin B_{17} and is promoted as a cure for cancer. It is not a vitamin at all and is one of a group of toxic substances which can release cyanide (a salt of hydrocyanic acid). The theory that amygdalin might cure cancer developed in the hope that the cyanide might kill cancer cells. Unfortunately, it is quite toxic to all cells. Eating apricot kernels or buying amygdalin on the black market are potentially deadly pursuits.

AMYLASES

Enzymes which break down complex carbohydrates. In saliva, an amylase called ptyalin mixes with food and begins the digestion of carbohydrate to maltose. Another amylase enters the small intestine to break down complex carbohydrates into maltose.

See also Enzymes; Digestion.

AMYLOPECTIN

A waxy starch molecule containing thousands of starch molecules in a branched configuration. Not as powerful a thickening agent as amylose. Some waxy corn or rice starches are almost entirely amylopectin and form very viscous solutions rather than firm gels.

See also Starch.

AMYLOSE

Another starch molecule which accounts for 25–30 per cent of the total starch in flour. Amylose forms a firm gel and so helps thicken liquids. It also causes shrinkage into a denser compact structure and thus contributes to the eventual separation of thickened sauces and the staling of products such as bread. This shrinkage takes place much more rapidly at refrigerator temperature and is the reason why bread should be stored frozen or at room temperature rather than in the refrigerator.

See also Starch.

ANABOLIC STEROIDS

Hormones used illegally by athletes in an attempt to build up muscle mass. The steroids used resemble the male hormone testosterone and have been shown to increase muscle mass in women when used in conjunction with strength training. Side effects also occur, including baldness, facial hair, coarsening of the skin and acne.

It has been difficult to test the effects of anabolic steroids on males because of the ethics of giving large doses of drugs known to cause atrophy of the testes, acne, baldness and an increased incidence of liver disorders, including tumours.

In an attempt to find a substitute for anabolic steroids, some athletes take growth hormone or extra quantities of amino acids. There is no evidence that these substances can increase muscle mass.

See also Hormones.

ANAEMIA

A number of conditions characterised by an inadequate number of red cells or misshapen red blood cells. Anaemias can develop from a chronic or acute loss of blood, from chemicals or diseases which destroy red blood cells, or if diseases of the bone marrow interfere with the production of red blood cells.

The most common form is iron deficiency anaemia which results in a lowered level of haemoglobin, the pigment in red blood cells which carries oxygen to all the body's tissues. Iron deficiency commonly occurs in women who do not eat enough iron-rich foods to meet the high needs of blood losses from menstruation and the demands of pregnancy and lactation. The average pre-menopausal woman needs twice as much iron as the average man. Ironically, the richest food sources of iron, such as meat, are usually given in larger quantities to men.

Deficiencies of vitamin B_6, folacin and B_{12} also cause various types of anaemia. In macrocytic anaemias (caused by a lack of B_{12} or folacin deficiency), there are larger red blood cells but a lesser number.

The usual symptoms of anaemia are due to a lack of oxygen being carried to the cells and include fatigue, irritability, dizziness and shortness of breath.

Any woman who has heavy periods and feels constantly tired and below par should see her doctor for a blood test to check for anaemia.

See also Iron; Copper.

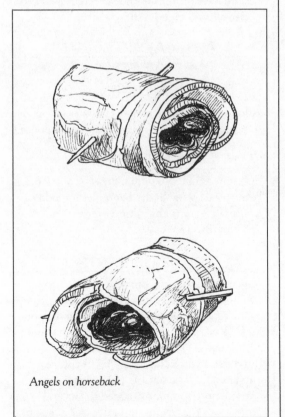

Angels on horseback

ANAEROBIC ACTIVITY

Takes place without oxygen. Short sharp bursts of physical activity occur anaerobically. The only fuel for anaerobic physical activity is glucose which is stored in muscles as glycogen. Short sprints, jumping, weight-lifting and throwing are examples of anaerobic activity.

See also Aerobic activity.

ANCHOVY
see Fish.

ANEURINE

Another name for thiamin.
See Vitamin B.

ANGEL CAKE

A cake made from egg whites, sugar and flour. Has no fat content (unless served with whipped cream). One average slice (75 g) has 775 kJ (185 Cals).

ANGELICA

A sweet dessert wine originally made in Spain.
See also Herbs.

ANGELS ON HORSEBACK

Oysters wrapped in bacon. Served either as an appetiser or at the end of a meal. Each angel on horseback has 340 kJ (80 Cals).

ANGINA PECTORIS

Pain in the chest or radiating to the neck, left shoulder or arm when insufficient blood reaches the heart muscle. Occurs in clogged or hardened arteries, usually at times of vigorous exercise or emotional stress. There is some evidence that the omega 3 fatty acids (see page 254) in fish oils may help angina sufferers. A low-fat diet and loss of excess weight are also important.

ANGOSTURA BITTERS
see Drinks, Alcoholic.

ANISE
see Drinks, Alcoholic.

ANISE
see Spices.

ANISE
see Vegetables, Fennel.

ANNATTO
see Colourings.

ANOREXIA NERVOSA

A condition of extreme thinness which is becoming more common in young women who diet excessively. Weight loss is substantial and menstruation stops as body fat levels fall to emaciation levels. Anorexics usually feel cold, are constipated and have hair loss; some die from their self-inflicted starvation. Those with anorexia often deny their condition and believe they are still fat. They may go to great lengths to avoid eating, or, if they do eat, they then induce vomiting or take large doses of laxatives.

Anorexia is much more common in middle to upper class families where the girls feel pressured to excel in most aspects of their lives. They are usually intelligent and do not 'rebel' in any other obvious way. Treatment is long and difficult.

See also Adolescents and diet; Bulimia nervosa; Calcium; Malnutrition; Undernutrition.

ANTACIDS
see Dyspepsia.

ANTIBIOTICS

A class of substances produced by micro-organisms and harmful to other micro-organisms. Antibiotics wipe out harmful bacteria and are thus beneficial in treating bacterial infections. Unfortunately, antibiotics can also destroy some of the useful intestinal bacteria which make vitamin K and the B complex vitamin, biotin. Short courses of antibiotics will not have a substantial effect but long-term usage may require supplementary biotin.

Antibiotics also come into the diet from some animal products such as meat, as they are used to prevent disease in the animals.

ANTIBODIES

Protective substances formed to fight allergens. A repeat dose of the allergen causes an immune response as the body produces many more antibodies. We make antibodies in response to a small dose of, say, measles or smallpox virus. On later exposure to the virus, we have the antibodies to fight it and thus prevent the disease. Some people also make antibodies to certain food proteins or polysaccharides.

See also Allergen; Allergies.

ANTI-CAKING AGENTS
see Additives, food.

ANTIGEN

A foreign substance which can cause the body to produce antibodies in an immune response.

ANTINUTRIENTS

Substances in foods which prevent nutrients being used by the body. Examples include tannin (prevents absorption of iron) and antivitamins (see page 25).

ANTIOXIDANTS

Prevent a substance combining with oxygen which would otherwise cause spoilage, either by making the food rancid, by discolouration or loss of flavour. Vitamins C and E are natural antioxidants, as are rosemary and sage. Butylated hydroxytoluene (BHT) and butylated hydroxyanisole (BHA) are antioxidants commonly added to fats and other foods to prevent rancidity (see page 36).

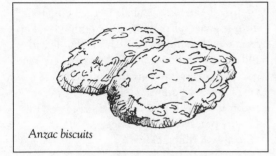

Anzac biscuits

Sulphur dioxide, or sodium metabisulphite (which produces sulphur dioxide), prevent oxidation and browning in fruits. The presence of antioxidants in foods is usually listed on the label. However, this can be hidden. For example, margarine contains antioxidants, but a food containing margarine will list the latter as an ingredient and will not repeat the ingredients in the margarine (see also page 199).

Some people believe that antioxidants will prevent oxidation of the polyunsaturated fats in the membranes around cells and that preventing this oxidation will delay the ageing process. They therefore take supplements of antioxidant substances such as vitamins C and E and sometimes BHA or BHT.

See also Ageing and diet, Free radicals and Antioxidants.

ANTIPASTO

A first course served before pasta. Generally includes a selection of dishes such as fresh or pickled vegetables, smoked, fresh or canned fish, shellfish, cheeses, hams, salamis, and melon.

ANTIVITAMINS

Substances which destroy or form complexes with vitamins. Examples include avidin in raw egg white which can destroy the B vitamin, biotin and thiaminase (in raw herrings) which can destroy thiamin. In general, antivitamins are not a problem in a varied diet.

ANZAC BISCUITS

An Australian biscuit containing rolled oats and golden syrup. Popular during World War I to send to the troops who became known as ANZACS (Australia, New Zealand Army Corps). An average-sized biscuit has 335 kJ (80 Cals).

APATITE

A crystalline form of calcium phosphate. The major mineral in tooth enamel.

APHRODISIAC

In spite of many hopes to the contrary, no food has ever been found to have aphrodisiac properties. Various foods may have an erotic effect on an individual, depending on his or her food preferences, but supposed aphrodisiac effects of foods such as fish, oysters and stout, are folklore not fact.

APOPROTEINS

Proteins which combine with fats to form lipoproteins (see page 210).

APPENDICITIS

The condition of inflammation of the appendix. Some claim that a low-fibre diet increases the risk of appendicitis. Since appendicitis hardly occurs in areas where fibre intake is high, this is likely to be correct.

APPENZELLER
see Cheese.

APPETITE

A desire for food including the sensation of pleasure which occurs at the thought, sight or smell of food. Not necessarily associated with hunger. Appetite can be increased or decreased in accordance with past experiences with particular foods.

APPLE
see Fruit.

APPLE JACK
see Drinks, Alcoholic.

APRICOT
see Fruit.

APRICOT KERNEL OIL
see Oils.

AQUAVIT
see Drinks, Alcoholic.

ARABINOSE
A sugar found in gums such as acacia gum.

ARACHIDONIC ACID
An essential polyunsaturated fatty acid found in some lean meats and some fish. Arachidonic acid is an important component of cell membranes, making up about one-third of the fatty acids in the cell's membrane. It is also used by the body to make prostaglandins, hormone-like substances which control blood pressure, blood clotting and the body's defence against foreign bodies. (See also page 281).

Most of the arachidonic acid in the body is made from linoleic acid in vegetable oils. Chemically, arachidonic acid has 20 carbon atoms and 4 double bonds and belongs to the omega 6 family. These fatty acids are classified according to their chemical structure. Each omega 6 fatty acid has the first double bond in its molecule located at the sixth carbon atom. Fatty acids belonging to the omega 3 family have their first double bond at the third carbon atom in their chain.

See also Linoleic acid.

ARGENTINE
see Fish.

ARGININE
One of the amino acids which make up proteins. It can also be made in the body from glutamic acid (see page 165). Arginine is taken by some body builders in the hope that it will build muscle and burn fat. It does neither. Very large doses of arginine given by injection may give a temporary stimulus of growth hormone but this is so small that it is not considered to have any practical significance.

See also Amino acids.

ARMAGNAC
see Drinks, Alcoholic.

ARRHYTHMIA
Any deviation from the normal heart rhythm.

ARROWHEAD
see Vegetables.

ARROWROOT
A starchy substance obtained from the fleshy root of a West Indian plant and used to produce clear, thickened sauces. It has little nutritional value. 100 g of arrowroot contain 1490 kJ (355 Cals).

See also Starch.

ARSENIC
Highly poisonous substance which may have some essential role in the human body in minute doses. Can be concentrated in shellfish from contaminated waters. Dangerous quantities are found in apricot kernels.

ARTERIOSCLEROSIS
Hardening of the arteries.
See also Heart disease.

ARTHRITIS
A condition of inflamed, thickened and painful joints. Some people with arthritis seem to be helped by omitting certain foods from the diet, but what upsets or benefits one person is not necessarily relevant to another. There is no

good evidence that foods such as tomatoes, eggplant, meat or dairy products cause or worsen arthritis. However, there are many anecdotal reports that a vegetarian diet is of benefit. Further research is needed to determine whether this is of definite benefit.

The omega 3 fatty acids (see page 254) found in fish and linseeds are currently being examined for a possible role in altering prostaglandins involved in inflammatory conditions. Early results with fish oils for rheumatoid arthritis show some relief of pain and stiffness.

Being overweight puts extra strain on joints and makes the symptoms of arthritis worse. Weight loss frequently brings relief.

ARTICHOKE
see Vegetables.

ARTIFICIAL SWEETENERS

Artificial sweeteners come in many varieties. The most common are saccharin, cyclamates, polyhydric alcohols such as sorbitol and mannitol, acesulfame K and aspartame. There are many other potential competitors to provide an alternative to sugar.

- *Saccharin* is a synthetic sweetener first made in 1879 and initially used because it was cheaper than sugar. Over the past 20 or 30 years, it has been used widely in low-kilojoule foods for overweight people or diabetics. Saccharin has an intensely sweet taste and is 300 times as sweet as sugar. Approximately 50 per cent of the population have a bitter taste in the mouth after eating saccharin; others can detect only its sweetness. The body does not digest saccharin — after tasting sweet in the mouth it is excreted by the kidneys.

  In 1977, saccharin was banned in the United States after a group of Canadian researchers found that it caused bladder cancer in mice. After an outcry from the general public (who wanted the sweetness without the kilojoules), from diabetic associations and from the soft drink industry, saccharin was permitted as long as the label on products containing it carried a warning.

  In other countries, such as Australia, medical and scientific experts looked at the issue and decided that the large doses of saccharin which would be necessary to increase the risk of bladder cancer could not be consumed (875 cups of artificially sweetened liquid a day!). Consequently, saccharin-containing products are still permitted in these places, in accordance with local food laws. In Australia, saccharin is only permitted in certain foods.

- *Cyclamates* are artificial sweeteners, found in 1937, usually occurring as sodium or calcium cyclamate. About 30–80 times as sweet as sugar and usually used in combination with saccharin. Cyclamates have been banned in some countries (such as the United States and the United Kingdom) because they were found to increase the incidence of bladder cancer in mice. The quantities required for this were much greater than could ever be consumed from foods which are artificially sweetened with cyclamates. Most substances are harmful in large doses, including the sugar which cyclamates replace.

- *Polyhydric alcohols* such as sorbitol, mannitol and xylitol are slightly less sweet than sugar and were introduced as sugar substitutes because they are absorbed more slowly from the digestive tract. However, these sugar alcohols do provide the same number of kilojoules as sugar. Large doses also cause diarrhoea and their use is inadvisable.

- *Acesulfame K* is made from acetoacetic acid and is 130 times as sweet as sugar. It appears to be a safe substance and is available in some countries, such as the United Kingdom.

- *Aspartame* is a new sweetener, made up of derivatives of two amino acids, phenylalanine and aspartic acid. It is 200 times as sweet as sugar and, unlike saccharin and cyclamates, it is digested in the body as a minute quantity of amino acids. Aspartame tastes so much like sugar that most people cannot distinguish between the two substances. It cannot be used in baked goods as the two amino acids break apart under heat and only taste sweet when they are joined together. Aspartame is probably the most thoroughly tested food additive ever released and appears to be perfectly safe. Those with the rare genetic disorder, phenylketonuria (PKU), cannot tolerate large quantities of phenylalanine and a warning for these people is usually placed on the label of products sweetened with aspartame (sold commercially as 'Nutra Sweet').

Other protein sweeteners also exist. An extract from serendipity berries which grow in West Africa is 2500 times as sweet as sugar. Another protein sweetener from a berry known as the 'miracle fruit' is 1600 times as sweet as sugar. It causes sour fruits such as lemons to taste delightfully sweet.

See also Sweetness.

ARUGULA
see Vegetables.

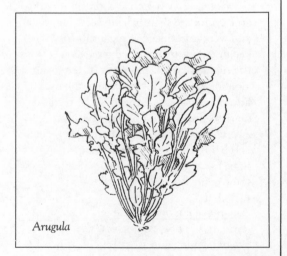

Arugula

ASAFOETIDA

A resin extracted from a plant and ground into a powder. Can be used in Indian cooking, especially in fish dishes.

ASCORBIC ACID
see Vitamin C.

ASPARAGINE

An amino acid first isolated from asparagus. It is not essential as it can be made from the amino acid aspartic acid.

ASPARAGUS
see Vegetables.

ASPARTAME
see Artificial sweeteners.

ASPARTIC ACID

An amino acid which is classified as non-essential since it can be made within the body from oxaloacetic acid, a substance which is produced during the metabolism of carbohydrates.

ASPERGILLUS

Mould which grows on peanuts, corn and certain nuts and produces a dangerous toxin called aflatoxin.

See also Aflatoxins.

ASPIC

A savoury, clear jelly made from stock from veal, chicken or fish bones. Naturally-occurring gelatine in the tendons of the bones dissolves into the stock and sets to a jelly when refrigerated.

ASPIRIN

Correctly called acetylsalicylic acid, aspirin is principally used as a pain killer. It also functions to prevent blood clots forming and is prescribed for some people at high risk of heart disease. It is absorbed from the stomach, and may cause indigestion. Related salicylates (see page 295) which occur naturally in fruits and vegetables cause a hypersensitive reaction (often in the form of hyperactivity) in a small number of people.

ASSAM TEA
see Tea.

ASTHMA

Asthma is a condition characterised by wheezing and shortness of breath caused by problems in the bronchi in the respiratory tract. Some foods will trigger an attack in some asthmatics. Products containing sulphites (additive nos. 221, 222, 223, 224) or monosodium glutamate (additive no. 621) are the most common offenders, although a variety of other naturally-occurring or added substances in foods may precipitate an asthma attack in susceptible individuals. Some commonly consumed foods such as processed orange juice, preprepared potato chips, wines and some dried fruits contain sulphites while packet soups, sauces, some frozen prepared meals, fast foods and Chinese meals contain MSG.

ATHEROSCLEROSIS

Hardening of the arteries due to a build up of plaque and fatty deposits, including cholesterol (athero means 'gruel', sclerosis indicates 'hardening'). As atherosclerosis becomes worse, it impedes the flow of blood and the heart is forced to work harder to pump blood through the arteries. If the fatty cholesterol-rich deposits build up sufficiently, blood flow may be blocked, causing the pain of angina. If a complete blockage occurs in one of the coronary arteries that feed the heart muscle itself, you have a heart attack. If a blockage occurs in an artery leading to the brain, you have a stroke. Arteries narrowed by atherosclerosis also mean that only a small

blood clot is needed to form a blockage. And to add insult to injury, those following the type of diet which contributes to atherosclerosis also have 'sticky' blood which easily forms clots.

Atherosclerosis is common in countries where the diet is high in fat, especially saturated fat (see page 119). There is now evidence that a change to a low-fat diet can remove some of the atherosclerosis from arteries.

See also Cholesterol and Heart disease.

ATHOLL BROSE

A Scottish dish made from milk simmered with rolled oats until thick, with honey, nutmeg, whisky and cream added. Served as a dessert. Any advantage the oats may have in reducing blood cholesterol levels will be wiped out by the cream.

ATKINS DIET

A high-protein, high-fat diet with very little carbohydrate, supposed to bring about effective weight loss. With this diet, you can eat all the meat, bacon, butter, cream, eggs and cheese you like, but you must not eat bread, cereals and grains, and only minimal quantities of fruit or vegetables. In practice, it is unlikely that most people will eat huge quantities of the permitted fats since there is little to eat with them and most people will feel nauseated if confronted with piles of fatty meat oozing with butter and cream.

In practice, the Atkins diet will usually have a reduction in kilojoules (see Energy) which may cause some loss of weight. Most of the initial weight loss, however, is due to the loss of glycogen from muscles and its accompanying water. With almost no carbohydrate in the diet, fats cannot be burned completely and ketones (see page 197) are produced. The theory is that these ketones will be lost in urine, leading to a loss of body fat. Ketone losses can only account for about 210 kJ (50 Cals) a day. They are highly toxic substances which can cause headaches, nausea, listlessness and, eventually, loss of consciousness. Such diets are not recommended.

ATP
see Adenosine triphosphate.

ATTA
A wholemeal flour used in Indian and Middle Eastern cookery.

AUBERGINE
see Vegetables, Eggplant.

AVIDIN
A substance present in raw egg white but destroyed when the eggs are cooked. In large quantities avidin can bind the B group vitamin, biotin. The risk of avidin deficiency is only likely if large numbers of raw eggs are eaten regularly.

AVOCADO
see Fruit.

AZAROLE
see Fruit.

AZUKI BEANS
see Legumes, Aduki beans.

B

BABA
A yeasted cake containing flour, eggs, butter, yeast and milk, often with added fruits or lemon rind. Once cooked, the cake is soaked with a flavoured syrup, usually containing rum and some type of fruit flavouring.

BABACO
see Fruit.

BABA GANNOUJ
A Lebanese dish made from the cooked flesh of eggplant pureed with garlic, tahini (ground sesame paste), lemon juice and cumin. Also called baba ganouj, it is usually topped with a little olive oil and served with flatbread. A 60 g serve has 590 kJ (140 Cals).

BACALAO
see Fish.

BACON
Made from various cuts of pork, bacon was traditionally cured by salting. The salt acts as a preservative by providing a high concentration of ions around any harmful bacteria, so that water is drawn out of the bacteria which then wither and die. Salt is now much less important as a preservative and is added mainly to provide the traditional flavour. Sodium nitrate is used to preserve the pink colour, contribute some flavour and, most importantly, kill bacteria, including the toxic variety which causes botulism.

Bacon is high in fat and contributes from 630−3150 kJ per 100 g (150−750 Cals).

See also Nitrates.

BACTERIA
The term bacteria covers a wide range of micro-

organisms which can be either beneficial or detrimental to human health.

'Good' lactic acid bacteria (see page 201) are used to thicken or curdle yoghurt, sour cream and buttermilk and to begin the process of making cheeses of all types. The distinctive flavour and texture of some cheeses is due to the particular bacteria which are introduced during their manufacture.

Bacteria reduce the tartness of wines and provide some of the wonderful complexities of flavour in good quality wines. Lactobacillus bacteria convert some of the tart-tasting malic and tartaric acids in grapes into a smoother tasting lactic acid (see pages 216 and 337).

Bacteria are also responsible for much of the flavour of sauerkraut, some types of pickles and sour-dough breads.

We also have millions of 'good' bacteria within our intestine. Some make vitamins for us (including biotin and vitamin K) while others digest dietary fibre and produce valuable acids in the process (see page 92).

Some bacteria, however, are quite incompatible with human health and may make foods go bad or cause diarrhoea, vomiting and even death. Others thrive on sugar caught in teeth and produce acids which eat through the enamel of teeth, causing decay.

Many bacteria which cause intestinal problems multiply to dangerous numbers at room temperature. For this reason, foods such as chicken, meats, fish, milk, any items with a mayonnaise or cream-based sauce or filling (including potato salad, custard tarts, cream-filled cakes) which can contain harmful bacteria, should be kept either hot or cold, since bacteria cannot multiply at extremes of temperature. It is also vitally important that community water supplies are not contaminated with harmful bacteria. Regular inspections are carried out to test water supplies.

Bacteria themselves also have potential as an animal or even a human food since 47—87 per cent of their dry weight is protein. In one day, 1000 kg of bacteria could produce 10 million kg of protein from energy sources such as petroleum by-products, the waste from fruit canning or from paper-pulp manufacture.

BAGASSE

The fibre which is left after the juice has been extracted from sugar cane. It can be used as a fuel or to make particle board.

BAGELS

Bagels are a traditional Jewish food made from a yeasted bread dough which is first boiled briefly and then baked. The initial boiling gives bagels their chewy texture. An average sized bagel has almost no fat and 630 kJ (150 Cals).

BAGNA CAUDA

A creamy garlic sauce served hot with raw vegetables.

BAGOONG

A shrimp paste made by cleaning small fish, mixing with salt (1 part of salt to 3 parts of fish), pressing into vats and colouring it with plant dyes. Bagoong is high in calcium.

BAKED BEANS
see Legumes, Haricot beans.

BAKER'S CHEESE
see Cheese.

BAKEWELL TART
see Tart.

BAKING POWDER

A mixture of alkali (sodium or potassium bicarbonate) and acid (such as calcium phosphate and tartaric acid). When used in baking, the mixture reacts and produces carbon dioxide which causes dough to rise. Baking powder can be made by mixing 1 part of bicarbonate of soda with 2 parts of cream of tartar.

BAKING SODA

The common name for sodium bicarbonate (or carb soda). When combined with acid ingredients such as yoghurt, soured milk, lemon juice or vinegar, carbon dioxide is formed. Baking soda is used to lighten scones and cakes.

BAKLAVA

A rich Middle Eastern or Greek pastry made with layers of buttered filo pastry, chopped nuts, sugar and cinnamon. Once cooked the pastry is steeped in a honey or sugar syrup. One small piece (60 g) has 840 kJ (200 Cals).

BALANCED DIET

This somewhat vague term means different things to different people. The best general description of a balanced diet is one which provides nutrients in the quantities recommended for good health and avoids excessive quantities of particular foods or their components (such as sugar).

Many countries have devised easy methods for the population to check the balance of their diets. Food groups are commonly promoted and consumers can check that they are having the recommended number of servings of food from each of four or five groups. For example, the five food groups used in Australia are as follows:

Group 1 — breads and cereals (at least 4 servings a day)
Group 2 — fruits and vegetables (at least 4 servings)
Group 3 — fish, poultry, lean meat, eggs, nuts, cheese, legumes (at least 1 serving)
Group 4 — milk or yoghurt (at least 2 servings)
Group 5 — butter or margarine (15 g)

These guides do not address the question of overconsumption of certain items (for example, meat or dairy products) which undoubtedly produces an unbalanced diet.

A balanced diet can also be described in terms of its macronutrients — protein, fat, complex and simple carbohydrates and alcohol. Common recommendations for a balanced diet, using this approach, are:

Protein — 10–15 per cent of energy
Fat — 20–30 per cent of energy
Complex carbohydrate — 40–50 per cent of energy
Simple carbohydrate — approximately 15 per cent of energy
Alcohol — 1 per cent of energy

This type of recommendation for a balanced diet then needs to be translated into specific foods.

The changes needed for a more balanced diet in Australia (and most Western countries) are encompassed in dietary guidelines such as those used in Australia:

- Eat more breads, cereals (preferably wholegrain) and more fruits and vegetables
- Avoid eating too much fat
- Avoid eating too much sugar
- Use less salt
- Drink less alcohol
- Eat a variety of nutritious foods

Most populations have traditionally managed to select a balanced diet from their native foods. This has become much more difficult in Western countries where the abundance of food items — some of which are nutritionally useless — can make it difficult for those with little knowledge of nutrition to select a balanced diet. This does not mean that people in Western countries need a variety of dietary supplements since these will rarely correct a diet which has been poorly chosen. The greatest impediment to a balanced diet in most Western countries is the high fat and sugar content of most foods and the low status given to sources of complex carbohydrate and dietary fibre.

See also Breads; Carbohydrates; Dietary fibre.

BALDNESS

see Alopecia.

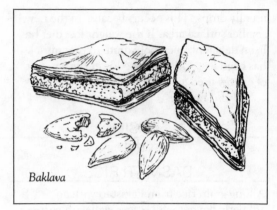

Baklava

BALM
see Herbs.

BALMAIN BUGS
see Seafood, Lobster.

BAMBOO SHOOTS
see Vegetables.

BANANA
see Fruit.

BANANA PASSIONFRUIT
see Fruit.

BANBURY TART
A sweet pastry from Banbury in England with a shortcrust pastry filled with a mixture of currants, candied peel and spices. One slice (100 g) has 1700 kJ (405 Cals).

BANNOCK
A Gaelic flat cake popular in Scotland. The dough is made from oatmeal, carb soda, lard or other fat. It is rolled out, cooked on a hot plate or griddle and served warm with butter and jam. One average bannock has 800 kJ (190 Cals).

BAP
A Scottish soft, breakfast roll, dusted with white flour and eaten hot with butter.

BARBADOS CHERRY
see Fruit, Acerola.

BARBARY FIG
see Fruit, Prickly pear.

BARBECUE
An outdoor meal in which meats, poultry or fish are cooked over a wood or charcoal fire. The barbecue originated with a group of Indians in the Caribbean who used a grating of green wood over a slow fire to cook strips of meat. If barbecued foods are cooked so that the food becomes charred, cancer-causing chemicals are produced. These are only likely to cause problems if eaten in large quantities. Barbecued foods which are not blackened are quite safe.

BARBECUE SAUCE
A thick sauce made from vinegar, mustard, tomatoes, salt, pepper, paprika, pepper and Worcestershire sauce. Used in place of tomato sauce and, naturally enough, at barbecues. One tablespoon (20 g) has 125 kJ (30 Cals).

BARBERRY
see Fruit.

BARLEY
see Grains, Cereals.

BARLEY WATER
A popular cure-all, barley water is made by soaking barley in water, boiling for several hours and straining off the liquid. It has no special curative powers, but the liquid contains much of the soluble fibre of the whole grain.

BARRAMUNDI
see Fish.

BASIC METABOLIC RATE (BMR)
The energy required for the basic process of maintaining body temperature and muscle tone

and to keep vital organs functioning when the body is at rest. Involves the energy to keep the heart beating, the lungs expanding and contracting, the kidneys filtering blood, the liver functioning and every cell in the body renewing its energy and getting rid of its wastes. BMR is measured while the subject is awake and resting and some time after eating. Energy used for basal metabolism is a little like the energy a car uses to idle.

The amount of energy used for basal metabolism varies with:

- Surface area (the larger the surface area, the greater the energy requirement)
- Amount of muscle (muscle is active tissue which burns energy; fat is largely inactive and uses almost no energy)
- Age (the body tends to slow down as it ages, especially if you exercise little and have less muscle)
- State of nutrition (the body slows down during dieting, fasting or starvation)
- How much time you spend asleep (the body slows down during sleep)
- The air temperature (the colder the air temperature, the more heat your body must produce to keep its internal temperature constant)

Pregnancy and fever increase the amount of energy being used by the body for basal metabolism. There is also some individual genetic variation.

Exercise uses up energy and also builds up muscle. The more muscle, the greater the energy used for basal metabolism. Thus exercise has a great effect on the body's ability to use energy, or burn kilojoules.

Even though it weighs much less, the brain uses about the same amount of the resting energy as the muscles. However, once the muscles begin to work during exercise, they use vast amounts of energy. By contrast, heavy thinking does not increase the amount of energy used by the brain to any extent.

After weight loss, the basic metabolic rate usually drops. This occurs because of the new smaller surface area. If the weight loss diet has been deficient in carbohydrate so that muscle has been lost, this will also lower the amount of energy used for basal metabolism.

See also Energy.

BASIL
see Herbs.

BASMATI RICE

A long grain rice from Pakistan with an aromatic flavour which goes well with curries and spicy dishes.

BATTER

A mixture of flour, eggs and liquid. Can be used to make crepes, pancakes or pikelets or for coating foods which are to be fried. Uncooked cake mixture may also be referred to as batter.

BAVARIAN CREAM

A custard with whipped cream and gelatine, flavoured either with fruits, coffee or chocolate. An average serving has 600 kJ (145 Cals).

BAY LEAF
see Herbs.

BEAN CURD
see Tofu.

BEANS
see Legumes; Vegetables.

BEAN SPROUTS
see Vegetables.

BEARNAISE SAUCE
see Sauces, Emulsion sauces.

BECHAMEL SAUCE
see Sauces, White sauce.

BEEF
see Meat.

BEEF TEA

The liquid which is left after beef is boiled in water and then strained. Beef tea was once given to invalids. Some of the meat nutrients do dissolve into beef tea, but much of the goodness remains in the meat.

BEE POLLEN

Pollen, collected from flowers by bees, is the main source of protein for bees and also contributes much of the minerals and vitamins needed by bees. The quantities of nutrients it contains, however, are too small to have any practical significance for humans.

BEER

see Drinks, Alcoholic.

BEETROOT

see Vegetables.

BEET SUGAR

Sucrose can be derived not only from sugar cane, but from the juice of the white vegetable, sugar beet. Sugar beet accounts for about 40 per cent of the sucrose produced in the world with Russia, Germany and the United States being the major growers.

BELL APPLE

Another name for the passionfruit (see page 152).

BEL PAESE

see Cheese.

BENEDICTINE

see Drinks, Alcoholic.

BENGAL GRAM

see Legumes, Garbanzos.

BENZOIC ACID

A preservative sometimes used as potassium, sodium or calcium benzoate (additive nos. 210, 211, 212, 213). Commonly added to soft drinks, juices and cordials. Some people are unusually sensitive to benzoic acid and suffer symptoms ranging from gastrointestinal pains to asthma if they consume products containing any of the benzoic acid additives. Most people have no problems with the levels used in foods.

BERGAMOT

see Herbs; Fruit.

BERIBERI

A disease which develops when the diet is deficient in thiamin (vitamin B_1). Nerve cells become inflamed and no longer function and fluid may accumulate in feet, ankles and legs and around the heart. Death can occur. Beriberi was common in parts of Asia when food supplies were inadequate and the protective thiamin in rice was removed by polishing. It is rare in Australia but can occur in alcoholics.

BERLINER

see Sausages.

BERRIES

see Fruit.

BESAN

The name given to flour made from ground chickpeas. Occasionally lentil flour is incorrectly labelled as 'besan'.

BETA CAROTENE

see Vitamins, Vitamin A.

BEURRE BLANC

see Sauces, Emulsion.

BEURRE MANIE

A paste made from butter and flour and used to thicken soups, sauces and casseroles. Generally added at the end of cooking.

BEURRE NOIR

see Sauces, Emulsion.

BEURRE NOISETTE
see Sauces, Emulsion.

BEVERLEY HILLS DIET

A popular gimmick diet which consists of individual fruits consumed singly, and in a particular order for the first ten days. Enzymes in these fruits are supposed to rid the body of fat. The rest of the diet consists of certain foods, eaten in unlimited quantity, but usually without accompaniments. For example, pasta may be eaten, but only on its own. The diet is nutritionally unbalanced.

BEVERLEY HILLS MEDICAL DIET

This diet is not connected with the Beverley Hills Diet (see above). It is somewhat more balanced than its predecessor and aims to reduce fats, cholesterol-containing foods, sugar, salt and animal protein foods, while increasing foods which provide complex carbohydrate and dietary fibre. It also encourages large quantities of vitamin supplements and promotes the virtues of 'wogging' — a combination of walking and jogging.

BHA

The abbreviation for butylated hydroxyanisole, another antioxidant used in margarines and cooking oils as a preservative. Like BHA, the effects of this antioxidant with cancer are dubious.

BHT

The abbreviation for butylated hydroxytoluene, an antioxidant which is added to foods such as nuts or margarines to prevent fats reacting with oxygen and becoming rancid. Some people are also taking BHA as a 'health food', in the hope it will offer protection against cancer, as has been demonstrated in some animal studies. Other experiments, however, have shown that BHA actually increases the chances of cancer.

BICARBONATE OF SODA

An alkaline substance commonly referred to as carb soda or baking soda. Used in baking to produce carbon dioxide and make cakes or scones rise. It is also added to green vegetables to produce an alkaline solution to restore the bright green colour of the vegetable by limiting the availability of the hydrogen ions which usually cause the natural chlorophyll in the vegetable to lose its colour. Unfortunately, carb soda also destroys vitamins B and C in vegetables.

BIERWURST
see Sausages.

BIJON

A noodle made in Southeast Asia from corn. Bijon looks like noodles but has some corn flavour.

BILBERRY
see Fruit.

BILE

Also called gall, bile is made in the liver, concentrated to about 20 times its original strength and stored in the gallbladder. When fat is present in the small intestine, bile is squirted from the gallbladder to assist in the digestion of the fats. About 250–1000 mL of bile are produced by the liver each day.

BILE ACIDS

Members of the steroid family which can be produced in the liver from cholesterol. In the intestine, bile acids combine with sodium or potassium to form bile salts which act a little like detergents to help break down fats into smaller particles. They also assist in the absorption of fat-soluble vitamins.

With certain types of dietary fibre, larger quantities of bile acids are excreted. This means that more cholesterol is used by the body to make more bile acids. This is one of the

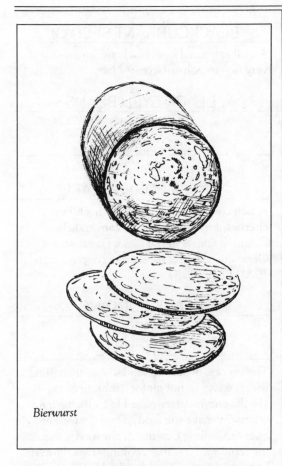

Bierwurst

major ways that a diet high in certain types of dietary fibre can reduce blood cholesterol levels.

BILE DUCT

The tube which carries bile from the gallbladder to the small intestine.

BILE SALTS

see Bile acids.

BILIRUBIN

A pigment formed from the breakdown of haemoglobin (see page 175). Normally excreted in bile but the level rises during jaundice, causing the whites of the eyes, the skin and urine to turn yellow.

BILLY

A tin in which tea is made, stews are cooked and vegetables are boiled. Billy tea refers to tea made in a billy over an open fire. The word 'billy' may have been from the Aboriginal word 'billa', meaning a creek or a river or it may have been a derivation of 'William'. During the reign of George IV, a big bush kettle had been called a 'royal George'. When William IV succeeded George IV, the kettle assumed the name 'royal William' or 'billy'.

BILTONG

Dried beef strips, originally made in South Africa. To make biltong, the meat is pounded and then smoked over a fire or left in the sun to dry. It is hard and chewy but useful in areas where there is no refrigeration.

BINGE EATING

see Bulimia nervosa.

BIOAVAILABILITY

The amount of any nutrient which is actually absorbed into the body in a usable form. Some nutrients come into the body in food but are present in a form which is not well absorbed. For example, spinach contains a lot of iron but this is of low bioavailability because it is bound up with oxalic acid and is thus not available to the body.

BIOFLAVENOIDS

Also known as vitamin P, these compounds include rutin and hesperidin, and are found in citrus fruits, other fruits and vegetables, buckwheat, tea, coffee, wine and beer. Bioflavenoids prevent vitamin C being destroyed by oxygen. They are widely found in the diet and there is no evidence that supplements are needed by most people.

BIOLOGICAL VALUE

Refers to the percentage of a protein which is

absorbed and retained by the body. Egg and breast milk protein have very high biological values since their protein is easily digested and assimilated by the body. Some proteins, such as gelatine, have almost no biological value and are fairly useless to the body.

BIOTIN
see Vitamins.

BIRYANI

An Indian dish made up of layers of spicy lamb and delicately perfumed rice.

BISCUITS

A baked, flat, crisp item which may be sweet or savoury. Sweet biscuits are made from flour (usually white), fat (usually beef fat or a saturated vegetable fat) and sugar. Savoury biscuits have less sugar and more salt.

What is known as a biscuit in Australia and England is called a cookie (if sweet) or a cracker (if savoury) in the United States. A biscuit in the United States is called a scone in England and Australia.

BISQUE

A cream soup, usually containing cream and egg yolks. Often made from seafoods, as in lobster bisque.

BITTERS
see Drinks, Alcoholic.

BLACHAN

A dried shrimp paste used in Indonesian cooking.

BLACK BEANS
see Legumes.

BLACKBERRY
see Fruit.

BLACKCURRANT
see Fruit.

BLACKCURRANT SEED OIL

An oil extracted from blackcurrant seeds and very rich in polyunsaturated fats.

BLACK-EYED BEANS
see Legumes.

BLACKFISH
see Fish.

BLACK FOREST CAKE

A rich chocolate layer cake with a filling of cherries, kirsch, whipped cream and chocolate. Originally made in the Black Forest area of Germany. An average slice has approximately 3000 kJ (715 Cals).

BLACK PUDDING
see Sausages.

BLANCHING

The process of placing food in rapidly boiling water, steam or hot air for a minute or two to kill the enzymes (see page 113) which would otherwise make the food go bad. Immediately after the boiling treatment, the food is plunged into cold water so that cooking stops. Frozen vegetables are usually blanched before freezing. This causes a small loss of vitamins.

BLANCMANGE

Originally, blancmange was a dish made from meat or fish boiled with sweetened almond milk and seasoned with sugar and salt. It was thickened with eggs. The blancmange of more modern French and English cuisine is made from sweetened milk, thickened with cornflour and flavoured with vanilla. An average serve of a modern blancmange has 670 kJ (160 Cals).

BLANQUETTE

A white sauce, usually served with meat as in veal blanquette. Also a variety of grape.
See also Wine, Varieties.

BLEACHING

A whitening process applied to flour to remove the natural yellow tinge. There is no real reason for bleaching other than to produce white bread. Flour left for some time will gradually lose its yellow colour, so the proponents of bleaching claim that they are merely speeding up a natural process and preventing the flour from sitting around risking insect infestation. Some countries ban the use of flour-bleaching agents and their populations suffer no ill-effects from eating creamy-coloured bread. Common bleaches used include chlorine or benzoyl peroxide.

BLINI

Small yeasted pancakes often made from buckwheat. Traditionally served with sour cream and caviar, but also used as a dessert with fruit or jam and cream. Recipe originated in Russia.

BLOATER
see Fish.

BLOOD ORANGE
see Fruit.

BLOOD PRESSURE

The pressure of the blood on the walls of arteries. Systolic blood pressure (the upper reading) shows the level of pressure when the heart is contracting; the diastolic pressure (the lower reading) represents the pressure when the heart relaxes between beats. It is particularly dangerous for this lower reading to be high. Blood pressure is related to the salt in the diet.

See also Salt, Hypertension.

BLOOD SUGAR

The level of glucose in the blood. All body cells use glucose for energy; the brain prefers not to use anything else. Normal blood sugar level after fasting is 60–70 mg/dL rising to 120 mg/dL after a carbohydrate meal and then remaining around 80–100 mg/dL between meals.

The body has various mechanisms to maintain its blood glucose within a certain range to protect the brain and other vital organs.

When we eat carbohydrates, they are broken down to glucose and absorbed into the blood. Some of this glucose is stored in the liver and muscles in the form of glycogen; the rest is used either by the tissues (under the influence of insulin), or converted to body fat (see page 56).

Some hours after eating, the blood glucose level falls and the body's first reaction is to send out a hunger signal. If we do not eat, the hormones adrenalin and glucagon will mobilise some of the liver glycogen to temporarily restore the blood glucose level. That is why a hunger pang lasts for a few minutes and then subsides.

If we continue to ignore the body's attempts to have us eat some food, the body begins to break down some of its protein tissue to form glucose. The process takes place in the liver and is known as gluconeogenesis (see page 164). It will restore the blood sugar level to normal, but will use up amino acids (from protein in the diet or in muscle). Fat cannot be turned into blood glucose.

The blood glucose level normally fluctuates during the day but it will generally right itself. The exception occurs in untreated diabetics where blood sugar may rise to very high levels and spill over into the urine leaving dangerously low levels in the blood.

Many people find that when their blood sugar level drops slightly (for example, just before meals or in the late afternoon), they become irritable, shaky and generally feel blue. Some believe they are suffering from low blood sugar (hypoglycaemia) although, technically, the blood sugar level is within the normal range. However, there is no doubt that for that particular individual, the temporary drop in blood sugar level is unpleasant. It can be avoided by eating more, eating carbohydrates which are more slowly digested (such as oats) or eating more frequently. It is not a disease, it is merely the body reacting a little more sensitively to the fact that it needs some food.

See also Hypoglycaemia; Insulin.

BLOODY MARY
see Drinks, Alcoholic.

BLUEBERRY
see Fruit.

BLUE EYE
see Fish, Trevalla.

BLUE GRENADIER
see Fish.

BLUE VEIN
see Cheese.

BMI
see Body Mass Index.

BMR
see Basic Metabolic Rate.

BOARFISH
see Fish.

BOCCONCINI
see Cheese.

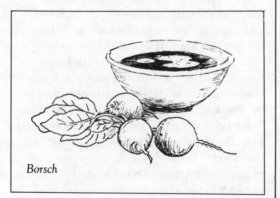

Borsch

BODY MASS INDEX (BMI)

Used as an indicator of overweight, BMI is calculated by dividing weight (in kilograms) by squared height (in metres). For example, a 1.8 m person weighing 72 kg would have a BMI of $\frac{75}{1.8 \times 1.8} = 22$. A value of BMI from $20-25$ has been found to be most consistent with good health. If your BMI is above 25, you are probably too fat; if it is below 20, you are probably too thin.

See also the chart on page 7.

BOK CHOY
see Vegetables.

BOLETUS
see Vegetables, Mushrooms.

BOLOGNA
see Sausages.

BOMBAY DUCK
see Fish.

BOMBE

A frozen dessert set in a high shaped mould. It may be made with layers of icecream or a coating of icecream and an inner layer of fruit mixture and cream. A bombe Alaska is made by placing a layer of sponge cake into a bombe mould, filling with icecream and, once frozen, turning the bombe onto a wooden board and completely coating it with a meringue mixture. The entire dessert (and board) is placed in a moderate oven for several minutes until the meringue browns. An average serving has 1800 kJ (430 Cals).

BONE

Bone consists of cells in a mixture of protein and minerals, predominantly calcium, phosphorus and carbonate. Bone serves a structural role, is the point of attachment for muscles, protects vital organs such as the brain and houses the bone marrow where important cells are made.

The bones are a storehouse of calcium and any time the body needs more calcium in the blood (where it is vital for the functioning of nerves and muscles), it can be withdrawn from the bone. The withdrawal and deposition of calcium in bones is under the control of a hormone produced by the parathyroid gland. Vitamin D is also essential for the movement of calcium into and out of bone.

If more calcium is being withdrawn from bones than is being deposited, the bones gradually become porous and weak and the condition known as osteoporosis develops (see pages 51, 256).

To keep bones strong and healthy, a number of factors are important. There must be an adequate supply of calcium from the diet, hormonal function must be normal, vitamin D and phosphorus must be present in the correct amounts, and the individual must have enough exercise to exert a pull of the muscles on bones. Excess sodium, caffeine or alcohol in the diet can also hasten the loss of calcium from bones.

Women have a special problem maintaining strong dense bones since the drop in oestrogen levels at menopause means less calcium will be retained by bones. Extreme thinness in women can also alter hormone levels and lead to loss of calcium from bones.

See also Calcium; Marrow bone.

BONITO
see Fish.

BORAGE
see Herbs.

BORAGE SEED OIL
see Oils.

BORDELAISE SAUCE
see Sauces, Brown.

BOREK
see Burek.

BORLOTTI BEANS
see Legumes.

BORON

A mineral required by plants but not known to be essential for humans. Found in small quantities in fruits, potatoes and other vegetables. Supplements containing boron are not advisable as it is highly toxic and safe doses have not yet been established.

BORSCH

A Russian or Polish soup made from beef stock and beetroot and served with sour cream. Other ingredients may include vegetables such as onions, carrots, parsley, or cabbage.

BOSTON BAKED BEANS
see Legumes.

BOTULISM

Food poisoning caused by the bacterium *clostridium botulinum* which live in soil. It can survive without oxygen and produce a toxin which can paralyse the lungs, heart and other organs. These bacteria can thrive in home-preserved fruits and vegetables which have not been properly sterilised. The more acid the food, the easier it is to destroy the spores of the bacteria. Alkaline foods require much higher temperatures to kill the spores than are generally available in the domestic kitchen, so adding an acid such as lemon juice, vinegar or citric acid, means that normal heat processing will kill the spores. Commercial canneries have strict regulations to prevent any growth of the bacteria. Throw out any food which you suspect may be contaminated with botulinum.

See also Food poisoning.

BOUDIN BLANC
see Sausages.

BOUILLABAISSE

A fish stew prepared in Mediterranean countries. A variety of fish and seafoods are cooked in a richly flavoured stock which generally includes olive oil, tomatoes, herbs and spices (including saffron).

BOUILLON

A clear broth made by cooking chicken, meat, fish or vegetables in water and straining off the flavoursome liquid. Used in soups, stews and sauces to provide more flavour than water. Has few kilojoules.

BOUQUET GARNI
see Herbs.

BOURBON
see Drinks, Alcoholic, Whisky.

BOURSIN
see Cheese.

BOWEL FUNCTION

The process whereby the large intestine propels its spent contents for excretion. Adequate bowel function depends on plenty of dietary fibre in the daily diet, as well as sufficient water. Since the wall of the bowel is a muscle, it can become slack with increasing age or, if not used, bowel function then deteriorates. The frequency of bowel motions is probably much less important that the consistency of the contents.

See also Dietary fibre; Digestion.

BOYSENBERRY
see Fruit.

BRACKEN
see Vegetables, Fiddlehead fern.

BRAIN, HUMAN

The human brain is nothing less than a marvel. Its development in the child depends on a good state of nutrition and those children who are malnourished during their early life may have impairment of brain function. Sufficient protein in the diet is particularly important for the normal growth of brain cells.

The brain's fuel is glucose from the blood. It cannot use fat as a fuel. During extreme starvation, the brain can use substances called ketones as fuel (see page 197).

The brain's function and one's mood may be influenced by diet if some agent interferes with the normal transmission of messages between the nerve cells within the brain. Various drugs, including caffeine, can do this. Certain amino acids such as tryptophan (a constituent of most protein foods) can also alter brain function (see page 349). Tryptophan promotes sleep. Milk contains tryptophan, and that's one of the reasons why we drink hot milk at bedtime. Although many parents maintain that their children's behaviour deteriorates after eating a lot of sugar, the biochemical evidence does not support the idea that sugar itself causes hyperactivity (although something else in the sugar-containing foods may). Sugar alters the metabolism of amino acids and actually promotes the entry of tryptophan into the brain, which should have a calming effect. Alcohol can also affect the brain by causing brain cells to shrink.

BRAINS

Lamb and calf brains are considered a delicacy by some. Before being eaten, they need to be soaked for an hour or two and the membrane removed. After a thorough washing, they can be simmered in water with a little lemon juice or vinegar.

Nutritionally, brains are a source of protein, most vitamins and many minerals. They have some fat and are very rich in pre-formed cholesterol. One set of brains has as much cholesterol as 10 eggs. This is only a problem if the diet is also high in fat. There is no special virtue in giving brains to invalids. 100 g steamed calf brains have 630 kJ (150 Cals); 100 g steamed lamb brains have 525 kJ (125 Cals).

BRAMBLE

see Fruit, Blackberry.

BRAN

The outside husk of a cereal grain. Wheat bran is the most commonly consumed bran. It has a high content of dietary fibre (44 per cent) and is valuable for preventing or treating constipation. However, only coarsely milled bran is useful in this regard; fine bran forms small hard faeces and may actually cause constipation.

Wheat bran also contains phytic acid (see page 266), a chemical substance which can form complexes with minerals such as calcium, iron and zinc, making them unavailable to the body. Since wheat bran itself contains quite high quantities of these minerals, the phytic acid only becomes a problem when people abuse bran by taking excessive amounts. A safe daily intake is 1−2 tablespoons. Larger quantities may have an undesirable scouring effect on the large intestine. Each tablespoon of unprocessed wheat bran has 60 kJ (14 Cals).

Oat bran is also popular and contains high quantities (about 16 per cent) of soluble fibre which has been shown to normalise fluctuations in blood sugar levels (for example, in diabetics). Oat bran may also lower levels of cholesterol in the blood.

See also Blood sugar; Constipation; Diabetes mellitus.

BRANDY

see Drinks, Alcoholic.

BRANDY ALEXANDER

see Drinks, Alcoholic.

BRASSICA

The family of vegetables which includes cabbage, cauliflower, broccoli, kohl rabi and Brussels sprouts. Each of these members is a descendant of the original wild cabbage which grew around the Mediterranean. There is some evidence that eating vegetables of the brassica family confers some protection against certain forms of cancer. Whether this is due to their content of vitamin C and carotene (see page 57), or to the presence of substances called indoles, or to a combination is not yet known.

BRATWURST

see Sausages.

BRAUNSCHWEIGER

see Sausages.

BRAWN

A mixture of meats stewed with spices and bones until the meat is tender. The bones are removed and the meat is cut up and allowed to set in the cooking liquor which forms a jelly. Any fat will rise to the top, forming a seal which prevents the meat drying out. The addition of pig's trotters or a veal knuckle provides plenty of natural jelly.

BRAZIL NUTS

see Nuts.

BREAD

Breads are made from some type of ground grain and water, with or without the addition of yeast, salt, milk and a variety of other ingredients. The original Stone Age breads were flat breads made from barley or wheat without leavening and baked on hot stones. Leavened bread was first made in Egypt about 4000 BC but the product was rather heavy because the parching used to separate the grain from its inedible hull destroyed the gluten (see page 165) which gives bread its light texture. It was not until several thousand years later that strains of wheat which could easily be dehusked were grown. These made leavened bread a much lighter, crustier product.

Grinding equipment gradually led to the production of finer flours and by 300 BC, making yeast for bread had become a recognised trade in Egypt. Indeed, baking bread was regarded as a worthy profession.

The Greeks were the first to equate superiority with the more expensive fine white breads. Only the poor and the peasants ate the cheaper, coarse wholegrain breads. Except in rice-eating countries, however, some type of bread became a staple part of the daily diet throughout the world.

Bread was considered so important that it acquired the title 'the staff of life'. Contrary to popular belief, this is not a biblical expression, but became commonly used from the pulpit in England during the seventeenth century to reflect the call for simplicity in all things.

Bread continued to be a staple food until about 20 years ago, when its consumption in countries such as Australia dropped dramatically as people picked up the somewhat absurd idea that bread was fattening. In most Mediterranean and European countries, bread continues to enjoy a greater status as a vital part of each meal.

In recent years, nutritionists have been recommending that bread should be given greater priority in daily food choices because it contains little fat and is an important source of complex carbohydrate. Eating more bread in place of fatty, sugary foods would restore some balance to the diet.

Increasing knowledge of the nutritional superiority of wholegrain breads is reinstating these loaves to an 'upper crust' position. In Western countries, there is now higher consumption of wholegrain breads among those with a higher level of education.

From the nutritional point of view, bread is an excellent product. Even white loaves contain some dietary fibre and a reasonable quantity of minerals and vitamins. The terms wholemeal or wholegrain are used for products made from the whole of the wheat grain; wholemeal means the grain is ground; wholegrain signifies that there will be bits of grain left. These have more dietary fibre and a higher content of minerals and vitamins than white breads.

Rye breads are generally made using some rye and some wheat flour. The latter is added to provide a higher content of gluten and thus produce a loaf with a better volume. Nutritionally, most rye breads rate about half-way between wholemeal and white, although some of the dark wholegrain rye loaves are nutritionally equivalent to wholemeal bread.

Multigrain breads are made from a mixture of white flour and whole grains of rye and/or wheat. Wholemeal multigrain loaves begin with wholemeal flour and add the grain pieces.

The idea that bread was fattening developed with the plethora of slimming diets which promised fast weight loss if the follower would avoid foods such as bread and potatoes. Such diets do indeed produce a rapid weight loss, but this is largely due to a depletion of glycogen (a storage form of glucose) and its accompanying water from muscles. Little body fat is lost with the 'no bread diets' and the apparent lost weight is soon regained. Such diets are useless for reducing body fat and have also given nutritious foods like bread and potatoes an undeserved reputation as being fattening.

Current guidelines in Australia suggest that a minimum of 4 slices of bread should be eaten each day.

See also Balanced diet; Carbohydrates.

BREADFRUIT

see Fruit.

BREAKFAST CEREALS

Australians are the world's largest consumers of breakfast cereals. To meet our voracious appetite for these products, the food industry has given us products which range from very nutritious single or combination grain products to those which are almost half sugar. Some

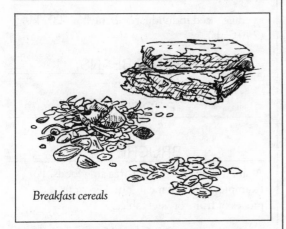

Breakfast cereals

breakfast cereal grains, such as oats or wheat or other grains used for porridge, have minimal processing. Others are heated, puffed, popped, toasted or extruded with a resulting loss of most of their original vitamins. The manufacturers usually replace a few of these; some also have added minerals such as iron.

In nutritional value, the top breakfast cereals are wheatgerm, rolled oats or oatmeal, or wheatmeal or mixed grain porridges. Wholewheat breakfast biscuits, bran cereals and some of the mixed cereals with added dried fruits come next. Products such as puffed corn or popped rice have little nutritional value apart from the few vitamins added to them. Unlike the products mentioned above, these have little dietary fibre.

The highly sweetened cereals may contain up to 48 per cent sugar — and virtually no dietary fibre. They are designed to appeal to children, the rationale for the pre-sweetening being that the child would have added sugar to most cereals. In reality, few children would add anything like as much sugar as comes in the highly sweetened products.

Mueslis range from being nutritionally excellent products to those which are more than 50 per cent fat and sugar. A careful reading of the ingredient list is needed to make a wise choice (ingredients are listed in their order of prominence in the product).

Some cereal manufacturers, however, circumvent the complete truth in ingredient listing by using several types of sugar. For example, if a product is 52 per cent sugar and 48 per cent rice, the ingredients would be listed as 'sugar, rice, salt, colouring, etc'. However, if the manufacturer uses 26 per cent each of two different sugars, the rice will be listed as the major ingredient. If you want cereal rather than sugar, avoid products with several types of sugar in the ingredient list.

See also Carbohydrates; Labels, food.

BREAM
see Fish.

BREAST CANCER

Recent studies show a definite link between breast cancer and diet, particularly in women over the age of 40. A high fat diet (any kind of fat) or gaining weight around menopause are significant risk factors.

BREAST FEEDING

Generally considered the ideal way to feed a baby. In the first few days after birth, the breasts secrete a thin yellowish fluid called colostrum (see page 79) which contains factors important for the baby's immunity to disease. By the third or fourth day, the milk 'comes in', in response to a hormone produced when the baby sucks on the nipples. This hormonal response may be sensitive to the mother's anxiety, embarrassment or lack of emotional support from those around her. Some mothers simply do not want to breast feed the infant. There is no justification for making such mothers feel guilty. Many women, however, find breast feeding an immensely enjoyable experience. Breast feeding also stimulates the uterus to contract, helping it return to its pre-pregnant state.

There are more than 100 biochemical differences between breast milk and cow's milk in the amounts and types of nutrients present.

For example, breast milk has more lactose (milk sugar), vitamins A, C, E and several of the B complex vitamins, more iron, cholesterol and essential fatty acids than cow's milk. The significance of all these differences is not yet fully understood.

The composition of breast milk also changes during the course of a feed. The baby gets most of the protein and lactose in the first few minutes and, as sucking continues, the fat content of the milk progressively increases. This tends to make the baby sleepy and the taste and texture also alter, reducing the infant's appetite. Breast-fed infants may thus have an inbuilt appetite control mechanism in their feed. Breast feeding can continue as long as it suits both mother and child. In general, once a child has a few teeth, foods which require chewing become more important in the diet and milk takes a lesser, but still important, role.

See also Lactation.

BREWER'S YEAST

The spent yeast from the brewing of beer is one of the richest sources of vitamins of the B complex. Live yeasts should not be consumed as they actually destroy some of the B vitamins within the body.

BRIE
see Cheese.

BRILLIANT (BLACK, BLUE, SCARLET)
see Colourings.

BRINJAL
see Vegetables, Eggplant.

BRIOCHE

A small, yeasted bread enriched with eggs and butter and usually coated with an egg and/or slightly sweet glaze. Often hollowed out and filled with a sweet or savoury mixture. An average-sized individual brioche has 1000 kJ (240 Cals).

BROAD BEANS
see Legumes.

BROCCOLI
see Vegetables.

BROCHETTE

A small skewer used for threading foods. For example, cubes of meat, chicken or fish, or pieces of fruits or vegetables.

BROILING
see Grilling.

BROWN FAT

More properly known as brown adipose tissue (or BAT), this form of fat is different from regular white body fat in that it is specialised for heat production. In rats and mice, brown fat has been shown to burn up kilojoules, either to provide extra heat in cold weather or to increase the number of kilojoules used if the animal overeats. Such effects have not been demonstrated in humans and the functions of brown fat remain the subject of research.

Brown fat makes up about 2—5 per cent of the body weight of newborn human infants and decreases with age.

BROWNIES

An American sweet which is somewhere between a rather moist, chewy cake and a biscuit. Often contain chocolate.

BROWNING (OF FOODS)

There are two major types of browning reactions: the desirable browning of meats, potatoes, breads and pastries; and the undesirable browning of fruits and vegetables.

The browning which occurs during cooking produces flavours which enhance a food. The reaction occurs either because of the caramelisation of a sugar in the food (for example, when marshmallows are toasted) or from an interaction between a carbohydrate and an amino acid (for example, when bread is toasted). This browning effect is called the maillard reaction (see page 216). It is responsible for the full flavour of a casserole when meat is browned before adding any liquid. It is also the maillard reaction which accounts for the difference in flavour between fried and boiled onions.

The browning of fruits and vegetables, on the other hand, comes from damage to the cells in the food and the consequent action of certain enzymes. If you cut an apple, for example, the knife will damage the cells and enzymes will then begin to oxidise chemical substances present in the apple. These substances (known as phenolic compounds) condense and join together until they form brownish-coloured compounds.

Adding a solution or powder containing sulphur dioxide will prevent the browning and development of off-flavours in fruits and vegetables. However, some people are sensitive to sulphur dioxide and its use is controlled by law.

BROWN SAUCE
see Sauces.

BRUSSELS SPROUTS
see Vegetables.

BUBBLE AND SQUEAK
Fried left-over vegetables, usually including cabbage and potato. Often served at breakfast.

BUCHU
A herbal tea which has a diuretic action. Safety not yet established.

BUCKWHEAT
see Grains.

BULGUR
see Grains.

BULIMIA NERVOSA
An eating disorder in which the victim eats large amounts of food, usually followed by self-induced vomiting or abuse of laxatives or unprocessed bran. With so much emphasis on slimness in women, and the profusion of fast weight loss diets, many women alternately diet and binge eat. After a binge, they usually feel depressed and hate themselves for what they see as their weakness. So they go back to yet another form of semi-starvation — until the next binge.

The behaviour is usually hidden and many sufferers go to great lengths to hide their food purchases and bingeing occasions. Most maintain a normal weight. Psychiatrists estimate that this type of eating disorder may afflict a considerable number of women, possibly up to 20 per cent.

See also Anorexia nervosa.

BULLOCK'S HEART
West Indian name for the custard apple.

BUREK
A savoury pastry, usually made with filo pastry wrapped around eggs, cream cheese and either spinach, pumpkin or meat. Sometimes called 'borek'.

BURKITT, DR DENIS
An eminent British physician who spent much of his working life in Africa where he noticed a striking lack of the diseases which afflict Western populations. In the 1970s, Burkitt proposed that the differences in disease patterns between rural Africans and Westerners were due to the lack of dietary fibre in the typical Western diet. After his observations, more research began into the effects of dietary fibre.

BURRITO
see Tortilla.

BUSH FOODS

Foods which are native to Australia and are still used by tribal Aborigines. The variety of bush foods may stagger those who believe Australia is largely desert. There are dozens of fruits — some, such as the green plum, being among the richest sources of vitamin C ever found. There are also many vegetables, tubers, roots, shoots, pods, nuts and wild grasses which provide an amazingly adequate diet. Animals (both large and small), birds, turtles and a variety of fish and other aquatic creatures also make up bush food.

See also Aboriginal diet; Insects, edible.

BUTTER

When cream is whipped, lumps of butterfat separate into a yellow mass. The remaining water is squeezed out to produce unsalted (or sweet) butter. 1−2 per cent salt may also be added.

Clarified butter or ghee has had even more of the water and any remaining milk solids removed. When heated, it does not burn or stick (see page 163).

The delicate flavour of butter is superb in cooking or as a spread. Unfortunely, however, butter is largely fat, about 60 per cent of which is saturated. 100 g butter have 3040 kJ (740 Cals).

See also Dairy products, Fats.

BUTTER BEANS
see Legumes.

BUTTER, BRANDY
see Hard sauce.

BUTTER CHEESE
see Cheese.

BUTTERFLY CAKES

Patty cakes which have a piece removed from the top, cream inserted in the cavity, and the top replaced in two halves to look like a butterfly's wings.

BUTTERMILK

Originally the milk left after cream was churned into butter. Bacteria would contaminate the buttermilk, making it slightly thick and turning it a little sour. Buttermilk is now made by adding a safe bacterial culture to skim or part-skim milk. It gives a rich, tangy flavour to scones, pancakes and cakes, and mixes to a smooth, refreshing drink with fruit juices.

The nutritional value of buttermilk varies according to the fat content of the milk. However, buttermilk is a good source of protein, calcium and riboflavin and provides small quantities of other vitamins and minerals. 100 ml have about 210 kJ (50 Cals).

BUTTERNUT PUMPKIN
see Vegetables, Pumpkin.

BUTTER, RUM
see Hard sauce.

BUTTERSCOTCH

A hard type of toffee which has a smooth creamy taste from added butter. With about 90 per cent sugar and 8 per cent fat, it is disastrous for teeth, and does nothing for the waistline! 100 g have 1760 kJ (420 Cals).

BUTYLATED HYDROXYANISOLE
see BHA.

BUTYLATED HYDROXYTOLUENE
see BHT.

CABANOSI
see Sausages.

CABBAGE
see Vegetables.

CABERNET SAUVIGNON
see Wine, Varieties.

CACAO
A tree native to the tropical parts of Africa and America. Its seeds are used to make cocoa and chocolate (see pages 71, 76).

CACTUS BERRY
see Fruit, Prickly Pear.

CADMIUM
This mineral has no known function in the human body. It does, however, have a number of toxic effects including fibrosis in the lungs, kidney damage and atrophy of the testes. Most of the cadmium in the body comes from cigarettes or from industrial sources. The highest food sources are kidneys and seafoods exposed to industrial contamination.

CAERPHILLY
see Cheese.

CAESAR SALAD
see Salads.

CAFFEINE
Caffeine comes in coffee, tea, cocoa or chocolate, and in cola drinks. One or more of these beverages is used by almost every community in the world, making caffeine the most commonly consumed drug. In Western countries, adults drink tea and coffee for their caffeine while children get theirs from cola drinks.

Caffeine is a stimulant and affects the brain, heart, nervous system, kidneys, the body's muscular co-ordination and the working of the respiratory organs. It may also relax smooth muscle in the respiratory system and this may be of benefit in dilating the breathing passages for those with asthma.

In the stomach, caffeine increases the production of acid, causing heartburn in some people, especially if they drink a cup of strong tea or coffee on an empty stomach.

Once in the bloodstream, caffeine acts as a stimulant on the central nervous system and the heart. Most people feel more wide awake and many report that they can think more clearly after coffee. These effects are apparent within 15−30 minutes after consumption and caffeine level in the blood peaks about an hour after ingestion.

From the blood, caffeine goes to the liver and is metabolised into substances which are excreted by the kidneys along with some water. Caffeine thus has a diuretic effect on the body. This can be a problem for those who also lose a lot of fluid through heavy sweating and find it difficult to drink sufficient water to replace their losses. Caffeine is not stored in the body and is excreted within 12−16 hours after intake.

Caffeine is an addictive drug and some people are more sensitive to it than others. If caffeine intake stops, most people will notice withdrawal symptoms such as headache, crankiness, a feeling of tiredness and even muscular discomfort. After a 'cuppa', the symptoms disappear. For many people, the need for a morning 'fix' is an essential start to the day.

In continued high doses (which will vary according to one's individual tolerance), caffeine causes a jittery feeling and may even cause headaches. It is also one of the most common causes of insomnia. If it were to be proposed as a new food additive, it is unlikely that any regulatory body in any country would allow caffeine to be added to foods.

However, in spite of its widespread effects on the human body, small quantities of caffeine probably do little harm to most people. In larger amounts, however, caffeine is likely to increase the heart rate and may raise the levels of some fats in the blood. Some early research linked high levels of caffeine intake with cancer of the pancreas but this is now thought to be due to other features of coffee rather than the caffeine.

For most people, 2—4 cups of coffee a day will cause few problems. Children are more sensitive to the effects of caffeine and probably should avoid it altogether.

Tea and cola drinks have less caffeine than coffee, but if tea is strong, it can have as much caffeine as coffee. Some herbal teas (see page 341) also contain caffeine. Cola drinks consumed by the can (the equivalent volume of about 2 cups of tea) can also contribute a significant amount of caffeine, especially in the diet of a small child. Low kilojoule cola drinks have the same caffeine content as the regular varieties.

Because of its effects on the stomach, those who are prone to stomach ulcers should avoid concentrated doses of caffeine.

Those who have trouble sleeping, should try avoiding tea, coffee, cocoa, chocolate and cola drinks and find out if caffeine is causing the insomnia. Some people find a single cup of coffee within 4 hours of bedtime is enough to cause tossing and turning. Others, especially those whose bodies are accustomed to a lot of caffeine, will sleep soundly after a good strong evening brew.

Cutting back on caffeine

- Learn to use water as a thirst quencher rather than relying on tea or coffee.
- Drink very weak tea as its caffeine content is quite low.
- Avoid cola drinks.
- Avoid chocolate and cocoa.
- Switch to decaffeinated coffees. The caffeine is removed from coffee beans either by steam or with chemical solvents. Most of the varieties of decaffeinated coffee beans or ground decaffeinated coffees use steam. The better quality instant decaffeinated coffees also avoid the use of solvents, although it is most unlikely that harmful quantities of residues of solvent would remain.
- Try cereal coffees. These are usually made from substances such as barley, rye, chicory and dandelions. They have no caffeine.

Caffeine content

BEVERAGE	CAFFEINE
Coffee, brewed, 1 cup	85 mg
Coffee, strong brew, 1 cup	120 mg
Coffee, instant, 1 teaspoon	60 mg
Tea, strong, 1 cup	80 mg
Tea, average strength, 1 cup	50 mg
Tea, weak, 1 cup	20—30 mg
Cocoa, 2 teaspoons	20 mg
Cola drinks, 1 can	35—55 mg

See also Chocolate; Cocoa; Coffee; Cola; Tea.

CAKE

A sweet bread batter, with or without added fat or other ingredients. Whipped fat (usually butter or margarine) or eggs or an aerating agent such as baking powder incorporate air into cake mixtures and produce a lighter cake. Nuts, dried or fresh fruits and a variety of other ingredients, may also be added. Nutritionally, most cakes do not rate highly since they usually contain both fat and sugar. Kilojoule values are generally high, the exact number depending on the type of cake. A slice of plain sponge cake might have as little as 840 kJ (200 Cals); a rich fruit cake might have 1470 kJ (350 Cals) in a 100 g slice; a slice of baked cheesecake can have 2730 kJ (650 Cals).

Commercial cake mixes produce very fine-textured results, due largely to the kind of chlorinated flour and emulsifiers used. The treated flour keeps the texture fine and tender while the emulsifiers stabilise the foam produced by whipping the fat. Some people prefer the fine texture of packet cakes; others like the coarser, moister texture of home-made products.

Cakes can be successfully cooked in a microwave if they are placed into a microsafe ring container (to allow more even heating) and placed on a special microsafe rack to raise them above the level of the bottom of the oven.

CALAMARI

see Seafood, Squid.

CALCITONIN

A hormone produced by the thyroid gland to control the level of calcium in the blood. If the level of calcium rises too high, calcitonin is released and prevents calcium being withdrawn from the bones into the blood. The action of calcitonin balances that of another hormone, parathyroid hormone. If the blood calcium level falls, parathyroid hormone causes calcium to be withdrawn from the bones to replenish the blood level.

CALCIUM

Calcium is a mineral which is essential for building strong bones and teeth (see also page 41). The body also maintains some calcium in the blood for the nervous system and muscles to function properly. This level cannot vary much. If it drops even a little, the body withdraws some calcium from the bones to make up the correct concentration of blood calcium. As far as the body is concerned, the bones are a reservoir of calcium.

If losses of calcium from the bones are greater than the intake from the diet, there is a slow but steady loss of bone calcium. The bones gradually become less dense, lose some of their strength and the condition known as osteoporosis, or porous bones, develops (see page 256).

Both men and women tend to lose calcium from their skeleton as they age, but women generally lose about twice as much as men. Porous bones and fractures are common in older women.

Around menopause, changes in the female hormone, oestrogen, accelerate the loss of calcium from the bones. The denser the bones are to start with, the less the chances of osteoporosis. It is therefore important for women to have built up sufficient calcium in their bones over the previous 20 or 30 years. The idea that calcium is not important after growth stops is incorrect.

The fashion for extreme thinness in women can exacerbate osteoporosis. Those women who either eat so little or exercise so much that their body fat level becomes so low that they stop menstruating have a double problem. They do not build up the strong skeleton which is needed for later life, and they begin to suffer the withdrawal of calcium which normally does not occur until menopause.

Large quantities of calcium are found only in a few foods and there are factors which interfere with the absorption of calcium. These include:
- *The amount of calcium in the diet* — you cannot absorb calcium unless you are taking it into the body
- *Vitamin D* — well supplied by the sun in countries such as Australia. In countries where the winter is so long and cold that skin is not exposed to the sun, vitamin D must be

obtained from butter, margarine or fish liver oils.

- *Phosphorus* — essential for strong bones, although excessive amounts can increase the loss of calcium from bones. We do not need to take phosphorus supplements as almost all foods supply it.
- *Hormones* — at different ages, a lack of oestrogen (see page 248) has two major effects on bones. During adolescence and the early adult years, a decrease in hormone levels reduces the accumulation of calcium. Around menopause, the normal decrease in oestrogen increases the amount of calcium withdrawn from the bones.
- *Exercise* — Western lifestyle discourages the weight-bearing exercise which is necessary for calcium to be absorbed into bones. Most people drive instead of walk, few do any heavy housework, work activities tend to involve sitting or standing and leisure activities rarely involve strenuous physical activity. Walking, carrying groceries or other items, dancing, running, walking up stairs, aerobics, skipping or active sports, will increase calcium absorption. Swimming generally has less benefits for bones. However, backstroke swimming may exert a pull on the bones in the spine which will encourage calcium deposition.

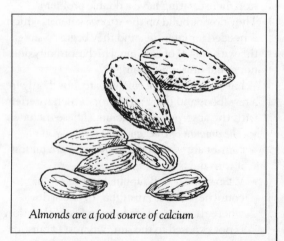

Almonds are a food source of calcium

- *Protein* — a high intake reduces calcium absorption. Doubling the protein from 50–100 g a day almost halves the amount of calcium absorbed. For this reason, very large serves of meat or other high protein foods are inadvisable. A well-balanced diet should contain enough protein, but not excessive quantities.
- *Salt* — a high salt intake interferes with calcium absorption.
- *Caffeine* — in large doses, the caffeine in foods such as coffee, cola drinks, tea and chocolate can interfere with calcium absorption.
- *Nicotine and alcohol* — both reduce calcium absorption.

Recommended calcium intake per day

Women	800 mg
after menopause	1000 mg
during pregnancy	1100 mg
during lactation	1300 mg
Men	800 mg
Girls, 12–15	1000 mg
16–18	800 mg
Boys, 12–15	1200 mg
16–18	1000 mg

Food sources of calcium

FOOD	CALCIUM
Milk (including skim), 1 glass, 250 ml	290 mg
Fortified low-fat milk, 1 glass, 250 ml	400 mg
Yoghurt, 200 g, natural	380 mg
fruit	305 mg
Cheese, 30 g slice	260 mg
Cottage cheese, 100 g	75 mg
Almonds, 50 g	125 mg
Sesame seed kernels, 4 teaspoons (10 g)	15 mg
Sesame seeds, with hulls, 20 g	200 mg
Sesame paste (tahini), made from whole sesame seeds, 20 g	190 mg
Sesame paste made from sesame kernels, 20 g	85 mg
Salmon, 100 g	185 mg
Tuna, 100 g	10 mg

Fresh fish fillet, 150 g	90 mg
Oysters, 6	145 mg
Soya beans, cooked, 1 cup	130 mg
Soya bean milk, 1 cup	55 mg
Fortified soya bean milk, 1 cup	290 mg
Soya bean curd (tofu), 100 g	130 mg
Egg, 1	35 mg
Orange, 1 medium	50 mg
Average piece of fruit	10 mg
Broccoli, 100 g	125 mg
Cabbage, 100 g	50 mg
Most vegetables, av. serve	35 mg
Baked beans, $\frac{1}{4}$ cup, 50 mg	20 mg
Most breakfast cereals, per 20 g serve	15 mg
Bread, per slice	10 mg

CALORIES
see Energy.

CALVADOS
see Drinks, Alcoholic.

CAMEMBERT
see Cheese.

CAMOMILE
see Chamomile.

CAMPARI
see Drinks, Alcoholic.

CANAPE

Bite-sized pieces of toast, bread, biscuit or pastry with a savoury topping. Usually served with drinks and designed to whet the appetite for the meal to come.

CANCER

Any of a group of diseases in which cells grow in an uncontrolled manner. Some types of cancer are at least partially related to diet. Some experts estimate this to be 65 per cent of all cancers in women and 40 per cent of those in men. These include cancers of the oesophagus, stomach, liver, pancreas, breast, bowel, uterus and prostate gland.

The mechanisms whereby diet influences cancer are not fully understood. Studies of epidemic diseases can provide clues as to possible causes of certain types of cancer. However, with many cancers being dependent on several factors, it can be difficult to distinguish between factors. For example, cancer of the bowel is higher in countries where red meat consumption is high. This could be due to the high content of protein or the fat, or to some other factor which also occurs in meat-eating communities. At this stage, there are certain known relationships between diet and cancer and many speculations. For cancers which are common in Western societies, a high fat intake is a prime suspect. Fat itself is unlikely to actually cause cancer, it simply makes it easier for cancer cells to proliferate.

There may also be some protective factors in foods. Vitamins A and C found in vegetables, as well as substances called indoles present in vegetables of the Brassica family (see pages 43, 189) may give protection against cancer.

Heavy consumption of alcoholic drinks may be related to certain types of cancer. Alcohol may act by altering the membranes around cells and allowing cancer-causing chemical substances greater access to the cell. Alcohol may also be a convenient solvent for cancer-causing chemicals.

Cancer of the oesophagus is rare in most affluent countries but occurs commonly in some parts of Asia (especially around the Caspian Sea) and Northern China. The diet in these areas is poor. Very few fruits and vegetables are eaten, and the soil lacks some minerals such as molydenum and selenium. Another possible clue comes from the habit in these areas of drinking scalding hot tea. The natural protection against consuming such hot foods is destroyed because of the dulling of the senses which results from the use of opium.

Cancer of the stomach was once common in Western countries; it is now rare in these areas, but still common in Japan, Iceland, parts of Russia and Eastern Europe. This type of cancer is thought to be related to a high intake of nitrites without a high intake of vitamin C. Nitrites are used in foods which are preserved by salting, smoking and pickling and are converted to cancer-causing nitrosamines in the stomach. This reaction does not occur if vitamin C is present. Refrigeration and more modern preservatives have dramatically reduced the use of salting, pickling and smoking as methods of preserving food. As a result, stomach cancer is becoming much less common.

Cancer of the large bowel (colon and rectum) is very common in Western countries and is showing no signs of decreasing. It is thought to be related to the high-fat/low-fibre diet, although which of these factors is the more important is not known. Vegetarians have much less bowel cancer, so a high meat intake may also be involved.

Liver cancer is much more common in heavy drinkers. It can also be caused by aflatoxins (see page 14), which are released from certain types of moulds which grow on peanuts, corn and some grains.

Breast cancer again shows very specific incidence, occurring mainly in Western countries. It is rare throughout Asia, although Asian women who migrate to countries such as the United States or Australia soon develop the high incidence of their new country.

There is evidence linking breast cancer with a high fat intake. It is certainly more common in women over 40 who are overweight, and this is usually related to a high fat intake. Fat also alters levels of certain hormones in the body, including oestrogen. It is clear that older women should avoid a high fat intake and weight gain in order to reduce their chances of breast cancer.

The ideal diet to give protection against cancer:
- Is low in fats (both saturated and polyunsaturated)
- Has plenty of fruits and vegetables
- Contains vegetables such as broccoli, cabbage, cauliflower, Brussels sprouts, turnips — see also page 43
- Has sufficient, but not excessive, quantities of protein foods such as meat
- Contains only small quantities of alcohol

CANDIDA

A yeast-like fungus, *Candida albicans* is normally found on body surfaces including the skin, mouth, vagina and intestinal tract. Candida infections can occur but are rare. Long-term treatment with antibiotics may kill off the normal antagonists of the fungus and allow it to grow to higher levels and produce candidiasis.

Candida is often falsely diagnosed as being the cause of a wide range of symptoms, including fatigue, depression, headaches, poor concentration or skin problems. The diagnosis is based on the theory that candida weakens the immune system. An anti-candida diet which omits sugars, white flour, dried fruits and yeast-containing foods such as bread, cheeses, wines, beer and yeast extracts, is prescribed. Supplements of vitamins, garlic, *Lactobacillus acidophilus* (see page 201), amino acids and some essential fatty acids, are also prescribed. There is no scientific evidence that this diet is of benefit in treating the symptoms listed above. Where the diet appears to be effective, it may be due to a sensitivity to food chemicals, such as amines, in some of the foods mentioned above.

There is also no evidence that the anti-candida diet is of benefit to those suffering from AIDS. At times, the restrictive nature of the diet can increase weight loss in these people and hasten the onset of weakness.

CANDY
see Confectionery.

CANNELLINI BEANS
see Legumes.

CANNING OF FOODS

Canning involves placing food into a hermetically sealed tin, and heating it rapidly to destroy harmful bacteria and deactivate enzymes which would make the food go bad. The high temperature kills all micro-organisms and their spores so that the canned product can then be kept safely at room temperature.

The first canned foods were produced by Nicholas Appert in France in 1810. Napoleon Bonaparte made use of canned foods for his armies during the nineteenth century.

Nutritionally, canned foods can contain almost the same level of nutrients as foods cooked in the home kitchen. There is some loss of vitamin C and thiamin (B₁) into any liquid in the can, so this should be used for stock or sauces. The major nutritional problem with canned foods is the quantity of salt added. The newer range of 'No Added Salt' products is solving this problem.

CANTELOUPE

see Fruit, Rockmelon, Melons.

CAPE GOOSEBERRY

see Fruit.

CAPERS

The pickled, unopened buds of a shrub which grows in Mediterranean regions, especially in Italy, Spain and Algeria. Commonly added to sauces served with fish or meat.

CAPON

A desexed male chicken, bred for its well-flavoured meat. Favoured because of its high proportion of white meat.

CAPONATA

A vegetable dish made with layers of eggplant, zucchini, mushrooms, onion and tomatoes cooked in olive oil, garlic and red wine and served cold.

CAPSICUM

see Vegetables.

CARAMBOLA

see Fruit.

CARAMEL

The compound formed during the reactions which occur when a sugar is heated to the point at which its molecules break. Various types of caramel are used as a brown colouring in foods. Additive no. 150.

Caramels are sweets made by boiling sugar syrup, butter and milk to approximately 115°C until it forms a brown, moist chewy solid. The characteristic flavour comes from a browning reaction between the milk proteins and lactose (milk sugar). 50 g have 850 kJ (200 Cals) and 8 g of fat.

CARAMEL SAUCE

see Sauces, Other.

CARAWAY SEEDS

see Spices.

CARBOHYDRATES

The most abundant organic compounds on earth, carbohydrates consist of simple sugars (monosaccharides and disaccharides) and complex carbohydrates (also known as starches or polysaccharides).

The most common of the simple sugars are:
- *Monosaccharides*
  glucose (also called dextrose or grape sugar)
  fructose (fruit sugar)
  galactose (formed during the digestion of milk sugar)
- *Disaccharides* (see page 95)
  sucrose (ordinary table sugar) made up of 1 molecule of glucose and one of fructose
  lactose (milk sugar) made up of 1 molecule of glucose and one of galactose
  maltose (malt sugar) made up of 2 molecules of glucose

Complex carbohydrates (polysaccharides) may

contain up to 10,000 simple sugars linked together and occur in grains and cereal products such as rice, wheat, breakfast cereals and pasta, and in vegetables, especially potatoes, corn and various legumes.

In many countries, complex carbohydrates contribute 70–80 per cent of the energy in the diet; in Western countries these important carbohydrate foods tend to be crowded out by foods high in fat, sucrose or protein.

Once eaten, carbohydrates are digested to glucose. This process occurs at different rates depending on the type of carbohydrate and whether or not it occurs in a food with dietary fibre. The glucose is available for use as energy by the cells. When more glucose enters the blood than is needed for the body's immediate energy needs, some of the excess is converted into glycogen, a form of glucose which can be stored in the liver and muscles as an energy reserve. If there is leftover glucose, it is converted into fat.

Glucose is a vital substance in the blood (see Blood sugar, page 39). Both sugars and complex carbohydrates can be broken down to supply glucose. However, there is a difference in other nutritional aspects of foods. Nutritionists generally prefer people to replenish their body's glucose from the complex carbohydrate foods or from the sugar in fruits (fructose) or milk (lactose) rather than from straight sugar because these foods also supply other important nutrients. Sugar is entirely lacking protein, minerals, vitamins or dietary fibre. There is also a difference in the rate at which glucose arrives in the blood from different foods. After eating sugar, blood glucose levels can rise fairly quickly. This causes the body to produce more insulin (see page 190) which can hinder the body's ability to use fats as an energy source.

Carbohydrates contribute 16 kJ (4 Cals) per gram — much less than is supplied by fats or alcohol. By themselves, therefore, carbohydrates should not be labelled

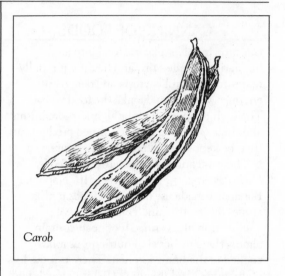

Carob

'fattening'. However, with carbohydrates such as sugar, it is easy to take in large quantities and overdo the body's requirements. The excess sugar is then converted to fat.

Nutritionists throughout the Western world are advising people to eat more carbohydrates, but in the form of fruit, grains, breads, cereals and vegetables. Sugar should form only a small part of a balanced diet.

See also Exercise; Fats; Glycogen.

Carbohydrate loading

A procedure used by some athletes to increase the amount of glycogen in muscles. Carbohydrate loading begins about a week before some endurance events. It involves first depleting the muscles of glycogen by eating very little carbohydrate and exercising hard. This phase takes several days and at the end of this time, many athletes feel awful. Some have headaches, others feel nauseated or dizzy as their muscles run out of fuel. A few researchers have reported disturbances to heart rhythm. The second phase involves eating lots of carbohydrates to replenish the glycogen stores. Exercise is kept to a minimum.

Carbohydrate loading certainly works to produce greater stores of glycogen in muscles. However, glycogen stores at almost this high level can be achieved by following a high-carbohydrate/low-fat diet all the time. Those athletes who insist on carbohydrate loading should follow a modified form in which the initial depletion phase still includes some carbohydrate to prevent the unpleasant side effects of a low carbohydrate diet.

CARBONATED BEVERAGES
see Soft drinks.

CARB SODA
see Baking soda.

CARCINOGENS

Substances which cause cancer.
See also Cancer.

CARDAMOM
see Spices.

CARDOON
see Vegetables.

CARIES, DENTAL
see Dental caries.

CARIGNANE
see Wine, Varieties.

CARMINE
see Colourings, Cochineal.

CARMOISINE
see Colourings.

CARNITINE (VITAMIN B–T)

Discovered in 1947, this substance was, at first, thought to be a vitamin. Carnitine plays a role in the way fatty acids are transported and used in the body. However, it does not fit the definition of a vitamin and is readily made in the body from the amino acids lysine and methionine. Some athletes take carnitine supplements, believing they will help them burn fat faster, but there is no evidence that they are of any value to athletes. A supplement is only needed if there is some reason why carnitine is not being made in the body. Further research into the role of carnitine is being carried out. In the meantime, it is unlikely that paying large amounts for carnitine supplements will be of any benefit.

See also Vitamins.

CAROB

The pod of the locust bean tree, also known as St John's bread, in the belief that the 'locusts' which St John the Baptist ate when he was wandering in the wilderness were carob pods. The pods can be eaten fresh but are more often dried and are often used as a chocolate substitute. Carob powder can be put to much the same uses as cocoa.

Nutritionally, carob is preferable to chocolate, as it contains dietary fibre and has less fat. 100 g carob powder have 755 kJ (180 Cals). Carob 'health' bars, however, usually have added sugar and/or fat. A 100 g carob bar has 1760 kJ (420 Cals), 53 per cent of which come from fat, most of it saturated.

CAROLINA RICE
see Grains, Rice.

CAROTENES

A group of substances (individually designated alpha, beta and gamma) which are converted into vitamin A in the membranes lining the walls of the small intestine. Beta-carotene has the greatest level of vitamin A activity. Carrots are particularly rich in beta-carotene, as the name suggests. Other orange or yellow fruits and vegetables such as pumpkin, mangoes, oranges, mandarins, pawpaws, rockmelons, yellow peaches and apricots are also rich in carotenes. Green and red products such as spinach, red capsicum, broccoli, watercress and parsley are also high in carotene; their orange colour is overpowered by the green pigment chlorophyll.

Within the human intestine, it takes 6

micrograms of beta-carotene to make 1 microgram of vitamin A. For this reason, the amount of beta-carotene in plants is divided by 6 to give the vitamin A equivalent.

See also Vitamin A.

CAROTENOIDS

Pigments which produce carotene. Carotenoids help trap certain wavelengths of sunlight to provide energy for the plant.

CARP

see Fish.

CARPETBAG STEAK

A thick piece of steak with a pocket cut into it which is stuffed with oysters before the steak is grilled. An Australian idea.

CARRAGEENAN

see Seaweed.

CARROTS

see Vegetables.

CASABA MELON

see Fruit.

CASARECCIA

A variety of pasta with 2 lengths of pasta twisted together at one end.

CASEIN

The major protein in milk which forms the curd in 'curds and whey' (see page 62). If acid is added to milk, the casein proteins clump together to form a curd. This occurs in making cheese, when bacteria which produce lactic acid are placed into warm milk together with some rennet. Sometimes extracted from skim milk in the form of sodium caseinate and used in coffee whitener, or as an additive to help keep fats distributed evenly throughout a food. Casein is also used in the manufacture of paper, glue and some plastics.

CASHEW APPLE

A pear-shaped swollen stem or 'false fruit' on top of the cashew nut. The plant originated in tropical Africa but is now grown mainly in India. The cashew apple is reddish/yellow in colour and several times larger than the nut. It is eaten raw, made into jams, jellies or a fruit soup. In Cuba, the cashew apple is fermented into a liqueur.

CASHEW NUT

see Nuts.

CASSATA

An Italian dessert originally made as an icecream 'case', filled with whipped cream mixed with glace fruits and almonds. Many cassatas these days are icecreams which contain chopped glace fruits and almonds.

CASSAVA

see Vegetables.

CASSIA

see Spices.

CASSIS

see Drinks, Alcoholic.

CASSOULET

A rich French stew containing beans, onions, garlic, a strongly flavoured sausage, pork, and duck or goose. The dish is cooked slowly so that the flavours blend well. At times, a mixture of fresh and preserved meats is used.

CATECHOL AMINES

see Pressor amines.

CATFISH

see Fish.

CAT'S TONGUES

You need not rush to protect your cat! Cat's tongues are crisp light biscuits often served with icecream. An average cat's tongue biscuit has 165 kJ (40 Cals).

CATSUP
see Tomato sauce.

CAULIFLOWER
see Vegetables.

CAVIAR

The eggs, or roe, of the sturgeon fish, salted to bring out the flavour. All true caviar is produced in the USSR and Iran, from fish caught in the Caspian and Black Seas. Caviar is graded according to the size of the eggs. Beluga caviar, the largest, is black. Osetrova is a little smaller and a grey, or grey-brown, colour. Sevruga, the smallest, is greenish black. The rarest caviar is the golden eggs of the sterlet fish. Cheaper caviar is usually made from eggs which have broken or are immature. Lumpfish and whitefish roe are dyed black with cuttlefish ink to resemble real caviar.

Nutritionally, caviar is high in protein, vitamin E and vitamins of the B group. It has little fat. A 5 g serve of caviar has only about 20 kJ (5 Cals).

CAYENNE PEPPER

A hot powder ground from dried red chillies. Used to flavour curries. Needs to be used sparingly.

CELERIAC
see Vegetables.

CELERY
see Vegetables.

CELLULITE

The name given to the dimpled fat which occurs on women's thighs and buttocks. Cellulite is simply fat which achieves its rippled appearance because the muscle fibres which normally hold thigh fat firmly have lost their elasticity. Women have greater fat deposits on their thighs than men and so the problem is rarely seen in males. It may occur in women of normal weight as well as in those who are overweight.

Contrary to the claims of some people, cellulite is not toxic wastes trapped beneath the skin. Nor is it the sign of a sluggish metabolism. It is merely fat which is not being supported by firm muscle.

Almost all women have fat deposits on their thighs for a reserve of energy. Studies have shown that thigh fat is remarkably stable except during pregnancy and lactation when there is a rapid turnover of fat from the thigh fat cells. It would appear that this thigh fat may have been an important survival mechanism to protect the offspring if a famine occurred during pregnancy or lactation.

Anyone who is overweight will lose fat from their thighs with a sensible diet and exercise program. Those who are not overweight will not find dieting effective in removing cellulite from thighs. Creams, various plastic wraps, spray-on materials and passive exercise machines are also ineffective for removing cellulite. Exercise, however, is valuable in firming thigh muscles so that the fat will not hang out in the familiar dimples or pockets. Along with exercise, there should be adequate amounts of carbohydrate in the diet to prevent breakdown of lean muscle tissue.

CELLULOSE

A form of dietary fibre (a polysaccharide) which occurs in vegetables and cereals, forming part of the structure of the plant. Cellulose is not broken down by the normal digestive enzymes but it is partially digested by bacteria in the large intestine. The extent of this digestion depends on the individual and on the total amount of cellulose being consumed. Those eating a lot of cellulose tend to digest less of it. Cellulose occurs in wheat bran, wheatgerm, processed bran and wholewheat

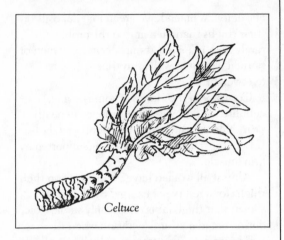

Celtuce

cereals and, to a lesser extent, in other cereals. It is also found in vegetables.

Cellulose is a valuable product to prevent constipation but it appears to have no effect on levels of blood cholesterol.

See also Dietary fibre.

CELTUCE
see Vegetables.

CEPE
see Vegetables, Mushrooms, Boletus cep.

CEREALS

Cereals are all plants from the grass family. They produce grains (or kernels) which are really dry fruits. The most commonly eaten cereal grains are wheat, rice, barley and oats. In some parts of the world, rye, corn (also called maize), millet and sorghum are important cereal foods.

Cereal grains are cheap to produce, relatively easy to transport and store, and provide an excellent base for the diet in most parts of the world. In Western countries, there has been a move away from cereal foods towards high protein, high fat and/or high sugar foods. This has proved detrimental to health and nutritionists now advise that more cereal foods be used in place of fatty or sugary foods.

CERVELAT
see Sausages.

CEVICHE

Raw fish which is marinaded in lemon or lime juice until the flesh becomes opaque. Popular in South Pacific Islands where it is often served with coconut milk. In Mexico, ceviche is served with avocado. Ceviche can also be made with raw scallops.

CEYLON TEA
see Teas.

CHABLIS
see Wine, Varieties.

CHACONINE

An alkaloid present in potato, along with solanine. In large doses, the substance can cause nausea, stomach cramps and vomiting.

CHALAZAE

The cords found in egg white which attach each end of the egg yolk to the shell and keep the yolk centred.

CHALLAH

A sweet bread dough, rich with eggs, made into a plait and traditionally served at Easter.

CHAMOMILE

Also called camomile. A plant with daisy-like flowers. The heads of the varieties *Anthemis nobilis* or *Chamaemelum* are dried and used to make a herbal tea. This tea does not appear to have any harmful effects although some individuals who are sensitive to plants such as goldenrod may also have a sensitivity to chamomile. The mild sedative action of chamomile helps some people sleep.

See also Tea.

CHAMPAGNE
see Wine, Varieties.

CHAPATI

An Indian flat bread generally made from wholemeal or chickpea flour and eaten with curries. Chapatis are cooked on a hot plate.

CHARCUTERIE

A place where meats are sold, especially in France.

CHARD

see Vegetables, Silverbeet.

CHARDONNAY

see Wine, Varieties.

CHARLOTTE

A baked dessert made by lining an ovenproof tin with buttered bread, filling with fruit puree then topping with more bread before baking. An average serve of, say, apple charlotte, has 1150 kJ (275 Cals) and 11 g of fat.

A cold dessert made by lining a mould with sponge fingers and filling the centre with a creamy mixture is also called a charlotte. An average serve has 1780 kJ (425 Cals) and 22 g of fat.

CHARTREUSE

see Drinks, Alcoholic.

CHASSELAS

see Wine, Varieties.

CHATEAUBRIAND

A large piece of fillet steak weighing 500–750 g. Usually cooked in butter, topped with Bearnaise sauce or butter and served for 2 people.

CHAYOTE

see Vegetables, Choko.

CHEDDAR

see Cheese.

CHEESE

See following pages

CHEILOSIS

A skin disorder of the lips characterised by a red, raw line where the lips close. Occurs with severe vitamin deficiency and may be confused with the chapping of lips due to sun and wind.

CHELATION

Process whereby minerals are formed into complexes with substances such as amino acids. Chelation therapy involves the injection of a chemical solution into the bloodstream and is supposed to remove unwanted minerals from plaque deposits in the arteries and hence clear the arteries. The solution used in chelation therapy is based on EDTA (see page 109). Heparin, an anti-coagulant substance may also be used. It is claimed that chelation therapy will help those with heart disease, arthritis, multiple sclerosis and many other conditions. There is no medical evidence that this is the case. Nor is there any guarantee that the treatment is entirely safe. In tests on animals, chelation therapy was found to remove calcium not only from plaque in the arteries but also from bones.

CHELSEA BUN

A sweet bread dough sprinkled with cinnamon and dried fruits before being rolled up into a series of buns which are baked touching each other. Often glazed with syrup and served with butter.

CHENIN BLANC

see Wine, Varieties.

CHERIMOYA

see Fruit.

CHERRY

see Fruit.

CHERVIL

see Herbs.

CHEESE

Since ancient times, milk from cows, sheep, goats or buffaloes has been used to make cheese. Records show that the Sumerians, Egyptians, Romans and Greeks all enjoyed cheese, the latter believing it to be the perfect food for athletes. That may not be quite correct, but since it takes about 10 l of milk to make 1 kg of cheese, there is no doubting the fact that cheese is a nutritious product. It is a way of keeping milk without refrigeration.

The first cheese was probably made by accident. Legend has it that a traveller carried some milk in a bag made from an animal's stomach and the enzyme rennin from the stomach turned the milk to curds and whey. The heat of the day caused the whey to evaporate and cheese was the result.

These days there are hundreds of different cheeses with variations being due to the enzymes used, the yeast and bacterial cultures, the degree of heating or physical processing and the time, temperature and environment used by the cheesemaker.

Basically, cheese is made by using the enzyme rennin to coagulate milk so that it separates into a thick curd and a watery whey. The whey is removed (although a few cheeses are made from it) and the curd undergoes further processing to produce the different cheeses.

The French are the world's greatest cheese eaters, munching their way through more than 200 varieties for a total per capita consumption of about 10 kg per year.

Nutritionally, cheese is a good source of calcium, protein and the B vitamin, riboflavin. It also supplies phosphorus and a range of other minerals and vitamins. The kilojoule value depends on the fat content of the milk used and ranges from 420 kJ (100 Cals) per 100 g for cottage cheese to 1930 kJ (460 Cals) per 100 g for cheeses such as stilton or parmesan.

The fat content of cheese varies from almost none in skim milk cheeses such as sapsago or quark to around 35 per cent in hard cheeses. Some figures for the fat content of cheese are confusing because they refer to the fat in the dry matter in the cheese. On this dry matter basis, cheeses marked double cream have 60 per cent fat while the triple creams have 75 per cent fat. However, these products contain a considerable amount of water and this reduces the fat content in the cheese as consumed. For example, cheddar cheese has 50 per cent of its dry matter as fat, but only 33 per cent of the actual cheese is fat when the water content is taken into consideration.

Creamier cheeses often have a higher water content. For example, cheddar has about 37 per cent water whereas the softer camembert has around 47 per cent. Cream cheeses have about 46 per cent water; the drier parmesan has around 28 per cent.

Cheese represents an excellent way for many people to obtain milk nutrients if they cannot digest lactose (milk sugar). Most mammals cease producing lactase, the enzyme needed to digest lactose, after they are weaned. Some humans are the same. For these people, the lactose is not digested and ferments, causing diarrhoea. Cheese is made from the milk curd. Since most of the lactose is left in the whey, cheese is an easier product for many people to digest. A lack of lactase is common among people from Middle Eastern countries, Southern Europeans and Asians.

Types

Hard (e.g. Parmesan)
Used mainly for grating. Generally aged for several years. Can be stored for long periods, preferably wrapped and in a cool place.

Semi-firm (e.g. Cheddar, Swiss, Edam)
All-purpose cheeses with flavours ranging from mild to robust. Keep best when refrigerated.

Semi-soft (e.g. Havarti)
Usually mild-flavoured, smooth-textured. Keep for several weeks if wrapped and refrigerated.

Soft-ripe (e.g. Camembert)
May be soft or have a soft creamy centre. Ripen quickly and last only a few weeks before developing a strong ammonia smell.

Blue (e.g. Roquefort)
Strong-flavoured and marbled with blue-green-grey moulds which originate from inoculation with various penicillium moulds.

Fresh (e.g. Cottage, Ricotta)
Usually taste slightly tart but should not be acidic. Keep only for a matter of days and require refrigeration.

Processed
Natural cheeses mixed with emulsifiers (see page 111) and extra salt to increase shelf life and produce a uniform product. Generally fairly elastic in texture and mild in flavour.

Different varieties

Unless otherwise mentioned, the cheeses have between 30–35 per cent fat (as consumed) and approximately 1680 kJ (400 Cals) per 100 g.

Ambrosia

A mild, semi-soft Swedish cheese, pale yellow with scattered irregular holes.

Appenzeller

A Swiss cheese, pale gold with small sparsely scattered holes and a smooth light brown rind. Similar to gruyere but with more moisture. When made, it is left for a few days in a mixture of cider, white wine and spices. May be made from full cream or partially skimmed milk.

Baker's cheese

A similar product to creamed cottage cheese but with a softer consistency.

Bel Paese

An Italian semi-soft rich, creamy and mildly tart cheese. Ripens in 4–6 weeks.

Blue Vein

There are over 50 varieties of these soft creamy cheeses with blue, green or grey veins of mould. Best known are roquefort, blue stilton. gorgonzola and bavarian blue. Fat ranges from 25–40 per cent.

Bocconcini

A fresh Italian mild-flavoured cheese a little like mozzarella. Usually served with olive oil and herbs such as basil. Fat content is 25 per cent.

Boursin

A triple cream French cheese with a smooth buttery texture and no rind. Often has added garlic, herbs or pepper.

Brie

Has been made in France since the eighth century. A perfectly ripe brie has a soft, even, creamy-coloured centre, bulging slightly inside the soft white rind. When cut, a ripe brie should ooze rather than run. When overripe, becomes ammoniated. Fat content is about 25 per cent.

Butter cheese

Semi-soft German cheese with a mild buttery flavour. Generally made in a sausage shape.

Caerphilly

A Welsh cheese with a white, smooth, moist, moderately firm texture and a slightly tart flavour. Best used fresh as it has a very salty flavour when overripe.

Camembert

A soft, ripe cow's milk cheese originally made in Normandy, France, using a *Penicillium camemberti* mould which produces a creamy internal texture and a white downy surface. Ripens in 6–8 weeks and has a mild, delicate flavour. Rather like brie. Fat content is 24 per cent.

Cheddar

Firm yellow cheeses ranging in flavour from mild to sharp. The curd is heated to hasten the removal of the whey and is cut into blocks and turned continuously in the process of 'cheddaring'. After pressing into moulds, it is left for 2–3 months for mild cheddar, 6–12 months for matured (tasty) cheddar and more than 18 months for vintage varieties. American cheddar cheese often has added colouring, making it a bright, almost orange, colour. Fat content is generally about 33 per cent.

Cheddar, processed

Pale yellow smooth cheese made by blending and heating cheddars and adding salt and emulsifiers to produce the smooth texture. Maligned by most cheese lovers, but has similar nutritional value to other cheeses. Fat content is about 26 per cent.

Cheshire

An English cheese which is available as red cheshire (contains annatto dye), white or blue (pale orange with blue veins). Loose textured and crumbly. Melts well in dishes such as Welsh rarebit.

Chevre

French white goat's milk cheeses with textures varying from soft, moist and creamy to dry. The flavour ranges from mild to tart. Sometimes coated in edible vegetable ash, herbs or cracked pepper.

Cottage cheese

Fresh, unripened cheese with soft, white particles and a brief shelf life. Flavour is generally bland but may be slightly acidic. Creamed cottage cheese has a small amount of added cream. Also available as bakers cheese, farm cheese or continental creamed cheese. Has less calcium than hard cheeses. Fat content is about 4 per cent. 100 g cottage cheese have 420 kJ (100 Cals).

Cotto

A fresh mild low-fat cheese, pale yellow and made from partially skimmed milk. Fat content is 12 per cent. 100 g have 890 kJ (210 Cals).

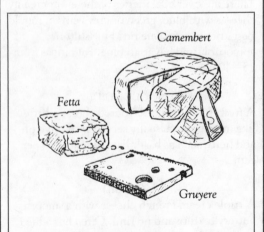

Camembert

Fetta

Gruyere

CHEESE

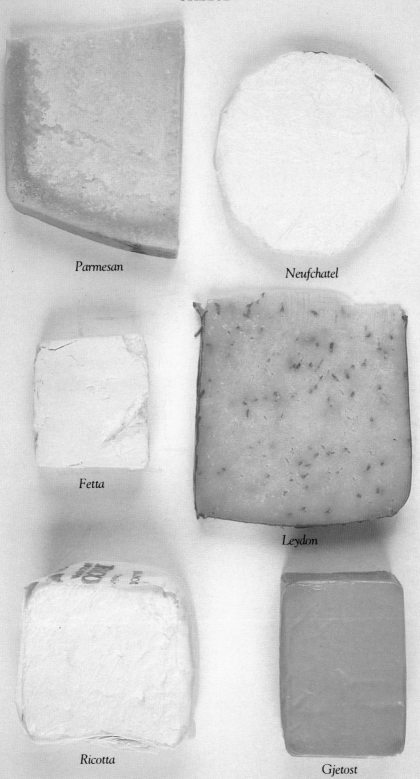

Parmesan

Neufchatel

Fetta

Leydon

Ricotta

Gjetost

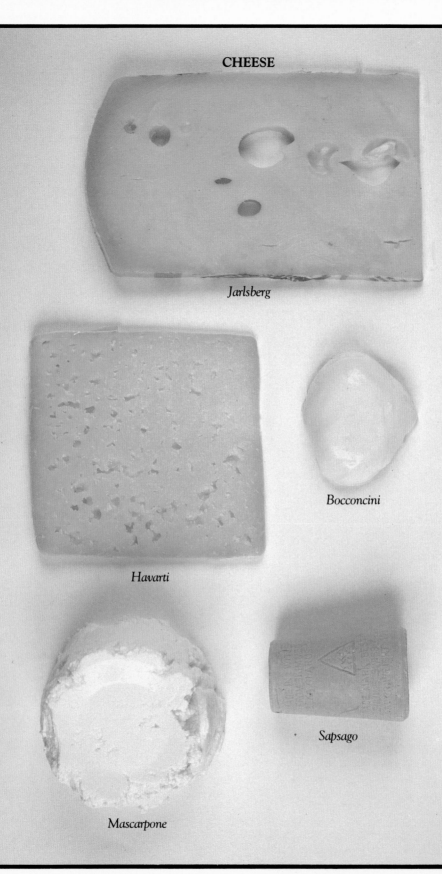

CHEESE

Jarlsberg

Havarti

Bocconcini

Mascarpone

Sapsago

Cream cheese

A soft, unripened smooth product with a rich but mild flavour. Some contain emulsifiers. Fat content is 33–45 per cent. 'Light' cream cheese is usually a mixture of cream cheese and cottage cheese and has about 16 per cent fat. 100 g have 820 kJ (195 Cals).

Edam

A traditional Dutch cheese with a smooth resilient body and mild mellow flavour. Some skim milk is used in edam giving a slightly less creamy texture than gouda. Usually sold in a red, wax-coated cannonball shape. Fat content is 24 per cent. 100 g have 1275 kJ (305 Cals).

Emmenthal

A French version of Swiss cheese (emmentaler) with a mild nutty flavour and holes which are larger than those in gruyere.

Farm cheese

A soft, unripened cottage cheese style with a slightly thicker texture. Usually made from low-fat milk. Fat content is 4–5 per cent. 100 g have approximately 500 kJ (120 Cals).

Feta

A Greek cheese traditionally made from goat's or ewe's milk, now commonly made from cow's milk, either full cream or partially skimmed milk. The flavour is rich, tangy and salty, the latter arising partly from the brine in which it is stored. The saltiness can be reduced by washing the cheese in water or soaking it in milk. Fat content ranges from 12–18 per cent.

Gammelost

A Norwegian cheese prepared from sour rather than fresh milk, surface-ripened with a blue-green mould throughout. While ripening, gammelost is stored on straw soaked with the juice of juniper berries. After 4–6 weeks, a furry mould covers the exterior. This is worked into the cheese and produces a very strong smell and an aromatic flavour. The fat content is extremely low; the taste must be acquired.

Gjetost

A Scandinavian cheese made from the whey of either goat's or cow's milk. The whey is heated until the lactose (milk sugar) caramelises to a brown paste. This provides a sweet, almost caramel-like flavour and a colour and texture resembling smooth peanut butter. The fat content is low but the cheese is unsuitable for those with a lactose intolerance.

Gorgonzola

One of Italy's oldest and most distinguished cow's milk cheeses with a rich, savoury, pungent flavour and blue-green veins throughout. Creamier than many blue cheeses and sometimes available in a white version without mould.

Gouda

The most popular Dutch cheese with a mild buttery smoothness which becomes stronger and firmer with ageing. Traditionally made in flat yellow wheels.

Gruyere

A Swiss cheese with holes about the size of a pea and a slightly sweet, nutty flavour. Less salt than most cheeses. 'Weeping eyes' in a Swiss cheese are a sign of maturity and quality. Excellent melting cheese and used in fondue.

Haloumi

A Greek cheese with a savoury, salty tangy flavour made from ewe's milk. Like feta, it is stored in brine, but has a much more pliable and almost stringy texture than feta due to the kneading and rolling it receives. Often served as cubes in lamb dishes or grilled. Sometimes flavoured with mint to counteract the saltiness. Fat content is about 18 per cent. Also called haloumy.

Havarti

A Danish, semi-soft cheese, originally known as tilsit. Has a mild, mellow to rich flavour.

Jack Cheese

A cheese made without rennet. Very mild,

rather bland and often made without the addition of any salt. Spreads easily.

Jarlsberg
A Norwegian cheese resembling Swiss. Delicate, buttery flavour, slightly sweet.

Kasseri
A Greek cheese made from ewe's or goat's milk. Similar to feta but with a harder texture which makes it more suitable for grating. Often fried and served hot.

Kishk
An Arabian cheese made from goat's milk.

Leicester
An English semi-firm cheese, deep orange in colour. Loose, flaky texture and a mellow flavour with a strong, smooth after-taste. Difficult to slice.

Leydon
A mild Dutch cheese spiced with caraway or cumin seeds. Often made from partially skimmed milk. Fat content usually about 24 per cent.

Limburger
A strong-smelling German cheese which is left in a humid atmosphere for 3 months to acquire its pungency and soft texture. Generally served with beer. Fat content is 28 per cent.

Liptauer
A mild, fresh Hungarian ewe's milk cheese, usually flavoured with paprika which produces a pinkish colour. Often mixed with mustard, anchovies, capers and beer.

Manchego
The best known Spanish cheese made from ewe's milk. Available in fresh, young, matured and vintage forms, the latter being left in olive oil for 12 months. Fat content is variable but may be high.

Mascarpone
A fresh, double cream Italian soft cheese with a smooth creamy texture a little like clotted cream or whipped butter. Usually served with fruit as a dessert. Keeps for only a few days.

Monterey Jack
Similar to cheddar but milder and with a smoother texture. Colour varies from very pale yellow to a rich orange, depending on the age.

Mozzarella
An Italian cheese made from cow's (or occasionally buffalo's) milk, usually available in a pear-shape. Has a smooth texture largely due to having been dipped in hot whey and kneaded during manufacture to produce a smooth consistency and the familiar stringiness when used in pizza. Fresh mozzarella, just a few hours old, is eaten in Italy with olive oil, salt, pepper and tomatoes. Fat content can vary from 12–25 per cent, the lower fat varieties being somewhat drier and more stringy.

Munster
First made in a monastery in Alsace in the Middle Ages, this semi-soft cheese can vary in flavour from mild to pungent. The American version is much milder than the French or German varieties.

Neufchatel
A soft ripened cream cheese originally made in Normandy in France. Best eaten fresh and excellent in cheesecakes.

Parmesan
A rich, full-flavoured, hard, Italian, cow's milk cheese which will keep almost indefinitely. First made in Parma in Northern Italy. Parmesan is a wonderful cheese for grating; some of the ready-grated versions are a far cry from the rich flavour of the real thing. The colour of a good parmesan is golden-yellow; lighter varieties have not been properly aged. Fat content is 25–35 per cent with the harder cheeses having the lower fat content. Calcium content is higher than most cheeses.

Pecorino Romano

An Italian cheese, similar to parmesan but with a slightly sharper flavour. The original Italian pecorino is made from ewe's milk. *Pecorina vacchino* is a similar cheese made from cow's milk.

Port Salut

A French semi-soft, smooth, savoury yellow cheese with an orange rind first made by Trappist monks in Brittany in the nineteenth century. Has a glossy texture with a few small holes and a flavour which gathers strength as it ages.

Provolone

An Italian cheese often seen hanging from the rafters of delicatessens in waxed cylinders of varying sizes with characteristic cord indentations. The flavour varies from mild to robust when aged. The curd of the cheese is kneaded in hot water to produce the rope-like strands which are gathered into a ball. When aged, the cheese becomes much harder and is often flaky. Fat content varies from 25–28 per cent.

Quark

A fresh, slightly acid cheese with a taste and texture somewhere between yoghurt and cottage cheese. Made from skim milk and may have a fat content as low as 1 per cent. Some varieties have a little added cream, bringing the fat up to 4 per cent. Also called quarg.

Raclette

A Swiss cheese similar to gruyere. The dish 'raclette' is made by holding a large piece of cheese near the fire and scraping the melted portion to serve with potatoes, gherkins and pickled onions.

Ricotta

Italian fresh cheese made largely from whey. The lactose in the whey produces a slightly sweet flavour. Texture is finer than that of cottage cheese. Salt content is low and fat varies from 6–14 per cent, depending on the proportions of whole and skim milk used. Often used in lasagne and Italian desserts. Keeps for only a few days.

Romano

A hard cheese, commonly made from cow's milk. Some of the fat is first removed from the milk to produce a harder cheese. Final fat content is about 25 per cent.

See also Pecorino Romano.

Roquefort

Probably the world's greatest cheese, this French bluevein inspired Casanova to the lines, 'Oh, how excellent is Roquefort, both to revive love and to bring to prompt maturity a budding love'. Made from ewe's milk, the snow white cheeses are skewered 36 times and aged in the cool, moist limestone caves of Roquefort. The flavour is rich, buttery and creamy-textured and has a piquant after-taste which has established its reputation. The rind is grey, the ripe cheese yellow and the blue veins are well marbled throughout.

Saint Paulin

A French semi-soft cheese something like Port Salut but with a milder flavour.

Samsoe

The national Danish cow's milk cheese with a mild nutty flavour. A little like Swiss cheese with some large holes and a yellow rind. Originally made on the island of Samsoe.

Sapsago

A Swiss cheese made entirely from skim milk. A special kind of clover is added which gives a greenish colour and a pungent flavour. Unlike most low-fat cheeses, sapsago is hard and can be grated. The only hard cheese allowed on some strict, low-fat diets.

Stilton

The king of English cheeses, white to pale yellow with a mellow but rich creamy flavour married to a slightly mouldy tang from the grey-green veins throughout. During manufacture, stilton is not pressed but is turned regularly until a brownish crusty rind forms. Sold in tall cylinders. The common practice of pouring port into the cavity of a stilton detracts from the flavour of both the port and the cheese. Fairly high in both salt and fat. White stilton is a young cheese in which the blue-grey veins have not yet developed.

Swiss
Light, yellow cheese with a sweet nutty flavour. Characterised by holes or 'eyes' which develop during its maturing process. The curd is salted and kept at 22°C (72°F) to stimulate

production of carbon dioxide which forms the holes in 6−8 weeks. Bacterial cultures control the development of the holes. The salt content of Swiss cheese is lower than in most cheeses. Fat content is 29 per cent.

Tilsit
German cheese rather like gouda.

Wensleydale
A semi-firm English cheese available in white or blue-veined forms. The white is fresh, young and ripened for only 3 weeks. The blue is robust, creamy and has a rich after-taste. These cheeses are considered ideal to eat with apples or apple pie.

CHESHIRE
see Cheese.

CHESTNUTS
see Nuts.

CHEVRE
see Cheese.

CHEWING
There was once a theory that every mouthful of food should be chewed 32 times. This is absurd, but it is important that foods be thoroughly chewed before being swallowed. Chewing is the first step in the process of digestion. Teeth grind and break food into smaller pieces making it easier for digestive juices to begin their work. The human mouth contains several types of teeth, indicating that we are, by nature, omnivores who eat both animal and vegetable foods. Chewing also allows saliva to moisten foods, making swallowing easier.

CHEWING GUM
The first chewing gum was made from spruce resin in 1850. Sweetened flavoured paraffin was also popular. In 1871, a New Yorker called Thomas Adams patented the process of making chewing gum from chicle, a product of the sapodilla tree which grows in rain forests of South America. Chewing gum is flavoured with various types of mint and has added sugar. Chewing gum is also now made synthetically. It is approximately 80 per cent sugars and 20 per cent gum. 100 g chewing gum have 1340 kJ (320 Cals). 1 pellet has 20−40 kJ (5−10 Cals). Artificially sweetened varieties with virtually no kilojoules are also available.

CHIANTI
see Drinks, Alcoholic.

CHICA
The product resulting from chewing ground corn so that an enzyme in saliva can split the

complex carbohydrate into glucose and maltose. In the sixteenth century, chica was used as a basis for making an alcoholic beverage.

CHICKEN

The most commonly eaten type of poultry, chicken is a valued part of the diet in most parts of the world. Chicken consumption is high in the United States and has been rising rapidly in countries such as Australia.

Chicken flesh is high in protein, low in fat and is a good source of many vitamins of the B complex as well as minerals such as iron, zinc and potassium. Much of the fat in chicken is found in or just under the skin. If this is removed, chicken becomes a very low-fat product with some cuts (such as the breast) having as little as 1.6 per cent fat — a much lower level than lean meat.

Of the fat in chicken, approximately 13 per cent is polyunsaturated, 52 per cent is monounsaturated and 34 per cent is saturated. This contrasts with meats where the percentage of saturated fat is much higher.

100 g cooked chicken breast have 660 kJ (157 Cals). For cooked chicken legs, 100 g (without bone) have 875 kJ (210 Cals).

CHICKPEAS
see Legumes, Garbanzos.

CHICORY

In addition to being used as a vegetable, the long fleshy taproot of chicory is roasted and ground for use as a coffee substitute.

See also Vegetables.

CHILDREN, GROWTH AND NUTRITION

Children have high requirements for most nutrients. Their rapid growth and development means that they need about twice as much protein per kilogram of body weight as an adult.

A lack of nutrients during growing periods not only prevents children achieving their full growth potential, but may affect the development of the brain. There is no way to compensate for malnutrition during a child's early years.

Within Western societies, most children are adequately nourished. Malnutrition is seen rarely and occurs mainly in those who are very poor or in children whose parents follow unusual dietary practices. For example, failure to grow is sometimes seen in children of very strict vegans (who eat no animal products) or fruitarians (who attempt to live on fruit and nuts). While adults may be able to survive on these diets, most children are unable to maintain the time and attention span which must be devoted to eating the large volumes of food necessary to provide adequate nutrition. If some of the limited range of foods are not liked by the children, their diets may be deficient in some nutrients (see Balanced diet, page 32). Growth may then be affected.

Some children appear to eat very little and yet seem to grow normally and to have plenty of energy. In reality, most of these children do eat, but usually not at mealtimes when parents are watching. It is also possible that those children who eat very little manage to absorb a greater percentage of nutrients from their food than other people.

Most cases of children refusing to eat certain foods are not due to a dislike of the food itself, but are a way of exercising power over parents. By not eating, the child is almost guaranteed attention — and often, the food of their choice! Most parents cannot help but react when a child refuses to eat the food which has been prepared. The reaction makes the problem worse.

Often, a child will eat a particular food when away from home, but flatly refuses to touch it when a parent is present. The best way to deal with this problem is also difficult: ignore the behaviour. Another way to deal with children who reject almost everything you put in front of them is to place serving dishes on the table and give everyone an empty plate. Now the onus is on the child to select some food — no-one is dictating what he or she will eat. Should the child choose to eat nothing, the only comment from parents should be that they will see the child at the next meal. If no food is given between meals, the problem is usually solved within a few days. A few difficult children may refuse to serve themselves anything for a week or two, but after that the problem generally disappears. No healthy child ever starved while food was available!

CHILLI

Spelled 'chili' in the United States. A small and very hot type of pepper or capsicum. Dried chillies are ground to make chilli powder.

Nutritionally, chillies are an excellent source of vitamin C, with red chillies supplying even more than the green varieties. They also have dietary fibre and many vitamins and minerals. In most cases, however, chillies are eaten in insufficient quantities to supply anything much except vitamin C. Hot-food lovers who eat a lot of chilli need not fear growing fat; 20 g chilli contain only 16 kJ (4 Cals).

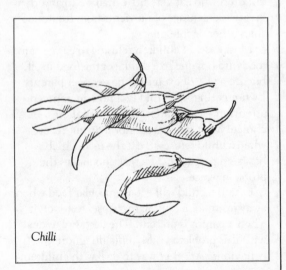

Chilli

CHILLI SAUCE

see Sauces, Other.

CHINESE GOOSEBERRY

see Fruit, Kiwi Fruit.

CHINESE LANTERN

see Fruit, Cape Gooseberry.

CHINOOK SALMON

see Fish, Salmon.

CHIPS

see Vegetables, Potato.

CHITIN

The material which makes up the cell walls of fungi. Plant cell walls are made up largely of cellulose while the chitin in fungi is a complex of carbohydrate and amines (a similar material to that of the outer skeleton of insects).

CHITTERLINGS

The intestines of pigs. Used in some Asian recipes or as sausage casings.

CHIVES

see Herbs, Vegetables.

CHLORINE

A mineral present in the body and foods as chloride. Helps maintain a balance of water in body cells and is an essential part of the digestive juices in the stomach. Chlorine is supplied by salt (sodium chloride) and also occurs naturally in meat, eggs, cheese and milk. Deficiencies only occur after prolonged vomiting or diarrhoea. There is no recommended daily dose but somewhere between 1700 and 5100 mg a day are considered safe and adequate.

Chlorine is used as a bleaching agent in flour to remove the slightly yellowish colour of the flour. There is no reason for this addition and it is banned in some countries.

CHLOROPHYLL

The green-coloured pigments in leaves (including vegetables) which trap solar energy so that the plant can use it in the process of photosynthesis to convert water and carbon dioxide into carbohydrate. The colours of chlorophylls are so strong that they often mask other red and yellow pigments in plants.

When green vegetables are cooked, the heat damages the structure of the cells, allowing the acids in the vegetable to come in contact with the chlorophyll. This permits hydrogen ions to replace the magnesium atoms in the chlorophyll, changing the pigments so that the vegetables lose their bright green colour.

Also used as a food additive (no. 140).

CHOCOLATE

Made from the cocoa bean, chocolate was enjoyed for centuries by people in Central America. During the sixteenth century, chocolate was introduced to Spain as a sweetened hot drink flavoured with cinnamon and vanilla. It was so highly prized that its composition remained a Spanish secret for nearly a hundred years before being introduced to France. Chocolate houses became the vogue for those wealthy enough to purchase the hot chocolate drink. Its stimulating effects (due to caffeine and theobromine) were well known.

It was not until 1828 that a Dutchman, van Houten, made a press to remove the rich chocolate liquor (which contains cocoa butter) from the cocoa beans. By adding cocoa butter to the chocolate liquor, along with sugar, a much smoother chocolate could be made. The Swiss then honed in on chocolate and developed a solid milk chocolate in 1876 and a filled chocolate in 1913.

To make milk chocolate, condensed milk is added and the mixture is kneaded in a conching machine to aerate and develop the flavour and smooth texture. Chocolate bars were first made in 1910 but became immensely popular when issued to the armed forces in World War I.

Chocolate is made as follows:
- Cocoa beans are roasted for a richer flavour
- Beans are cracked open to free the kernels from the shells
- Kernels are ground to form a thick chocolate liquor
- Further grinding, pressing and mixing with cocoa butter produces a smooth silky texture in the chocolate
- Sugar is added
- For milk chocolate, milk solids are added
- The emulsifier, lecithin, is added to keep the fat and solids evenly spread throughout the finished product
- Chocolate is shaped

Nutritionally, chocolate is something of a disaster since it is high in both fat and sugar, contributes many kilojoules and does little for the waistline. Of the large quantity of fat in chocolate, more than 62 per cent is saturated, 34 per cent is monounsaturated and only 3 per cent is polyunsaturated. On a slightly more positive note, chocolate contributes some potassium and small quantities of other minerals and some vitamins. Chocolate is also less damaging to teeth than other sweets, possibly because it contains some anti-decay factor. 100 g of chocolate have 2205 kJ (525 Cals) making it one of the richest sources of food energy. Some people interpret this as a good thing, and so it may be — for those who need to carry a compact source of kilojoules. It should be remembered, however, that energy which is not used is quickly converted to body fat.

The Swiss are the world's greatest chocolate eaters, munching their way through an average of 10 kg a year, that is, about 200 g a week for every man, woman and child in the country. The Norwegians eat 8 kg a year, followed by the English, Germans and Belgians. Australians eat about 4 kg of chocolate a year.

See also Caffeine; Cocoa.

CHOCOLATE BROWN HT
see Colourings.

CHOCOLATE PUDDING FRUIT
see Fruit, Sapote.

CHOKO
see Vegetables.

CHOLECALCIFEROL
Another name for vitamin D.

CHOLECYSTOKININ (CCK)
A hormone produced in the small intestine when food arrives from the stomach in the duodenum (the first part of the small intestine). Cholecystokinin also stimulates the gallbladder to send some bile into the intestine to digest fats. Also found in the brain and may assist in the transmission of impulses in nerves.

CHOLESTEROL
A fatty, waxy substance which looks something like the wax which accumulates in the ears. Cholesterol is a vital part of cell membranes and certain hormones. It is used by the body in making vitamin D, is found in the brain and nerve cells and is a vital part of the membranes which surround all body cells. Cholesterol is also used to make bile salts which are important in the digestion of fats.

Cholesterol is certainly not an undesirable substance. However, we don't need to eat it since the body is able to make its own supplies. Each day the liver produces about 1000 mg of cholesterol; individual cells can also make their own supplies. Problems with cholesterol arise when some people make far too much cholesterol and the excess builds up (with other substances) in the arteries. Clogged arteries can impede blood flow and also provide an ideal site for blood clots to lodge (see Atherosclerosis, page 29).

Most of the excess cholesterol in the blood arises when the diet is high in saturated fats.

These are found not only in animal products such as fatty meats and some dairy products, but in many vegetable fats, especially coconut and palm oils (used in processed foods, fast foods and for commerical frying). The idea that animal fats are responsible for high levels of cholesterol in the arteries is thus inadequate.

Cholesterol also exists ready-made or pre-formed in some foods. Confusion over animal and vegetable fats has arisen because only animal products contain pre-formed cholesterol. Brains, liver, kidneys, egg yolks, meats (including lean meats), poultry, seafoods and dairy products all contain pre-formed cholesterol. However, high levels of cholesterol in the blood are far more likely to arise from eating saturated fats than from taking in pre-formed cholesterol. This means that foods such as prawns or eggs which have been damned because of their relatively high content of pre-formed cholesterol are not so bad after all since they do not contain large quantities of saturated fats. Have your eggs cooked with bacon or batter and fry your prawns, however, and you have foods which are high in saturated fats.

Some foods, such as oysters and crab, were once thought to have a high content of pre-formed cholesterol. More refined techniques for measuring cholesterol showed that much of this actually consisted of other sterols. (Cholesterol is only one of a family of sterols and the only member which has a significant effect in the human body.) This is the reason for inconsistency in recommendations regarding shellfish. Only prawns and squid have higher levels of pre-formed cholesterol. Since the saturated fat content of prawns and squid is low, they really do not present any problems.

To lower blood cholesterol levels, the most important action is to reduce saturated fats in the diet (see page 119). A small number of hypersensitive people also need to reduce their intake of pre-formed cholesterol. A preoccupation with reducing foods containing pre-formed cholesterol, while ignoring many foods with a high content of saturated vegetable fats, has hindered efforts to reduce blood cholesterol levels in Western populations.

The excretion of cholesterol is also important. Recent research with foods such as oats and legumes shows that these foods can increase the excretion of cholesterol in the faeces. This reaction may occur because of the particular types of fibre in foods (soluble fibres work best) or it may be due to other factors in the food. It has been clearly shown that unprocessed wheat bran does nothing to reduce blood cholesterol levels whereas oats, legumes and certain fruits and vegetables are effective. Initial medical research suggested that the reduction of blood cholesterol with these foods was due to an increased excretion of bile acids. Since cholesterol is used by the body to produce bile acids, their removal should mean that more cholesterol is diverted from the blood to make a fresh supply of bile acid. Further research is needed to clarify the issue.

See also Fats, Saturated fatty acids.

HDL and LDL Cholesterol

Cholesterol in the blood is attached to protein molecules, in compounds known as lipoproteins. Three important lipoproteins are high-density lipoprotein (HDL), low-density lipoprotein (LDL) and very-low-density lipoprotein (VLDL).

HDL is often called 'good' cholesterol since it removes cholesterol from the artery walls, returning it to the liver. LDL and VLDL cholesterol are 'bad' since they deposit cholesterol in cells. Ideally, this should mean that the cells stop producing their own cholesterol. In practice, however, it appears that large quantities of LDL and VLDL dump too much cholesterol in the cells, which, in some people, continue to also produce their own supplies. The result is a build up of cholesterol. HDL cholesterol is protective against coronary heart disease; LDL promotes it. People from long-living families, endurance athletes and some young women, have high levels of HDL cholesterol.

Saturated fats in the diet increase the bad LDL cholesterol and decrease the good HDL. Polyunsaturated fats decrease the bad LDL but also reduce the level of the good HDL. Monounsaturated fats decrease the bad LDL and increase the good HDL (see page 210 for further details).

Until recently, only total cholesterol levels in blood were measured. This does not provide a complete picture. However, most people who have high levels of blood cholesterol have too much of the bad LDL.

CHOLINE

Once thought to be a vitamin of the B complex, choline is a part of the compound lecithin. As such it is widely distributed in foods including eggs, fish, grains, vegetable oils and legumes. Lecithin is also used in many processed foods including icecream, chocolate, desserts, mayonnaise, margarine and baked goods. Choline has several important functions in the body. It plays a role in the way the body uses fats and prevents fats accumulating in the liver. It is also important in nerve cells in relaying information between nerve fibres and from nerves to muscles. Choline is not regarded as a vitamin because it can easily be made in the body. Some benefits from extra choline have been found in people with neurological disorders. However, large doses taken as a supplement cause dizziness, nausea, diarrhoea, abnormalities in heart rhythm and a fishy odour.

See also Lecithin.

CHORIZO
see Sausages.

CHORON
see Sauces, Emulsion.

CHOUX PASTRY
see Pastry.

CHOWDER

A thick soup, often containing seafoods, salted pork or bacon, potatoes, onions and milk. The word 'chowder' is a corruption of the French term for 'cauldron'. Various types of chowder are popular in parts of the United States.

CHROMIUM

An essential mineral for humans. Chromium is part of an organic compound, called the 'glucose tolerance factor', which is involved in the chemical reaction by which insulin helps the body cells absorb glucose. It is thought that there may be some defect in this mechanism in some diabetics. Chromium is highly toxic in large doses so self-medication is not advisable. The richest food sources are egg yolk, fish and shellfish, wine, beef, wholemeal bread, wholegrain cereals, potatoes, oysters and brewer's yeast.

Daily requirements are estimated as:

	mg chromium
Infants	0.01–0.06
Children, 1–3 years	0.02–0.08
4–7 years	0.03–0.12
7 + years	0.05–0.2
Adults	0.05–0.2

Like all minerals, excess chromium is harmful.

CHURRO

A deep fried puff of choux pastry, served sprinkled with icing sugar.

CHUTNEY

Originally an Indian accompaniment to curries. Chutneys consist of a mixture of fruits, vegetables, sugar, spices and some type of acid cooked until thick. Often eaten with cold meats. Nutritionally, chutneys will vary with the ingredients. In general, chutney provides about 40 kJ (10 Cals) per teaspoon.

CHYLOMICRONS

The form in which fat is transported from the intestine through the lymph glands to the blood. They form in the small intestine following the absorption of fats. Chylomicrons of fat can be used as a source of energy or stored in body fat depots.

CHYMOTRPYSIN

An enzyme in digestive juices which helps break down proteins into their component amino acids.

CIDER
see Drinks, Alcoholic.

CIGUATERA
see Food poisoning.

CINNAMON
see Spices.

CINSAUT
see Wine, Varieties.

CIRRHOSIS

A condition or irreversible changes to the liver in which the normal soft tissue is replaced by hard fibrous tissue. Major causes include chronic high alcohol intake and malnutrition. Contrary to popular belief, however, cirrhosis is not confined to the alcoholic who eats little. Large amounts of alcohol can cause cirrhosis, even in the presence of a good diet.

In the early stages of cirrhosis, symptoms are jaundice and nausea. If all alcohol is avoided and the diet contains plenty of protein and carbohydrate (but little fat), some regeneration of the liver is possible at this stage. Later there is increased jaundice, infection, haemorrhage, high blood pressure, coma and, finally, death.

A doubling of the safe alcohol intake to 4 drinks a day for men and 2 for women is associated with a higher incidence of cirrhosis. The safe level for women is lower since women

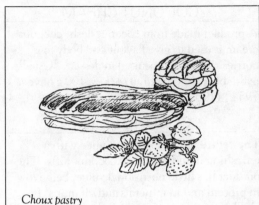

Choux pastry

are generally smaller than men and have a lower muscle content, and so cannot metabolise alcohol to the same extent.

See also Alcohol.

CITRANGE
see Fruit.

CITRIC ACID

An organic acid found in almost all plants, and especially in citrus fruits, strawberries, raspberries, pears, pineapple, tomatoes and bananas. Commonly used as a flavouring in sweets and soft drinks to provide a tartness to offset the sugar used. Also used as an additive (number 330) in jams and jellies to provide a gel-like consistency. When combined with an antioxidant, citric acid helps prevent foods going bad from exposure to oxygen. Quantities used as a food additive are small and are less than amounts usually found in foods.

CITRON
see Fruit.

CITRUS FRUITS
see Fruit.

CLAM
see Seafood.

CLARIFIED BUTTER
see Ghee.

CLOBASSY
see Sausages.

CLOUDBERRY
see Fruit.

CLOVE
see Spices.

CLUSTER BEAN

The bean from a leguminous plant which grows in India and looks rather like a soya bean. The bean has many seed pods, each containing many seeds. From these guar gum, a viscous fibre, also known as galactomannan, can be extracted (see pages 159, 174).

COBALAMIN
see Vitamin B_{12}.

COBALT

A mineral which is essential for humans since it forms part of the vitamin B_{12} molecule. The discovery that cobalt was an essential nutrient was made by Australian researchers in the 1920s. Only very small quantities are required and these are easily obtainable from green leafy vegetables and meats. Cereals and dairy products have little cobalt. A normal Western diet contains anything from 10−200 mcg a day. The actual cobalt intake is relatively unimportant — it is the vitamin B_{12} content of foods that matters.

Humans absorb far more cobalt from foods than is needed for vitamin B_{12}. This may mean that there is some other function for cobalt that is not yet known.

Cobalt was once used to improve the foaming qualities of beer but was found to have toxic effects on the heart in those who were heavy drinkers. It is no longer used. The toxicity may have been due to the combination of alcohol and cobalt.

COBNUTS
see Nuts, Hazelnuts.

COCHINEAL
see Colourings.

COCKTAIL

A drink containing a mixture of ingredients, with or without alcohol. First described in the eighteenth century, cocktails were originally associated with outdoor social or sporting occasions. Cocktails are popular in the United States and, until recently, places selling cocktails in London were known as American bars.

The 1920s and 1930s were times of major inventiveness in producing drinks which did not obviously contain alcohol. Many cocktails began at this time. In the 1980s, cocktails seem to be enjoying a new wave of popularity.

See also Drinks, Alcoholic and Non-alcoholic for individual cocktails.

COCOA

The word 'cocoa' is an eighteenth century corruption of the original 'cacao' (see page 49). Cocoa is a concentrated powder made from the seeds of the cocao tree. After grinding the seeds to make chocolate liquor, the mixture is pressed to remove much of the cocoa butter. The resulting cocoa cake is pulverised to form cocoa powder. Since cocoa tastes fairly bitter, it is usually sweetened with sugar in drinks. It is also used in cakes, biscuits and as a flavouring for desserts.

Nutritionally, cocoa powder contains about 22 per cent fat plus some protein. It also contains iron, potassium and zinc quantities and small amounts of some of the B complex vitamins. One teaspoon of cocoa contains 65 kJ (15 Cals).

See also Caffeine; Chocolate.

COCONUT
see Nuts.

COCONUT CREAM

A product made from coconut flesh, coconut cream is used to give flavour and body to curries. It can also be used in desserts. Usually available canned or in a packet, 100 g have 795 kJ (190 Cals).

COCONUT MILK

The centre of the coconut is filled with a refreshing liquid known as coconut milk. The product has little nutritional value, being low in protein and in minerals and vitamins. It is also low in fat. A 250 mL glass of coconut milk has only 220 kJ (52 Cals).

Coconut milk is also the term applied to the liquid expressed after boiling water has been poured over desiccated coconut. The fat and kilojoule content of this type of coconut milk will vary with the degree of pressure applied to the coconut.

COCONUT OIL
see Oils.

COD
see Fish.

COD LIVER OIL
see Oils.

COELIAC DISEASE

A condition in which the protein in some types of grain damages the lining of the small intestine. It occurs in one in 2500 of the population and is usually diagnosed in young children who have diarrhoea and fail to gain weight normally. Once the intestine becomes inflamed with the condition, other nutrients are not absorbed and a picture of generalised malnutrition occurs. Adults can develop coeliac disease although this occurs only rarely.

Treatment of coeliac disease is the removal of the protein gluten from the diet for life. Since gluten occurs in wheat, rye and barley, all these grains and products made from them must be omitted. This includes most breakfast cereals, pasta, breads, cakes, biscuits, scones, pizza and pies. Rice, corn and buckwheat products can be used as replacements. Many crackers, pasta, breakfast cereals, bread and biscuits made without gluten are now available.

Some people with coeliac disease can tolerate small quantities of oats; others cannot. Coeliacs should be careful that recipe books they use have been checked by a dietitian as there are some available which do not omit all sources of gluten. Lists of processed foods free of gluten are available from government health departments.

See also Gluten.

COFFEE

The earliest coffee beans came from the *Coffea arabica* shrub of Arabia and were used as a food as well as a stimulant. The use of the coffee bean as a drink began in Ethiopia about AD 1000 when the beans were roasted, pulverised and whipped into hot water. It was not until many centuries later that coffee became popular and coffee houses sprang up in the old cities of Constantinople and Mecca. Gradually coffee became a favoured brew throughout the Middle East. Soon coffee trees were being planted in India and Latin America.

Europeans became aware of coffee by the middle of the sixteenth century but most considered it too expensive and too stimulating for general acceptance. Gradually this changed and first the Dutch, and then the rest of Europe, accepted the new beverage. Coffee was planted in Brazil and production increased rapidly.

The original *Coffea arabica* is still grown but has been joined by the high-yielding, hardy *Coffea robusta*. The latter variety has a higher content of caffeine than the more expensive arabica. *Coffea arabica* grows wild in Ethiopia and is cultivated in Indonesia, East Africa and South America. It has a richer, tastier and more aromatic flavour and is considered the finest type of coffee. *Coffea robusta* grows mainly in Africa and is much more flexible in its climatic requirements. It also produces a much larger crop, making it cheaper. Robusta has a higher caffeine content than the Arabica bean and is commonly used for instant coffee.

The average annual yield of coffee from a single tree averages about 450 g. Since coffee is consumed all over the world, there are a great many coffee shrubs.

The coffee beans are removed from the berries in which they grow and are dried and shipped. They are not roasted until they reach their destination. The degree of roasting affects the flavour with longer and hotter roasting producing stronger flavoured coffee.

Espresso coffee (Italian for 'pressed out') is a strong coffee made by forcing a combination of steam and hot water through a large portion of highly-roasted ground coffee.

Instant coffees are made by brewing the coffee with water and then evaporating the water by spraying a mist of concentrated coffee into a stream of hot air. To freeze dry instant coffee, the concentrated coffee is cooled to a temperature of −60°C. The temperature is then raised slightly under high vacuum. Then the coffee crystals go directly from ice to vapour.

Decaffeinated coffee is made by first steaming unroasted coffee beans, causing the caffeine to move to the outer layers of the beans. The caffeine can then be removed by using a solvent, steam or vegetable oil, or by rubbing away the outer layer of the bean. Robusta coffees have almost twice the caffeine level of the arabicas.

Making coffee is considered an art in some parts of the world. It can be made by the following methods:

- *Jug* — Warm a pot (preferably china or earthenware), dry it and add medium or coarsely ground coffee (1 dessertspoon per person). Pour hot water over the grounds, stir and leave in a warm place for 5 mins before serving.

- *Plunger pot* — Basically a refined version of the jug, but has an inbuilt strainer which prevents the grounds landing in the cup. A heaped spoonful of coffee is placed in the jug for each cup of boiling water. Pour the water over the grounds and leave to stand for a few minutes before serving.
- *Filter* — Place finely ground coffee into a filter paper which is in a specially shaped filter paper holder over a jug. When the water boils, leave it for a few seconds and then pour a little slowly over the grounds to wet them. Then pour the remaining water over the coffee.
- *Automatic filter machine* — Place finely ground coffee into a filter paper and add fresh cold water to the flask in the machine. The machine will heat the water and automatically drip it through the coffee grounds.
- *Espresso machines* — These force steam and water under pressure through the coffee. Finely ground dark roast coffee is used to produce a strong and slightly bitter brew.
- *Vacuum machines* — Cold water is poured into a glass bowl which fits into another bowl on top containing a filter which holds the coffee. As the water boils in the lower bowl it rises up the funnel and mixes with the coffee in the upper bowl. When the heat is removed from the lower bowl, the coffee drips into the lower bowl and is ready to serve.
- *Copper saucepan* — Turkish coffee is made in a long-handled one. A heaped teaspoonful of pulverised coffee is placed into the saucepan with each tiny cup of water. Sugar is usually also added at this stage. The mixture is stirred and heated. As soon as it boils it is removed from the heat. This is done 3 times. No milk is ever served with Turkish coffee.

Different coffees are consumed in various parts of the world. In America, the coffee is made mainly from robusta beans which are highly roasted and made by filtering or using an espresso machine. A lot of instant coffee is also consumed. To most other people, American coffee has little subtlety. However, some excellent coffees are available if one searches.

A variety of coffees are available in Australia, from very good to quite poor quality. All methods of coffee making are used. Belgians drink large quantities of coffee, taking it with milk and sugar in the morning. In Brazil, the home of coffee, the beverage is consumed in large quantities — usually with half milk in the mornings and black with lots of brown sugar in the afternoon.

In Denmark, coffee is also very popular, a light to medium roast being most popular. It is sometimes drunk with aquavit, the national clear spirit. Their neighbours, the Finns, have the world's highest coffee consumption. The Germans also take their coffee drinking seriously and consume more coffee than they do beer. Most of their coffee is made by the filter method and high quality, medium roast beans are used. Cream or milk is added. The French give coffee drinking pride of place in their daily rituals, drinking it strong and rather bitter, with half milk in the mornings and black at other times. Perhaps the greatest reverence for coffee is given by the Italians who like their coffee to be of high quality and strong.

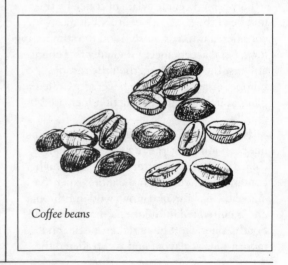

Coffee beans

The Egyptians have made coffee their drink, consuming many cups of Turkish coffee (finely powdered) each day. The Greeks also drink Turkish coffee, occasionally adding cardamom pods for a different flavour. Mexicans add cinnamon or other spices to their brew. The Swedes also like cardamom in their strongly brewed coffee. The English have never really taken to coffee although it is now drunk mid-morning and after dinner. To most Europeans and Americans, the English brew is somewhat lightly roasted and weak.

See also Caffeine.

COGNAC
see Drinks, Alcoholic.

COINTREAU
see Drinks, Alcoholic.

COLA
see Drinks, Non-alcoholic.

COLCANNON
An Irish dish made by frying a mixture of cooked cabbage and mashed potato. Similar to 'bubble and squeak'.

COLD, COMMON
The common cold comes into contact with nutrition because of the theory that it may be prevented or alleviated by taking extra vitamin C and, possibly, vitamin A. Of the well-controlled studies which have examined this theory, most have found no evidence to support it. The only positive results have shown that vitamin C reduces the duration of a cold by slightly more than 1 day so that it lasts 5 days instead of the usual 6.

COLESLAW
see Salads.

COLLAGEN
A structural protein in connective tissue which accounts for 30 per cent of the protein in the human body. Collagen is in skin, muscles, blood vessels, tendons, cartilage and in young bones. Within the body, collagen requires vitamin C for its formation. When collagen is heated in water, it forms gelatine. In fact, the word 'collagen' comes from a Greek word meaning 'glue producing'. When meat is cooked, the tough fibres soften as the collagen fibres respond to the heat of cooking.

See also Protein.

COLLARDS
A green vegetable of the cabbage family. Good source of vitamins A and C and may have a protective role against cancer.

COLLOIDS
A suspension of tiny particles in some other medium. Sauces which are thickened with egg or oil (as in mayonnaise) depend on fats breaking into small fragments and forming an emulsion with the water part of the sauce. Such a system is a colloidal one with tiny particles of one liquid dispersing into another with which they cannot mix.

COLON
The large intestine from the ileum to the rectum. By the time food residues reach the colon, most of the proteins, fats and carbohydrates will have been digested by enzymes. In the colon, bacterial digestion of dietary fibre occurs and much of the water which has entered the colon is reabsorbed.

Cancer of the colon is common in Western countries. Whether this is due to the high content of fat or the lack of dietary fibre is not yet clear. Probably both factors are involved.

COLOSTRUM
A clear fluid secreted by the mammary glands immediately after birth. Colostrum contributes proteins, minerals and vitamins and also

contains important anti-infective agents which protect the young from disease. After a short period, the colostrum ceases and milk is produced. For human babies, even those mothers who do not want to breast feed should try to allow the infant to take the protective colostrum.

See also Breast feeding.

COLOURINGS

Substances added to foods to make them look more appealing. There is no nutritional reason for their use, although there may be good marketing reasons for their inclusion in foods. Colours may be natural or synthetic but each country allows only specific substances to be used to colour foods. Permitted colourings differ between countries, depending on their individual assessment of any potential hazards and the need for the particular colouring. If one colour is already in use, permission to use another will not necessarily be granted. Some of the more commonly used colourings are described below.

Amaranth

A red colouring material used in the United Kingdom and Australia but not permitted in the United States. Additive no. 123.

Annatto

The yellow- or red-coloured seed pod of a tropical tree which is used to colour foods such as margarine, cheese and other foods. Additive no. 160 (b).

Brilliant black

Also known as brilliant black BN or black BN. Not permitted in the United States. Additive no. 151.

Brilliant blue

A colouring permitted for use in some cakes, desserts, certain jams, jellies, margarine, sauces, toppings and some other food categories. Not permitted in the United Kingdom. Additive no. 133.

Brilliant scarlet

A colouring also known as ponceau 4R in the United Kingdom. Not permitted in the United States. Additive no. 124.

Carmine

see Cochineal.

Carmoisine

A red colouring used in Australia and the United Kingdom, but not in the United States. Additive no. 122.

Chocolate brown HT

A brown colouring used in Australia, but not in the United Kingdom or the United States. Additive no. 155.

Cochineal

A bright pink-red extract obtained from a scale insect *Coccus cacti* which grows on cacti. When they are laying eggs, the insects are removed, killed and dried and the red colour extracted. The red colour is due to a pigment called carminic acid. Both substances have additive number 120.

Erythrosine

A red colouring widely permitted throughout the world. Additive no. 127.

Green S

As its name implies, a green colouring. May cause hyperactive reactions in susceptible children. Additive no. 142.

Indigo carmine

A blue colouring used in foods. Widely permitted. Additive no. 132.

Sunset yellow FCF

A widely used yellow colouring. Additive no. 110.

Tartrazine

A yellow colouring, widely used, but sometimes criticised, for causing asthma and hyperactivity in susceptible children. However, recent evidence indicates that other colourings in foods are much more likely to cause problems than tartrazine. Often found in snack foods, sweets and drinks but is increasingly being replaced by carotenoid colourings. Additive no. 102.

COMFREY
see Herbs.

COMPLEX CARBOHYDRATES
see Carbohydrates.

CONFECTIONERY

Also called candy, lollies or sweets, the first types of sweet confectionery were made by the Egyptians from honey and fruit concentrates. Confectionery remained a rare treat until sugar became more widely available in the fourteenth century. Sugar, gum arabic and various nuts were used to produce sweet gums, jellies and candies which were sold by pharmacists ('a little bit of sugar to make the medicine go down').

Confectionery became very popular in the seventeenth and eighteenth centuries but it is only in the twentieth century that it has become cheap enough to achieve widespread consumption. Nowadays, children in most countries of the world are given sweets, and the popularity of these products extends to people of all ages. In those areas where there are no dentists to repair the damage from these products, dental decay and its associated pain is becoming a grim reality.

Basically, confectionery is made by boiling sugar and cooling it to varying degrees to produce products from hard candy to softer caramels. A variety of other ingredients are added, including butter, chocolate, other sugars, nuts, flavourings and colourings. Apart from providing kilojoules, most types of confectionery have little nutritional value. Because of their effect on the teeth, and the fact that they frequently replace other more nutritious foods, they have little to offer apart from the pleasure they provide in the mouth (before the tooth decay becomes apparent).

Boiled sweets have about 1380 kJ (330 Cals) per 100 g; toffees have 1780 kJ (430 Cals) per 100 g; chocolate has 2220 kJ (530 Cals) per 100 g.

CONGEE

A rice porridge in which both the rice and the watery liquid in which it is cooked are eaten. Commonly eaten in Asian countries as a bland counterpart to spiced and fermented dishes.

CONGENERS

Various higher alcohols (that is, with more carbon atoms) and other substances present in small quantities in wines and some other alcoholic drinks. They are produced by the action of yeast on amino acids in grapes or cereal grains and are present in larger quantities in alcoholic drinks of low quality. Congeners are quite toxic and contribute to the hangover experienced after drinking, especially if the alcoholic beverages were of poorer quality. See also page 105.

CONSTIPATION

A condition of infrequent and/or hard bowel motions. True constipation is related much more to the consistency of the faeces than to the frequency. Constipation is common in Western countries where the diet lacks dietary fibre due to the high percentage of refined foods eaten. An increase in a variety of types of fibre, including those from wholegrain cereal and bread products, vegetables, legumes and fruits, helps cure constipation. Drinking sufficient water is also important.

See also Bran; Laxatives; Dietary fibre.

CONTRACEPTIVES

Oral contraceptives can affect nutritional status. Some women, but not all, have a greater need for vitamin B_6 and folic acid (another of

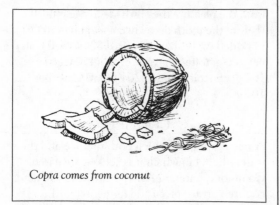

Copra comes from coconut

the B complex vitamins) and possibly for vitamin C, riboflavin and zinc. The Pill also decreases the losses of iron from the body and may help prevent anaemia in many women. Those taking the Pill also have higher than usual quantities of vitamin A in the blood; supplements of this vitamin are therefore not recommended.

The fact that some women need more of some vitamins has been used to justify large doses of extra vitamins for women on oral contraceptives. This is unnecessary and potentially hazardous.

COOKIE

An American term for biscuit (the latter is the American term for the English scone). In Scotland, a cookie is a small bun.

COOKING

The process of cooking involves some type of heat. This helps soften tissues, increase some flavour components and make some foods more palatable. All cooking methods cause some loss of nutrients, but in many cases this is minimal. The idea that only raw foods are nutritious is nonsense. A mixture of raw and cooked foods generally produces the healthiest diet. Raw foods become monotonous to some people, and cooking may even increase the bioavailability of some nutrients such as carotene.

Boiling, baking, barbecuing, frying (with or without fat), grilling, microwaving, moist baking as in casseroles, pressure cooking, steaming and stewing, all have their place in increasing the palatability of various foods.

As a general rule, foods which are overcooked lose more nutrients. This applies particularly to vegetables and to some methods of meat cookery. Microwaving and steaming vegetables give a much better retention of nutritional value than boiling. The greater the volume of water added to foods, the larger the losses of nutrients. In a soup or stew, this may be less important since the liquid is consumed.

Foods which are cooked with dry heat (as in barbecuing or grilling) will lose some of their nutrients with moisture loss. Adding salt to the food enhances this so that sprinkling steak with salt and then barbecuing it will cause not only a loss of extra moisture but also more nutrient loss. Barbecued foods should not be subjected to such a high heat that the surface turns black as this can lead to the production of cancer-causing substances.

COPPER

A mineral which is essential (with iron) to prevent anaemia, copper is also needed for healthy connective tissue, strong bones, for making elastin in skin and also to keep the aorta of the heart and the central nervous system in a healthy condition. It is also involved in making the brown pigment, melanin, in hair and skin.

Copper is found widely in foods, especially in liver, oysters, crab, legumes, wholegrain cereals and bread, vegetables, Brazil nuts, chicken, peanut butter, dried apricots, bran, meats and cocoa.

Only small quantities of copper are needed (approximately 2 – 10 mg/day is considered safe). Large quantities are extremely toxic to the liver, kidney and brain. It is inadvisable to use copper cooking utensils unless they have a protective coating covering the copper.

Vitamin C, too much zinc, sulphides and raw meat decrease the absorption of copper while fresh vegetables increase its absorption.

COPRA

The dried white flesh of coconut.
See also Nuts, Coconut.

CORAL TROUT
see Fish.

CORIANDER
see Herbs; Spices.

CORDIAL
see Drinks, Non-alcoholic.

CORN

The second most commonly grown grain, also known as maize. Originally important in the diet in Central and South America, corn is also a major crop in the United States. Different varieties of corn are consumed as a vegetable (sweetcorn), ground for use in cakes and breads, popped for the familiar snack food 'popped corn', taken as corn or maize oil, or used as a major animal feed.

Corn created great problems in some of the southern parts of the United States where it made up the major part of the diet. All cereal grains lack one or more of the amino acids which make up protein. Corn is especially deficient in lysine and also in tryptophan. This latter amino acid is used to make niacin, one of the B vitamins. To make matters worse, the niacin present in corn is chemically tied-up so that it is unavailable to the body. This resulted in large areas of the southern States suffering from pellagra, a disease caused by a lack of niacin. The symptoms — diarrhoea, dermatitis and, eventually, dementia — brought great human misery (see also page 382).

Pellagra had not been a major problem in South America simply because the Aztecs had always used lime or ashes when preparing corn.

Later technology was able to identify that this process not only made the husk much easier to remove but improved the availability of the amino acids, lysine and tryptophan, as well as releasing niacin from its chemical bonds. Early Aztec civilisations made this remarkable discovery without the aid of modern biochemistry. These days corn is boiled in a 5 per cent lime solution for about an hour before being washed, drained and ground. All corn is treated this way before being sold. Where corn is grown on the home farm, local people know to also use this processing method. As a result, pellagra has disappeared.

Nutritionally, once treated, corn provides complex carbohydrate, iron, some vitamins of the B complex and some dietary fibre. Fat content of cornmeal is 3.5 per cent, which is more than in wheat or rye but less than the fat in oats. 100 g cornmeal have 1510 kJ (360 Cals).

See also Cereals; Grains.

CORN CHIPS

The latest addition to the packets of crunchy snack foods, corn chips are at least made from corn and do contain dietary fibre. They are made by boiling corn and allowing it to stand for about 10 hours so that water can penetrate the hard grain. The cooked, moistened corn is then washed to remove the skin (which includes some dietary fibre). The corn is then ground using stone-grinding wheels which allow a dough to be made without much heat being generated, as this would make the dough too sticky. The dough is then fed into large rollers which cut it into small pieces which are then toasted at a high temperature to dry out the corn chip and make the characteristic marks on the surface. The corn chips are allowed to cool and are then fried in vegetable oil (usually a saturated vegetable fat). To complete the change from a healthy cob of corn to a popular snack food, salt is added. A 25 g packet of corn chips has 815 kJ (195 Cals) and

220 mg of sodium from salt (which is 10–24 per cent of the average maximum recommended daily sodium intake). They provide some iron and a little calcium.

CORNFLAKES

A breakfast cereal first made in 1902 from flakes of corn flavoured with barley malt. The success of Cornflakes © eventually led to the Kellogg Company being set up in the United States.

Nutritionally, cornflakes provide complex carbohydrates and have several vitamins added. They also have far more salt than is apparent to the taste buds and a 30 g serving has as much salt as a 30 g packet of salted potato crisps. Cornflakes have around 11 per cent added sugars and almost no dietary fibre. A 30 g serve has 475 kJ (113 Cals) before milk is added.

CORNFLOUR

The starchy portion of the corn once all the dietary fibre has been removed. Most brands of cornflour have added wheat starch and may be unsuitable for those on gluten-free diets who must avoid wheat products. Used for thickening sauces, soups and casseroles. Cornflour has only very small quantities of nutrients. A 10-g tablespoon of cornflour has 145 kJ (35 Cals).

See also Starch.

CORNISH HEN

A small hen, popular to serve as a whole or half bird in the United States.

CORNISH PASTY

Coming from Cornwall in England, the Cornish pasty is a pastry encasing meat and vegetables. Potatoes, turnip and carrots usually share their pastry bed with beef and kidney, all ingredients being cooked inside the pastry.

CORN OIL
see Oils.

CORN SYRUP

A syrup made by extracting the starch granules from corn and treating them with acid or enzymes so that the starch is fermented to form sugars. The resulting syrup is very sweet and this is determined by the degree of breakdown of the starch. By controlling the kinds of sugars, and hence the viscosity, in corn syrup, it has many uses in maintaining moisture in various sweet products. 100 g of corn syrup have 1220 kJ (290 Cals).

CORONARY ARTERIES
see Heart disease, Atherosclerosis.

CORONARY HEART DISEASE
see Heart disease, Atherosclerosis.

COTECHINO
see Sausages.

COTTAGE CHEESE
see Cheese.

COTTAGE PIE

A dish made from cooked minced meat topped with mashed potato and browned in the oven.

COTTO
see Cheese.

COTTONSEED OIL
see Oils.

COURT BOUILLON

A liquid prepared for poaching fish. Usually made from water with vinegar or lemon juice, peppercorns and some herbs. Has virtually no kilojoules.

COUSCOUS

A form of semolina made from the endosperm of hard durum wheat, couscous is steamed several times until it is light and fluffy. In Western countries, couscous grain is usually purchased already steamed and needs only to be placed in a steamer above a simmering stew for a few minutes. Alternatively, you can cover the grain with boiling water and leave it to stand for about 10 mins by which time it will be light, dry and fluffy. Served in North Africa with a chickpea and vegetable stew, in some other countries couscous is steamed, sweetened with sugar and eaten with fruit or honey.

Nutritionally, couscous is quite a good source of iron, contains some B complex vitamins and has 950 kJ (227 Cals) per 100 g.

CRAB
see Seafood.

CRABAPPLE
see Fruit.

CRANBERRY
see Fruit.

CRAYFISH
see Seafood, Lobster.

CREAM

The fat portion of milk, cream comes in different thicknesses. In the United Kingdom, single cream has 21 per cent fat, whipping cream has 35 per cent fat and double cream has 48 per cent fat and is very thick indeed. Single cream will not whip. In Australia, cream has 35 per cent fat, except for reduced or light

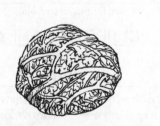

Crepinette

cream which has half this level.

Sour cream is made by adding a bacterial culture to cream to thicken it and give a slight tang. It usually has 35 per cent fat with light sour cream having half this level.

Clotted cream is made by heating creamy milk (preferably from a Jersey cow) and skimming off the cream from the top. When left to cool, this cream becomes very thick and is quite yellow in colour. It may have about 50 per cent fat.

Cream contains vitamin A and carotene (which is converted to more vitamin A in the body) and small quantities of vitamins E, D and the B complex. It has little calcium. Regular cream has 1380 kJ (330 Cals) per 100 g.

CREAM CHEESE
see Cheese.

CREAM OF TARTAR
see Tartaric acid.

CREATININE

A waste product formed when muscles are used in physical activity. The greater the muscle mass, the greater the excretion of creatinine in the urine.

CREME BRULEE

A traditional French dessert, creme brulee is a rich custard topped with sugar which is caramelised under a griller. An average serve has 1315 kJ (315 Cals).

CREME DE BANANE
see Drinks, Alcoholic.

CREME DE CACAO
see Drinks, Alcoholic.

CREME DE CASSIS
see Drinks, Alcoholic.

CREME DE MENTHE
see Drinks, Alcoholic.

CREME FRAICHE

Cream which has been treated with a special culture to make it thick and slightly tangy. Available in France but can be made by stirring cream with a spoonful of yoghurt and keeping warm for about 8 hrs. Chill before serving.

CREME PATISSIERE

A thick, rich custard used to fill French pastries.

CREOLE

The cooking style of New Orleans which reflects influences of Spanish, French and Indian cuisines.

CREPE

A thin French pancake, served on its own or filled with a sweet or savoury filling.

CREPES SUZETTE

Sweet crepes, simmered in a sauce of orange and lemon juices with Curacao, Grand Marnier or Cointreau, and served flaming with brandy.

CREPINETTE

see Sausages.

CRESS

see Vegetables.

CRETINISM

see Hypothyroidism.

CROISSANT

A French crescent-shaped yeasted roll. The dough for croissants is interleaved with butter, providing a light flaky texture but a high content of fat. One average-sized croissant has 840 kJ (200 Cals) — the same number as 3.5 slices of bread.

CROQUE MONSIEUR

A French sandwich with a filling of ham and cheese, fried in butter before serving.

CROQUETTE

A combination of a thick sauce mixed with some type of vegetable, chicken, seafood or meat, dipped in egg and breadcrumbs and fried.

CROTECIN

An orange colour obtained from saffron which is extracted from the stigmas of the crocus flower (native to Greece but also grown in parts of Asia). The intense colour of saffron comes from crocin and crotecin.

CROWN ROAST

A specially prepared lamb dish made up of two racks of lamb cutlets bent to form a crown. Roasted before being served hot.

CSABAI

see Sausages.

CUCUMBER

see Vegetables.

CUMBERLAND SAUCE

A sauce made with red currant jelly, port, finely shredded orange rind and some mustard. Served with game or ham.

CUMIN

see Spices.

CUMQUAT

see Fruit.

CURACAO

see Drinks, Alcoholic.

CURDS AND WHEY

see Cheese.

CURRY

A spicy dish which includes a variety of flavours from spices (both mild and hot). Commonly used spices include turmeric, chilli, coriander, cumin and pepper. For the best flavour, the spices are roasted or dry fried before adding meat, fish, chicken, or vegetables, and then simmered with some type of liquid (water, coconut milk or yoghurt). Curries are usually accompanied by flat bread, cucumber (to cool the heat of the curry), yoghurt and various sambals (see page 298).

CUSTARD

A mixture of milk, eggs and sugar, usually flavoured with vanilla. The mixture may be stirred on top of the stove or baked in an oven until it sets into a smooth creamy consistency. Half a cup of custard has 630 kJ (150 Cals).

CUSTARD APPLE
see Fruit.

CUSTARD SAUCE
see Sauces, Other.

CUSTARD TART
see Tart.

CUTTLEFISH
see Seafood.

CYANOCOBALAMIN

The correct name for vitamin B_{12} (see page 385).

CYCLAMATES
see Artificial sweeteners.

CYSTEINE

A sulphur-containing amino acid which is useful in diets which are partially deficient in the essential amino acid methionine (lacking in most legumes).

CYSTINE

A sulphur-containing amino acid which can be made in the body from other amino acids. An important component of hair and of the hormone insulin.

DAIQUIRI
see Drinks, Alcoholic.

DAIRY PRODUCTS

Dairy products include milk, cheeses and yoghurt, as well as cream and butter. Humans have been using these products for thousands of years. Sheep and goats were domesticated first, probably around 8000–9000 BC. Cave paintings show that dairy animals were well used by 4000 BC, and traces of cheeses have been found in Egyptian tombs dating back to 2000 BC.

Dairy products have been widely used throughout Europe but are not common in Asia. With a few exceptions, milk is the most commonly used product in Northern Europe with cheeses dominating the dairy foods of Southern Europe.

Today, dairy products are still not used to any extent in Asia or the smaller Pacific Islands. Australia and New Zealand, however, have well-established dairy industries.

Refrigeration has altered dairying, making milk much more popular. Yoghurt and cheeses still dominate areas where there is little refrigeration.

In general, the non-fat part of dairy products is a valuable source of calcium, protein and several minerals and vitamins, especially riboflavin (one of the B vitamins). Cream and butter have much less nutritional value.

For discussions of individual dairy products, see under categories such as butter, cream, cheese, icecream, milk, yoghurt etc.

DAMPER

A bread, rather like a scone dough, which was frequently eaten by early European settlers in Australia. The name may have been derived from that of the explorer William Dampier.

A true damper is made by combining flour, water and salt, mixing it into a cake and baking it in the hot ashes of a fire. The ashes are knocked off before the bread is eaten.

Australian children have traditionally made damper by moulding the bread dough around a green stick and leaving it in a fire until cooked (by which time, the outside is usually well-blackened).

DAMSON
see Fruit, Plum.

DANDELIONS

This ubiquitous plant grows almost everywhere. Its leaves are blanched and eaten as a salad vegetable or steamed. It is best to eat the leaves before the plant has flowered when they are less bitter. The root can be roasted and ground to use as a coffee substitute.

DANISH PASTRY

A rich, flaky, yeasted pastry with a variety of sweet fillings which may include jam, nuts, custard or dried fruits. Usually glazed with a sugar syrup. Generally eaten at breakfast or during the morning. A small (75 g) Danish pastry has about 13 g of fat (mainly saturated), 21 g of sugar and 1175 kJ (280 Cals).

DARJEELING TEA
see Tea.

DATE
see Fruit.

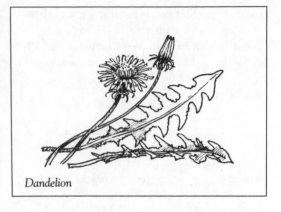

Dandelion

DAVIS, ADELLE

A popular American nutritionist, whose ideas about the need for large quantities of protein, mineral and vitamin supplements as cures for many diseases, brought her into disrepute with qualified nutritionists. In spite of her claims that various foods and supplements could cure cancer, she herself died of cancer.

DDT

Common abbreviation for dichloro-diphenyl-trichloroethane, an insecticide first made in 1874. During World War I, DDT was found to be effective against mosquitoes, fleas, lice and various insects which attack food crops. Unfortunately, DDT has been so widely used throughout the world that, even though it is no longer used, traces can be found in almost every food we eat, in human body fat and even in breast milk. The effect of this is unknown. The higher up the food chain you go for food, the greater your chances of accumulating DDT as each animal accumulates the residues from its food. Since DDT was banned in most countries, residue levels are beginning to fall.

DECAFFEINATED COFFEE
see Coffee; Caffeine.

DECAY, TOOTH
see Dental caries.

DEHYDRATED FOODS

Removal of water from foods is one of the oldest methods of food preservation. Once water is removed, bacteria which normally attack food cannot survive. Dried fish, dried meat and even dried eggs have been used in Asia for centuries, while dried fruits and vegetables have also been popular throughout the world. Dehydrated foods are also a boon to hikers and explorers.

In general, the shorter the drying time, the more acceptable the resulting food. Drying in a vacuum is especially good for fruits, vegetables and coffee. Spray drying entails atomising a product (such as milk) and exposing it to hot air to produce a dried powder. Freeze drying simultaneously freezes and dries foods.

Drying of foods causes some loss of vitamins, especially vitamin C and thiamin (B_1). There is also some loss of lysine (an amino acid) from the protein of dried milk. Freeze drying results in a good retention of nutrients.

DEHYDRATION

A loss of water from the body which occurs from not drinking sufficient fluid to make up for losses. The average person loses 2.5 l of water a day, not including obvious sweating. If this is not replaced, the body soon becomes dehydrated and most people can survive only a few days without water.

Dehydration occurs in endurance athletes who fail to drink sufficient water to make up for their heavy losses. It also accompanies repeated diarrhoea and vomiting, high body temperature, taking diuretics (see page 96) or kidney failure. With a loss of 3−5 per cent of normal body water, physical performance falters; with more than 5 per cent loss, the muscles become flabby, the skin wrinkles and the eyes begin to shrink; 15 per cent loss of water is fatal.

As dehydration progresses, the blood volume decreases and the output of the heart is reduced so that there is less blood flow to the skin. Sweating decreases and, with no way to dissipate heat from the body, the temperature rises rapidly. At this stage, the blood becomes thicker, the kidneys fail to function and waste products accumulate. As the body temperature rises, the output of the heart decreases and cardiac shock causes death.

DEHYDROASCORBIC ACID

An oxidised form of ascorbic acid (vitamin C) which acts in the same way as ascorbic acid. Early reports that vitamin C disappeared very quickly from oranges once they were picked were due to the vitamin being present in its oxidised form.

See also Vitamin C.

DEMERERA SUGAR

A raw sugar with some light molasses added to provide colour. If unavailable, substitute raw sugar.

DENTAL CARIES

Tooth decay (dental caries) is the most common health problem in Western countries. It occurs when bacteria feed on sugars in the mouth and form acids which attack the enamel on teeth, causing the caries lesion.

Bacteria accumulate in plaque; sugars come from foods or from the plaque itself. Prevention of dental caries involves removing plaque, avoiding sugars which stick between teeth and cleaning teeth straight after eating. Chewing foods such as carrots or apples stimulates the flow of saliva and helps dilute sugars. Fluoride also makes the tooth enamel stronger and more resistant to decay.

See also Plaque.

DEOXYRIBONUCLEIC ACID (DNA)

A nucleic acid which carries the genetic information for cells. A sugar called ribose, and various vitamins, are required for the synthesis of DNA. Charring foods may damage the DNA and cause changes to cells.

See also Nucleic acids.

DEPRESSION

A condition with many causes which may result in changes to eating habits. Some people eat much more when they are suffering from depression; others lose interest in food and eat very little. Many people become depressed during fasting or when trying to follow very strict diets. This may well be due to an alteration in chemical substances present in the brain (see Tryptophan, page 349). A lack of carbohydrate may also cause temporary fluctuations in the blood sugar level which cause mood changes in many people (see page 56). Eating a little more food will fix this situation.

Some drugs used to treat depression influence nutrition. Monoamine oxidase inhibitors, for example, are designed to improve mood by allowing greater quantities of a particular chemical to build up in the brain. These same drugs also allow large quantities of an amino acid called tyramine to be absorbed through the wall of the intestine, causing headaches, nose bleeds, increased blood pressure and even stroke. When these drugs are being used, the diet must be as low as possible in tyramine (see page 350).

Other drugs used to treat depression alter the appetite, making it easier for weight gain. In some people, this may increase the depression.

A feeling of fatigue and lack of energy is technically not the same as true depression. Feeling constantly tired may be due to a lack of sleep or too many problems, or it may have a nutritional basis. Contrary to popular belief, a lack of vitamins is not a common cause of this problem. A lack of iron is much more common, especially in women, and causes lethargy. A lack of food (for example, with many strict weight reduction diets) also causes a lack of energy.

DERMATITIS

Various skin disorders, occasionally related to a sensitivity to particular food ingredients (either naturally present or added). Some rare types of dermatitis may also be due to vitamin deficiencies. If it is suspected that some food is causing dermatitis, the elimination diet (see pages 19, 110) should be tried, under the guidance of a qualified dietitian.

See also Allergies.

DEXTRINS

Chains of starch with anything from 4 to several hundred glucose molecules.

DEXTROSE
see Glucose.

DEVILS ON HORSEBACK

Prunes wrapped in bacon and grilled. Commonly served as an hors d'oeuvre. Each one has 275 kJ (65 Cals).

DEVON
see Sausages.

DHAL

The name given to a puree made from various legumes, including lentils, Bengal gram (also known as garbanzos or chickpeas), green gram (also known as mung beans), red gram and pigeon peas. Eaten with rice, dhal is a major part of the diet in India. 100 g of cooked dhal have 605 kJ (145 Cals) and is high in dietary fibre, protein and iron.

DHOSAI

Pancakes made from lentils and ground raw rice. Commonly eaten in India.

DHUFISH
see Fish.

DIABETES MELLITUS

A condition characterised by variations in

blood glucose levels caused by a lack of insulin. In Type I diabetes (also called 'insulin dependent' or 'juvenile onset diabetes'), there is little or no production of insulin by the pancreas. The condition usually occurs in childhood, adolescence or in early adulthood. The early symptoms are great thirst, excessive passing of dilute, sweet urine and loss of weight. If untreated, coma and death can result. Long-term complications include changes to the eyes, blood vessels and heart, nerves and kidneys.

Type II (or 'non-insulin dependent' or 'maturity onset diabetes') is far more common and occurs in older people, most of whom are overweight. Early symptoms are mild but long-term damage is just as likely as in Type I diabetes. In particular, diabetics have a higher incidence of coronary heart disease.

In Type II diabetes, insulin may be produced but there is some resistance to its action. When the underlying weight problem is solved, the condition often disappears. Even though there is a genetic component to this type of diabetes, it usually only becomes apparent in the overweight. Unlike Type I diabetes, Type II is largely preventable.

Diabetes may also arise during pregnancy. This is called gestational diabetes and is detected by sugar in the urine and a higher than normal sugar level in the blood. This type of diabetes needs to be controlled to avoid damage to the baby. A diet high in dietary fibre and complex carbohydrate, and low in refined sugar, is often sufficient. Gestational diabetes may disappear after the pregnancy but may return with any subsequent weight gain. The same type of diet should be continued throughout life.

Diabetes is not caused by eating sugar, but those who have the condition need to avoid refined sugar. Instead, they should opt for a diet high in dietary fibre and the complex carbohydrates found in wholemeal bread, wholegrain cereals (especially oats), legumes,

vegetables and fruit. Fats should be kept low and alcohol strictly limited, or avoided altogether. The current diabetic diet is rather similar to the pattern of healthy eating which nutritionists advise for everyone.

The aim of treatment is to keep blood sugar levels as normal as possible. The soluble fibres in oats and legumes help in this regard, as does the regular spacing of meals and snacks throughout the day. Diabetics should never miss meals.

Type I and some Type II diabetics are given insulin by injection. The types used generally give a sustained release of insulin and this requires regular meals with approximately equal quantities of carbohydrate. Should the insulin level rise too high (due to an inadequate meal being eaten), the blood glucose level may drop too low. At such times, a rapidly absorbed form of sugar (such as fruit juice or barley sugar) is required to restore the blood glucose level.

The old style diabetic diets were so low in total carbohydrate that fat levels were inadvertently high. Since diabetics have a greatly increased risk of heart disease, these diets were abandoned in favour of the high complex carbohydrate/high dietary fibre diets which provide much better control.

DIARRHOEA

The frequent passing of loose, watery stools which occurs as a symptom of food poisoning, emotional upset, bacterial or viral infection of the intestine, use of laxatives or some disease state. In cases of food poisoning or infection, the best treatment for diarrhoea is to eat nothing and drink only clear fluids such as clean water. Fluid intake is vital to avoid dehydration.

DIELDRIN

A chlorine-containing compound used as an insecticide. Residues may remain in the food chain and governments set limits as to tolerable levels since it stimulates the central nervous system and is toxic.

DIETARY FIBRE

Dietary fibre is defined as those parts of food which are not digested in the stomach and small intestine by normal digestive acids and enzymes (see page 113). However, it is not correct to think of dietary fibre as being indigestible. Dietary fibre is digested, but its breakdown takes place mainly in the large intestine during its fermentation by bacteria. In this process, the bacteria multiply by the million and once they die, their bodies contribute substantially to the faeces which are excreted.

Dietary fibre is not one substance. Just as there are a variety of vitamins, so there are a number of different types of dietary fibre, each with its own type of action within the body. Unprocessed bran, commonly considered to be almost synonymous with dietary fibre, contains some types of dietary fibre but is totally lacking in others.

Dietary fibre exists only in the vegetable kingdom and is found in grains, breads, cereal products, vegetables, fruits, legumes, seeds and nuts. It also occurs in gums which are used in food processing.

The two major categories of dietary fibre are:

Soluble fibres

Insoluble fibres

Until recently, a measurement of fibre in a food took account only of the insoluble fibre, cellulose. This factor was referred to as the 'crude fibre' and represents only a small fraction of the total dietary fibre present in a food.

Soluble forms of dietary fibre include gums (present in oats and legumes, and added to some foods), pectin (in fruits and citrus peel) and some polysaccharide substances in legumes and oats. These types of fibre are 100 per cent digested by bacteria, producing valuable acids during this process.

Cellulose and a range of hemi-celluloses present in vegetables, nuts, seeds, fruits and grains, are also digested. The extent of this process depends on the individual, the particular food and the total fibre content of the diet.

Lignin is a type of dietary fibre which appears to undergo very little change in the human intestine (see page 208). This does not make it a useless type of fibre since it appears to help remove some unwanted substances, such as excess cholesterol, from the body.

The best known function of dietary fibre is its ability to prevent and cure constipation. Even this process is not a simple cause of fibre going in one end of the intestine and eventually emerging from the other. Fibres which are totally soluble still prevent constipation. This action occurs firstly from the contribution of the bodies of millions of dead bacteria, and secondly, because one of the acids produced during the digestion of the soluble fibre stimulates the intestinal wall to propel faeces (see pages 42, 115).

Insoluble fibre, such as is found in unprocessed wheat bran, is also valuable in the treatment of constipation because of its ability to absorb water and form softer faeces. This action is confined to coarsely milled bran; fine bran forms hard faeces and may increase constipation.

Soluble fibres, but not the insoluble types, also help control blood sugar levels and, possibly, cholesterol levels. The fibre in oats, barley and legumes, for example, forms a gel in the stomach and slows down the rate at which sugars from foods enter the blood. These foods have proved valuable in better control of diabetes.

Oat fibre also helps lower blood cholesterol levels. Some of this effect is attributed to the soluble fibre's ability to remove bile acids from the intestine. Since one of the major uses of cholesterol is to make bile acids (which help in the digestion of fats), removing these bile acids means that more cholesterol must be diverted from the blood to make more bile acids. This action cannot account for all the increased excretion of cholesterol which occurs with oat fibre. Whether a waxy type of fat also helps remove cholesterol, or some other mechanism is at play, is not yet known.

There is also some evidence that dietary fibre may be important in preventing bowel cancer. Early medical reports assumed that this occurred because more frequent defecation with a high-fibre diet meant that any potential cancer-causing substances would spend less time in contact with the bowel wall. Later research suggests that one of the acids produced during the bacterial digestion of dietary fibre may have anti-cancer properties. It is also possible that the benefits of fibre in combating bowel cancer may reflect the fact that a diet which is high in fibre is also low in fat. (A high-fat diet is known to increase cancer risk.)

There is no doubt that people in Western countries will benefit from increasing their dietary fibre intake from the current low level of around 15 g a day. A desirable level is estimated to be 30−40 g a day. However, it is important that this fibre comes from a variety of sources. Eating heaps of unprocessed bran in an effort to raise fibre intake is undesirable and can cause deterioration of the cells lining the large intestine. 1 to 2 tablespoons of bran a day is considered safe.

See also Cellulose; Polysaccharides.

DIETARY GUIDELINES

Recommendations issued to improve the diet of any group of people. Many Western countries, plagued by diet-related health problems, have issued dietary guidelines designed to alter the diet. Most Western countries' dietary guidelines emphasise reductions in fat, sugar, salt and alcohol and increases in cereal, grain and vegetable products.

DIET FOODS

Foods which have reduced energy. May include low-kilojoule jams, jellies, soft drinks, cheeses, breads, cereals or other foods modified to reduce their energy.

DIETS, SLIMMING

Weight loss diets abound in Western countries where excess weight is a real problem for a large percentage of the population. However, it is also a problem that many young women in Western countries follow slimming diets when they are not overweight in the first place, while many others, especially men, totally ignore the health risks which arise from their excess body fat.

Most popular diets may reduce weight in the short term but they are usually ineffective for permanent weight control. Body weight can be manipulated by reducing the amount of carbohydrate consumed and this is the basis for most slimming diets. Without carbohydrate, the muscle stores of glycogen (see page 165) are used to supply energy. Each gram of muscle glycogen is stored with almost 3 g of water, so the use of the 600 g or so of muscle glycogen in the average body is accompanied by a loss of 1.5−2.0 kg of water. This shows up on the scales as a weight loss but merely represents a temporary drop in fluid and glycogen supplies. As soon as carbohydrate is reintroduced into the diet, glycogen stores return — usually in slightly larger quantities!

Very low kilojoule diets of less than 4200 kJ/day (1000 Cals) are ineffective for weight control, since the body which is being fed insufficient food will slow down the rate at which it burns energy. Studies have shown that people can reduce body fat stores better with a well-balanced diet of 5000−6300 kJ/day (1200−1500 Cals) than with energy intakes half this level.

For successful slimming, the following facts are important:
- There is no miraculous way to dissolve body fat. No supplements, pills, injections,

drinks, biscuits or formula diets can melt away fat. There are also no special combinations of foods, or fat-dissolving substances in fruits or any other food, which will remove fat.

- Body fat can only be lost slowly. Fat accumulates slowly and that is the only way for it to be burned up by the body. A fat loss of 0.5 − 1.0 kg/week can be achieved with a sensible diet plus increased exercise. Except in cases of severe disease or high fever, greater losses of weight are due to losses of glycogen, water and lean muscle tissue.

- Going 'on' a diet for 8 days or 8 weeks will not solve a weight problem. Going 'on' a diet implies that one will go 'off' the diet. The only way to permanent control of body fat is a permanent change in eating and/or exercise habits. In practice, a combination of a good eating pattern plus increased exercise is the best recipe for losing and controlling body weight.

- Basic body shape cannot be changed by dieting. The world's top diet and exercise program cannot change your basic bone structure or body type. However, many people blame their skeleton for a large body size when the real problem is not the underlying bone structure but the fat layers covering it. Many women have a basic pear-shaped body. Weight loss will not change this basic body shape; it simply turns these people into smaller 'pears'.

- There is no way to reduce weight in just one part of the body. A sensible eating and exercise pattern will remove excess fat from the whole body in keeping with the basic body shape.

A sensible weight reduction diet should include:

- At least 4 slices of bread, preferably wholemeal (6 slices would be more appropriate for those who exercise a lot)
- Plenty of vegetables — at least 4 per day, but as many as desired
- 2 − 4 pieces of fruit (3 − 5 for those who exercise a lot)
- A moderate serving of some type of protein food such as fish (not fried), chicken or turkey (without skin), very lean red meat (small serve), eggs, cheese (small piece), legumes (dried peas or beans)
- 500 mL milk (low-fat) or non-fat unsweetened yoghurt (200 g yoghurt = 250 mL milk)
- As little fat, alcohol and sugar as possible. Where some fat is unavoidable, a small quantity of olive oil is the best choice.

Increasing daily exercise is also important. A daily walk of 30 mins is ideal.

See also Balanced diet; Fasting.

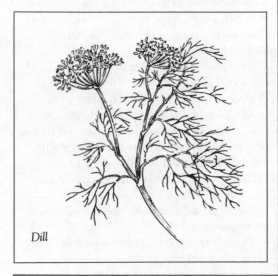

Dill

DIGESTION

The process of breaking down foods, so that their nutrients can be absorbed and used by the body. Digestion occurs in the gastrointestinal or alimentary tract — a tube about 10 m long.

Digestion begins in the mouth when foods are chewed and mixed with saliva. An enzyme present in saliva (an amylase) also begins to break down complex carbohydrates. Broken into smaller pieces by the teeth, food passes through the oesophagus to the stomach. See page 22.

The stomach acts as a large holding chamber where food is mixed which acid and gastric juices into a thick acid mixture called chyme (pronounced 'kyme'). An enzyme, pepsin, begins breaking down proteins into smaller units, but fats and carbohydrates have to wait for their digestion in the small intestine.

The production of gastric juices is influenced by nerve impulses; if you are upset or angry, more or less gastric juices can be produced. The cells lining the stomach also produce a special mucus which prevents the stomach wall being damaged by the strong acid.

Alcohol can be absorbed from the stomach, especially if carbon dioxide is present, as is the case with champagne or spirits mixed with soda or other soft drink. Alcohol is also absorbed more rapidly if there is no food in the stomach. From the stomach, food gradually passes into the upper part of the small intestine, the duodenum.

In the small intestine, bile from the liver neutralises the acid from the stomach and creates an alkaline environment. Again mucus is secreted to protect the intestinal walls from the strong alkali.

In response to the presence of food in the duodenum, the pancreas sends out pancreatic juice containing a wide range of enzymes to break down protein, carbohydrate and fats. The pancreatic juices and intestinal secretions contain enzymes to break down proteins, fats and carbohydrates so the current fad that the body cannot digest proteins and carbohydrates at the same time is nonsense.

In the small intestine, proteins are broken down to amino acids, carbohydrates are digested to simple sugars, and fats are broken down to monoglycerides, fatty acids and glycerol. Dietary fibre is separated from other nutrients, but very little digestion of fibre occurs. The presence of fibre, however, slows down the rate of digestion at this stage. This can be important in promoting satiety and reducing the rate at which sugars are ready for absorption into the blood. Diabetics, for example, find blood sugar levels much easier to control when they eat plenty of dietary fibre.

The next step is the absorption of the sugars, amino acids, fatty acids, minerals, vitamins and water into the bloodstream, to be taken to the liver and redirected to appropriate sites. Most absorption of nutrients occurs from the small intestine through the tiny projections called villi which cover the folded surface of the intestine. The total area for absorption is of the order of 300 sq m. As we have seen, alcohol can be absorbed directly from the stomach, while water and the products of dietary fibre digestion, are absorbed from the large intestine.

The 'leftovers' after digestion and absorption from the small intestine consist of dietary fibre, water and some complex carbohydrates which escape the action of the starch splitting enzymes. These substances pass to the large intestine where water is re-absorbed and dietary fibre and undigested carbohydrates are fermented by bacteria. The final residue for excretion consists of some unfermentable fibres, the bodies of millions of bacteria (which make up about 70 per cent of the faeces) and some water (see also page 42).

See also Enzymes.

DIJON MUSTARD
see Mustard.

DILL
see Herbs.

DILL PICKLES

Cucumbers pickled in vinegar flavoured with dill seeds.

DISACCHARIDES

Sugars made up of 2 simple sugar molecules. Examples include:
- Lactose — 1 molecule of glucose and 1 of galactose

- Maltose — 2 glucose units
- Sucrose — 1 molecule of glucose and 1 of fructose.

Once disaccharides enter the small intestine, enzymes split them into their component sugars.

See also Carbohydrates; Monosaccharides.

DIURETICS

Drugs which increase the flow of urine. Caffeine and other methylxanthines in coffee, substances in some herbs (such as dandelion and buchu), and alcohol, have a diuretic action on the kidneys. These drinks are therefore not a good way to replenish losses of water from the body.

A variety of drugs (commonly called 'water pills') are also used to remove excess fluid in those whose high blood pressure is preventing their kidneys from excreting the normal volume of water. Diuretic drugs act by removing excess sodium from the body; inadvertently they also remove potassium and magnesium. These important minerals must be replaced to avoid muscle weakness.

Diuretics are sometimes prescribed for those who are overweight. They are totally useless to reduce body fat, and since overweight people have too much fat rather than too much water, diuretics are inappropriate fat reduction aids. Any weight loss is merely water which will soon return. Diuretics can also cause a loss of minerals and result in muscle weakness and dehydration. The only justification for their use is in cases of severe sodium retention, usually accompanying high blood pressure or kidney damage.

DIVERTICULAR DISEASE

A condition where pouches form in the wall of the intestine. When these are inflamed, the condition is known as diverticulitis. It is relatively unknown except in Western countries and is caused by a lack of sufficient dietary fibre. Eating more fibre throughout life is important to prevent the diverticula forming. Those with the condition are advised to eat more high-fibre foods but to avoid foods such as passionfruit which contain pips. Some studies indicate that one-third of older people in Western countries have diverticular disease.

DNA

see Deoxyribonucleic acid; Nucleic acids.

DOCOSAHEXAENOIC ACID (DHA)

A polyunsaturated fatty acid belonging to the omega-3 family. Important in the nervous system, brain and retina. Found in fish liver oils, fish such as cod, mackerel and herring, and also in turkey, chicken and some plants.

See also Omega 3 fatty acids.

DOLMADES

Stuffed vine leaves (or occasionally stuffed cabbage or lettuce leaves). Commonly eaten in Greece and Turkey where the young grape vine leaves are stuffed with rice, minced lamb, herbs, lemon and olive oil, cooked and served either hot or cold.

DOLOMITE

This substance is made from ground limestone and contains calcium bicarbonate and magnesium. Most often used as a form of garden lime, but ground dolomite powder is sometimes sold as a source of calcium for humans. However, the form of calcium present is not well absorbed by the body.

DORADILLO

see Wine, Varieties.

DORADO

see Fish.

DOUGHNUT

A yeasted dough which is fried and then rolled in sugar. Hardly a nutritionist's delight, a 75 g donut has 11 g of sugar, 16 g of fat (mainly

FISH

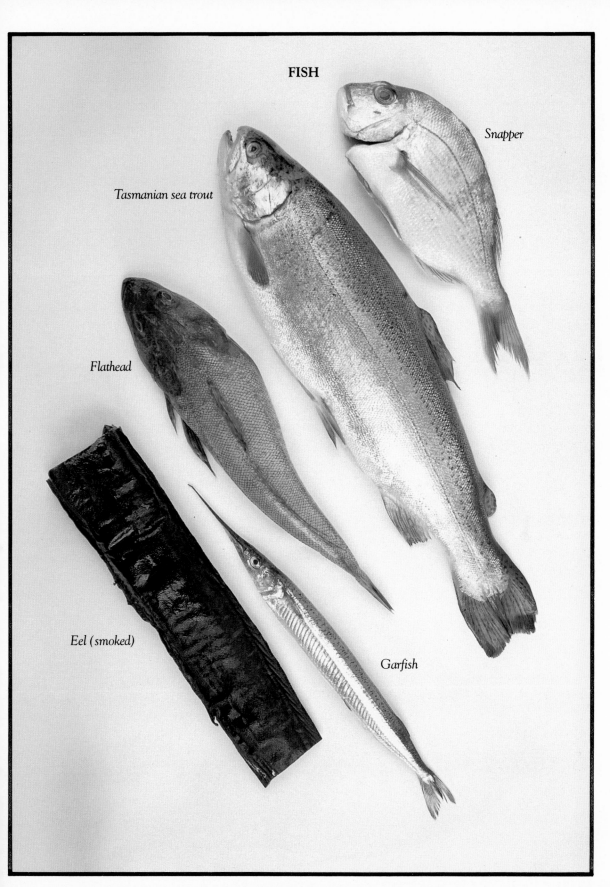

Snapper

Tasmanian sea trout

Flathead

Eel (smoked)

Garfish

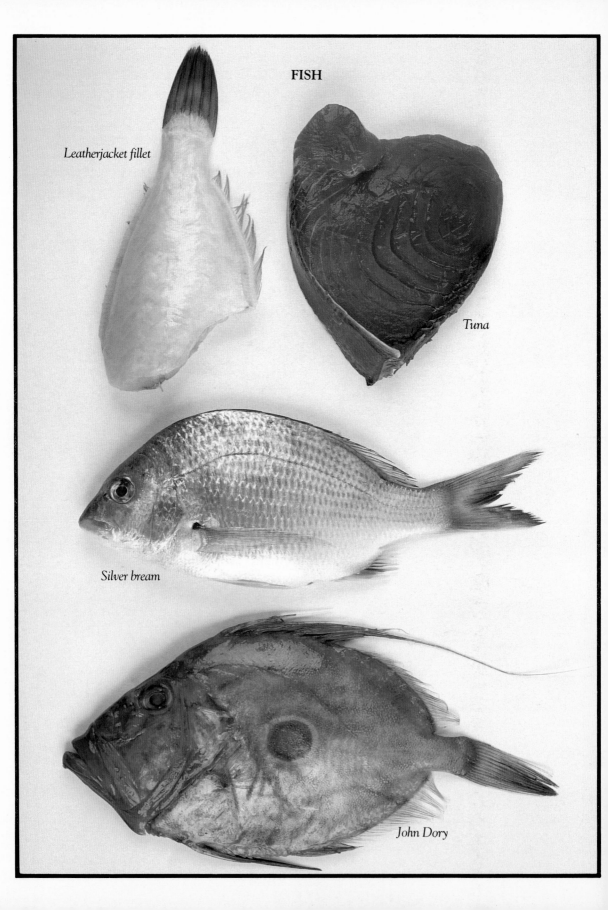

FISH

Leatherjacket fillet

Tuna

Silver bream

John Dory

saturated) and 1255 kJ (300 Cals). Iced and jam-filled donuts have even more sugar.

DRAMBUIE
see Drinks, Alcoholic.

DRIED FOODS
see Dehydrated foods.

DRIED FRUITS

Apples, apricots, bananas, currants, dates, figs, grapes, nectarines, peaches, pears and plums are commonly dried, mostly as they have been for thousands of years — by the sun. Raisins are dried purple grapes while sultanas are dried green, seedless sultana grapes. A few fruits, such as prunes, may be dried in a drying chamber. As fruits dry, enzymes may cause some discolouration, particularly in those which are a lighter colour. The addition of sulphur compounds prevents the natural darkening and allows the final product to retain more moisture as well as more vitamins.

Dried fruits do not contain added sugar, but since they have a lower moisture content than their fresh counterparts, they have a higher concentration of their natural sugar. This gives them a sweet taste but does not increase the sugar content per unit of fruit. For example, 6 dried apricot halves have the same quantity of sugar as 3 whole fresh apricots. However, since dried fruits have less water, they are less filling and so have the potential to be consumed in larger quantities than their fresh counterparts. This can be useful when a more concentrated food is required.

For details about the nutritional value of particular dried fruits, see individual entries under Fruits.

DRINKS, ALCOHOLIC; NON-ALCOHOLIC
See following pages.

DRIPPING
The fat which comes from meat. Beef dripping is almost pure fat and 100 g have 3740 kJ (890 Cals). Of its fat, 45 per cent is saturated; 51 per cent is monounsaturated and 4 per cent is polyunsaturated. It is not a nutritionally desirable product.

DRUGS AND NUTRITION

A number of drugs affect the absorption of certain nutrients, just as foods can alter the absorption and usefulness of some drugs. Drugs can also affect nutrition by altering the appetite; some, such as oral contraceptives, increase appetite, while others, such as morphine or levodopa, may decrease appetite. A few drugs make particular foods taste unpleasant. Some drugs do not mix with foods (for example, some anti-depressants must not be combined with foods rich in amines) and a few drugs are actually used as foods (for example, tea, coffee, alcohol). To complicate matters further, some nutrients, when taken in large doses, act more like drugs than nutrients. This applies to large doses of vitamins.

The effects of many drugs on nutrients can be rectified by having a nutritious diet. However, with drugs which are used for prolonged periods, such as anti-convulsants, the effect on vitamins is such that a supplement may need to be prescribed with the drug. Some long-term cholesterol-lowering drugs also affect the absorption of vitamins E and folacin and this may need attention.

Antibiotics wipe out not only harmful bacteria but may destroy some of the useful bacteria which manufacture vitamins such as biotin. If used for a only a few days, the normal intestinal bacteria will soon re-establish themselves, but with long-term antibiotic treatment, a biotin supplement may be necessary (see page 24).

The dosage of drugs should always be based on body weight, and the pharmacist may need some information on a person's dietary intake. To date, these factors have only rarely been considered.

DRINKS, ALCOHOLIC
see also Alcohol; Drinks, Non-alcoholic

Alcoholic beverages have been used by human civilisations for as long as recorded history. Wild wheat or barley left in water until it formed a bubbling brew probably represented the first alcoholic beverage.

Alcohol can be produced by the fermentation of grains, fruits, sugars, vegetables or the sap from some trees. The alcohol is produced, as a by-product, when naturally-occurring yeasts break down the sugar in the particular food. The content of alcohol varies from 4−6 per cent in beer, 10−15 per cent in wine, 20 per cent in fortified wines to 40 per cent in spirits and liqueurs.

Absinthe

A greenish, flavoured distilled alcoholic drink originally made by Henri-Louis Pernod. The alcohol content is 68 per cent and the flavouring comes from wormwood (banned in some countries because it is believed to contain toxic oils), plus licorice, fennel, angelica root, hyssop and aniseed. The classic 'absinthe drip' is made by dripping water through a sugar cube into the liquor which turns a cloudy white. Similar drinks, but with lower alcohol and no wormwood, include ouzo, raki, and pernod.

Advocaat

A popular Dutch liqueur made from brandy, sugar and egg yolks. 50 mL has 570 kJ (136 Cals) and 8 g of alcohol.

Ale

see Beer.

Amaretto

An Italian drink, made in Saronno (Italy), and flavoured with almonds. Used in mixed drinks and Italian desserts.

Amontillado

A dark-coloured, aged fino sherry.

Angostura bitters

West Indian concoction consisting of cloves, cinnamon, quinine, nutmeg, prunes, rum and gentian (the root of a blue-flowered plant which grows in mountainous areas). First made in 1824 and named after an old Venezuelan town. A few drops of bitters are added to some drinks and also used in desserts.

See also Bitters.

Anise

An alcoholic drink made in Spain, France and The Netherlands and flavoured with anise, fennel seeds and coriander.

Apple jack

An apple brandy made in the United States from fermented cider.

Aquavit

A flavoured distilled liquor with over 40 per cent alcohol which is made from fermented potato or grain and is filtered through charcoal. Its colour ranges from clear to pale yellow. Sometimes called schnapps, its name comes from *aqua vitae* (Latin for the 'water of life'), originally used for liquor distilled from wine. A traditional part of the Scandinavian smorgasbord.

Armagnac

A very dry brandy from the southwestern region of France. It has no sugar added and is aged in sappy black oak casks.

Beer

Beer is a brewed and fermented beverage made from water, barley, hops and yeast. The brewing begins with dry barley which is soaked and allowed to germinate.

After soaking in water, the barley grains swell and their cells begin to grow. About a week after this germination process begins, sufficient enzymes have accumulated in the barley grain to convert the stored starch (or complex carbohydrate) in the grain into maltose (a simple carbohydrate or sugar). The resulting malt is heated and dried to halt the action of the enzymes. The skill of the brewer is to heat the malt sufficiently to produce flavour and colour compounds without actually killing the enzymes. Pale ales and lagers are produced from more gentle heating to make a light malt. Dark, strong beers are made by using a more intense heat to give a darker malt. Once dried, the malt is stored as a powder.

Traditional beer (still made in Germany) used only the malt and warm water. Most modern breweries add cane sugar to boost the carbohydrate content.

To produce beer, the malt is soaked in water to form a mash and the enzymes once again begin working to convert the complex carbohydrate into sugars. The final material is called the 'wort'. The darker malts used have fewer enzymes and so will not produce as much of the sugars as the lighter malts. The greater the amount of complex carbohydrate left, the more body the beer will have.

The wort is filtered through the malt husks and then boiled with hops (or hop extract) so that the resins and oil from the hops will contribute a bitterness and aroma. Finally, yeast is added to transform the sugar into alcohol.

Some strains of yeast clump together, trap the carbon dioxide they produce and rise to the surface (top-fermenting yeasts), while others stay separate and gradually fall to the bottom when fermentation is over (bottom-fermenting yeasts). With plenty of oxygen at the top of the mixture, top-fermenting yeasts produce slightly acidic, stronger-flavoured ales (such as brown ale, stout or porter ale). Bottom fermentation produces lagers and lighter-flavoured beers such as many of the German beers.

Controlling the conditions of the quantity and type of yeast, the amount of oxygen, motion and temperature, produces the different varieties of beer.

Beers generally have 4–5 per cent alcohol. Very few of the original B complex vitamins from the yeast remain in the finished product. Since the metabolism of the sugar and alcohol in beer in the body requires some B complex vitamins, heavy beer drinkers can become deficient in these, especially thiamin (B_1).

A 375-mL can of beer has 650 kJ (155 Cals). Low-alcohol beers range from 0.9–3.2 per cent alcohol and a can has 300–480 kJ (72–115 Cals).

Benedictine

A liqueur flavoured with honey, thyme and myrrh, first made by the Benedictine monks at the Abbey de Fecamp in Normandy in 1650.

Bitters

An aromatic (usually alcoholic) liquid containing bitter substances extracted from roots, herbs and bark. The aromatic ingredients may include juniper, cinnamon or other spices or camomile. The alcohol content is generally around 40 per cent, but since only small quantities are used, the amount of alcohol consumed is very small. Bitters were first made in France in the sixteenth century.

See also Angostura Bitters.

Bloody Mary

A drink made from tomato juice, vodka, Worcestershire sauce and lime or lemon juice. An average bloody Mary has 295 kJ (70 Cals) and 8 g of alcohol.

Bourbon

see Whisky.

Brandy

An alcoholic beverage distilled from wine, and usually aged in wooden containers to develop an amber colour. Ageing improves brandy but once bottled it does not improve further. The most famous brandies are Cognac and Armagnac, both produced in France. Marc brandies are distilled from the material remaining in the wine press after the grapes have been pressed. Fruit brandies (such as cherry brandy) may be fermented from a fruit mash. Cheap brandies are made by adding sugar, colouring and flavouring to various distilled wines.

A 30 mL nip of brandy has 275 kJ (65 Cals) and approximately 10 g of alcohol.

Brandy Alexander

A cocktail made from brandy, cream, creme de cacao and ice, shaken vigorously together. An average brandy Alexander has 795 kJ (190 Cals) and about 14 g of alcohol.

Cabernet sauvignon

see Wine, Varieties.

Calvados

An apple brandy distilled from apple cider. Made in Calvados, an apple growing area in northern France.

Campari

A liqueur made from grape spirit with herbs, quinine bark (which produces much of its distinctive flavour) and the peel from bitter oranges. Usually mixed with soda water or used in cocktails.

Cassis

Blackcurrant syrup made from sugar and blackcurrants.

Chablis

see Wine, Varieties.

Champagne

see Wine, Varieties.

Chardonnay

see Wine, Varieties.

Chartreuse

A basil-flavoured liqueur originally made by the monks in a Carthusian monastery in Chartreuse, France, in the seventeenth century. Also contains honey. Available as green or yellow Chartreuse, the green having a higher alcohol content than the yellow.

Chenin blanc

see Wine, Varieties.

Chianti

see Wine, Varieties.

Cider

A drink fermented from apples. Popular in many countries, sometimes as a 'dry' cider and sometimes as a 'sweeter' product. The sweetness comes from the sugar present. Vintage cider with a much higher alcohol level is also available. A 250 mL glass of sweet cider has 440 kJ (105 Cals); dry cider has 375 kJ (90 Cals). Vintage cider has 1045 kJ (250 Cals) per 250 mL glass.

Cocktail

see Cocktail.

Cognac

A superior quality brandy produced in France and named after the town of Cognac. It was first made in the seventeenth century by double distillation in pot stills followed by ageing in oak. It is now produced in 7 designated areas and aged in oak until it is smooth, complex and well-flavoured. The age is shown by various symbols: Three Star has been aged for 2 years; V.S.O.P (very superior old pale) has had 4 years; and Napoleon has had 5 years.

Cointreau

A French liqueur flavoured with bergamot oranges. Popular in cooking, especially in desserts and also used in drinks or as an after-dinner liqueur.

Creme de banane

A liqueur made from bananas, sugar and spirits. Used in drinks or over icecream.

Creme de cacao

A West Indian liqueur made from a distillation of cocoa beans, sugars and some vegetable extracts.

Creme de cassis

A French liqueur made from blackcurrants.

Creme de menthe

A liqueur made in France and containing peppermint, cinnamon, ginger, orris (a species of iris) and sage. Used in cocktails and sometimes served over icecream.

Curacao

A Dutch liqueur made from brandy flavoured with the dried peel of oranges from the island of Curacao.

Daiquiri

A cocktail made from white rum, fruit juice, sugar, ice and fruit. Kilojoules vary according to the type of daiquiri, but a typical drink would have about 670 kJ (160 Cals) and about 16 g of alcohol.

Drambuie

A Scottish liqueur made from Highland malt whisky, honey, herbs and spices. Its name comes from an old Gaelic phrase meaning 'the drink that satisfies'. Most Scots would agree.

Egg nog

A drink made from eggs, beaten with sugar, cream and brandy, rum or whisky.

Traditionally drunk at Christmas in the northern hemisphere. The kilojoules vary according to the mixture used, but will be in the vicinity of 2300 kJ (550 Cals) per serve.

Galliano

An Italian liqueur named after an Italian soldier, Guiseppe Galliano. Flavoured with herbs and commonly used in the cocktail called a Harvey Wallbanger.

Gimlet

A drink made from gin, lime juice, sugar, soda water and ice. A typical drink would have about 585 kJ (140 Cals) and 16 g of alcohol.

Gin

A distilled liquor made from a grain mash and flavoured with juniper berries. First made in Holland in the seventeenth century, its name comes from the French word for the juniper berry. Gin quickly became popular, especially in England. By the eighteenth century, gin drinking had become a great vice and gave rise to the temperance movement.

There are two major types of gin, Dutch and English. The first is made from a mash of barley fermented to a beer which is then distilled to a spirit called a malt wine. This is distilled again and juniper berries and other herbs are added to produce the distinctive Dutch gin.

English gin is made from a mash of corn and malt and distilled to a spirit with over 90 per cent alcohol. This is diluted with distilled water, combined with the flavouring agents (which might include orris root, angelica, liquorice, orange and lemon rind, various barks and spices), and distilled again. The resulting product is dry and has a higher alcohol content and more flavouring agents than the Dutch gin.

Most gins are not aged. Dutch gin tends to be served alone, or with water. English gin is commonly mixed with tonic. In the United States, gin forms the basis for cocktails such as the martini or gin sling (see below).

30 mL of gin has 275 kJ (65 Cals) and approximately 10 g of alcohol.

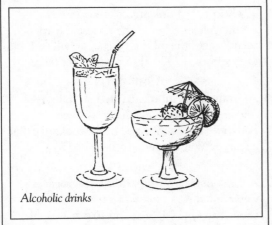

Alcoholic drinks

Gin sling
A cocktail made from gin, lemon juice, sugar, ice, bitters and mineral or soda water. A typical drink would have 545 kJ (130 Cals) and 12 g of alcohol.

Glogg
Also known as glüwein, this is a drink made from red wine, heated with orange peel, cloves, cinnamon and sugar. Dried fruits such as raisins or apricots are sometimes added. Served hot. The exact kilojoule value will depend on the ingredients.

Grand Marnier
A French liqueur made from brandy and the peel from bitter bergamot oranges. Used in drinks, in cooking (especially with poultry) and a major ingredient in the sauce for crepes Suzette.

Grasshopper
A green cocktail made by shaking together equal quantities of creme de cacao and creme de menthe. 1 grasshopper would have about 740 kJ (175 Cals) and 18 g of alcohol.

Harvey wallbanger
An American cocktail containing vodka, Galliano, orange juice, sugar and ice. A typical drink has about 840 kJ (200 Cals) and 24 g of alcohol.

Irish coffee
A drink made by adding Irish whiskey to hot, freshly brewed coffee and topping the mixture with cream. The whiskey is gently heated so that the drink is hot as it is sipped through the cool cream. Traditionally served in tall heatproof glasses. Irish coffee has about 800 kJ (190 Cals) — not counting any sugar you may add.

Kirsch
A liqueur distilled from crushed cherries. Kirsch is used as a drink or is added to dishes such as cheese fondue, various apple desserts or cherry cakes. The liqueur contains very small amounts of cyanide which come from the cherry pips.

Kummel
A German liqueur flavoured with caraway seeds, cumin and fennel.

Lager
see Beer.

Lamb's wool
see Fruits, Crabapple.

Liqueurs
These are alcoholic drinks produced by distilling fermented sugars and flavouring with various substances. Alcohol content ranges from 25–60 per cent by volume. Most liqueurs are made by combining a spirit such as brandy with sugar, fruit or fruit extracts, herbs, cacao, vanilla beans or other flavouring agents. Many liqueurs were first made by monks.

Individual liqueurs include advocaat, Benedictine, campari, Chartreuse, cointreau, creme de banane, creme de cacao, creme de cassis, creme de menthe, Curacao, drambuie, Galliano, Grand Marnier, kirsch, kummel, maraschino, pernod, sambuca, Southern Comfort, strega.

Madeira
A sweet dessert wine, usually fortified with brandy and made on the island of Madeira. It differs from sherry in being made with more

acidic grapes which produce its distinctive tang.

Mai tai

A cocktail made from white rum, orange and lime juices, ice and fruits such as cherries or pineapple. A typical mai tai has 545 kJ (130 Cals) and 16 g of alcohol.

Maraschino

A liqueur made from fermented maraschino cherries and sugar. Used in many desserts.

Margarita

A cocktail made from tequila, cointreau, lime or lemon juice and ice. The rim of the glass in which the margarita is served is dipped in water and then into salt so that the salt forms a crusty frosting through which the drink is sipped. An average margarita has 470 kJ (110 Cals) and 17 g of alcohol.

Marsala

A sweet dessert wine, fortified with brandy and made in Sicily. Used in many Italian desserts, and an essential ingredient in the dessert zabaglione (see page 407).

Martini

A drink made from ice, gin and vermouth, usually garnished with an olive. The usual ratio of gin to vermouth is 5 parts of gin to 1 of vermouth. The dryness of the martini depends on the amount of gin and the type of vermouth used. An average martini has 530 kJ (125 Cals) and 20 g of alcohol.

Mint julep

A drink made from crushed mint, sugar, ice and either whisky, brandy, gin or bourbon. An average mint julep has 545 kJ (130 Cals).

Mirin

A Japanese wine made by fermenting rice. Very pale in colour and with a mild flavour. Similar to Chinese sake.

Muscat

A sweet dessert wine, fortified with brandy. Made from muscatel grapes. Has similar kilojoule value to port.

Ouzo

A spirit flavoured with anise. Popular in Greece.

Pernod

A liqueur which includes pernod flavouring, an oil from aniseed. Mainly drunk around the Mediterranean regions and in parts of Asia.

Port

Originally, the term port meant a Portuguese wine. Now it means a sweet wine fortified with brandy. To make port, the fermentation process is halted when half the original sugar of the grape remains. This wine is then poured into a barrel with brandy: about 75 per cent wine and 25 per cent brandy. With such a short fermentation process it is essential to extract all the flavour from the grapes. This was once done with continuous treading but mechanical means have now taken over from the human foot.

Vintage port is bottled after 2 years and then aged for up to 20 years in the bottle. Tawny port is aged longer in the barrel and picks up a brown colour during this time.

60 mL of port has 400 kJ (95 Cals) and 10 g of alcohol.

Retsina

A Greek wine flavoured with the resin from pine trees. Its somewhat astringent flavour is said to blend well with Greek food. It has no special nutritional properties.

Rum

A drink made by taking the residues from sugar refining and mixing them with molasses, allowing the mixture to ferment and then distilling it. The resulting product is then diluted. Rums are also aged; light rums for 1 year, heavier varieties for up to 6 years.

Jamaican rum undergoes a longer fermentation and is not distilled to the same degree of purity as other rums. It has a stronger taste.

Rum was the first mass-produced spirit. Unlike brandy or whisky, the raw materials for rum were available for nothing — they were a by-product in the production of white sugar.

This spirit became popular in the West Indies in the seventeenth century when it became the most prosperous aspect of sugar growing. It became standard ration for sailors and was responsible for much of the drunkenness for the next few centuries.

Rum is now used as a drink, in cocktails and in cooking, especially in desserts and fruit cake. 30 mL of rum has 275 kJ (65 Cals) and 10 g of alcohol.

Rusty nail

A drink made from 2 parts whisky to 1 part drambuie, stirred with ice and garnished with lemon peel. An average rusty nail has 550 kJ (130 Cals) and 19 g of alcohol.

Sake

A Chinese wine made from fermented rice. Although it tastes 'light', sake has a similar alcohol content to wine.

Sambuca

A clear Italian liqueur with a slight aniseed flavour. Usually served with a whole coffee bean in the glass. The bean is chewed at the end of the drink. Used as an aperitif or a liqueur.

Sauterne

see Wine, Varieties.

Schnapps

see Aquavit.

Screwdriver

A mixture of orange juice with vodka and ice. A typical drink has 400 kJ (95 Cals) and 8 g of alcohol.

Sherry

A fortified wine which may be dry or sweet. The name is derived from the Spanish city Jerez which was anglicised to sherry in the seventeenth century. The major grape used to make sherry is the palomino (see page 402). Fino sherry is a young, dry sherry with a light, delicate flavour. The sweetness or dryness of sherry is determined by the grapes used, the length of fermentation and how long it is aged. A 60 mL glass of dry sherry has 295 kJ (70 Cals) while sweet sherry has 335 kJ (80 Cals). Both have 10 g of alcohol.

Slivovitz

A dry white brandy made from plums. Hungarian or Serbo-Croatian origin.

Southern Comfort

A liqueur made in the southern states of the United States from whisky and a variety of fruits, including peach and orange.

Spirits

The general term for concentrated alcoholic drinks made by distilling various types of alcoholic liquors. The alcoholic liquor (with about 5−15 per cent alcohol content) is heated until it boils. Since alcohol has a lower boiling point than water, the vapour will be much more concentrated than the original liquid. The concentrated vapour is then condensed and collected and will have an alcohol content of 50−70 per cent. If the distillation is repeated, the alcohol content can rise even higher.

Strega

An Italian liqueur which includes oranges and a number of herbs. Used in drinks and also poured over some Italian cakes to form a moist syrup through the cake.

Tequila

The juice from the leaves of a Mexican cactus, the agave, fermented and distilled to produce a spirit which has become the national drink of Mexico.

Tia Maria

A Jamaican liqueur made from rum, spices and coffee extract.

Vermouth

A concentrated wine which may be sweet or dry (the sweet variety has a higher sugar content). Available in white, pink or a dark-coloured variety. It has an alcohol content of about 18 per cent (approximately 1.5 times that of wine). 60 mL of sweet vermouth has 345 kJ (82 Cals) while dry vermouth has 295 kJ (70 Cals). Both would contribute 9 g of alcohol.

Vodka

A clear spirit distilled from rye, malt or potatoes and commonly made in the Soviet Union and Poland. It is filtered through powdered charcoal and this removes impurities and most of the flavour. Its processing also removes most of the congeners (see page 81), so that it is less likely to cause a hangover than most other alcoholic drinks. Like most spirits, vodka is about 32 per cent alcohol. 30 mL has 275 kJ (65 Cals).

Whisky

Spelt 'whiskey' in the United States and Ireland, this is a spirit distilled from grains which may be malted, unmalted or a mixture of both types. Scotch whiskies are made from barley which has been malted to a pale colour so that there is maximum sugar present for the growth of yeast. Scotch is then kept in casks which have been used to store sherry. Over years of storage, the Scotch picks up some colour and flavour from the wood. Top quality Scotch whiskies are made purely from 1 malt distiller and have a strong flavour. They are known as 'single malts'. Some Scotch derives a unique flavour from the peat smoke which is used to dry the malt. The majority of Scotch produced these days consists of a blend of the malted product (about 30 per cent) with neutral grain alcohol which is more cheaply produced from corn.

Irish whiskey is made from a mixture of 40 per cent malted barley and 60 per cent unmalted. No peat smoke is used. It is also triple distilled and has a milder flavour than Scotch.

In the United States, bourbon is a whisky made from barley malt and ground corn mashed together and fermented for several days. After distillation, bourbon is aged in oak barrels which have been charred on the inside. This contributes colour and flavour.

The average alcohol content of whisky is 33 per cent. A nip (30 mL) has 275 kJ (65 Cals) and 10 g of alcohol.

Whisky sour

A combination of whisky, orange and lemon juices, sugar, ice and a garnish of orange, lemon and cherries. An average whisky sour has 695 kJ (165 Cals) and 16 g of alcohol.

Wine

see Wine.

Tom Collins

A cocktail made from lemon juice, sugar, ice, gin and soda water. A typical drink has 460 kJ (110 Cals).

DRINKS, NON-ALCOHOLIC

A variety of beverages based on fruits, dairy products or a collection of flavourings and colourings. Those containing juices or yoghurt will have a positive contribution to make to nutritional needs. Others, such as carbonated soft drinks, contain large quantities of sugar (approximately 40 g per 375 mL can) and no useful nutrients.

Cassis

Blackcurrant extract blended with sugar to form a syrup.

Cola

Cola drinks contain water, sugar, colouring, flavouring and an essence made from the kola nut. Some also contain added caffeine, as well as that found naturally in the kola.

The world famous beverage, Coca-Cola © (also known as Coke), was first formulated in 1886, and, like other formulas of that time, is said to have contained cocaine. It was marketed as an 'ideal brain tonic' and as being good for 'headache and exhaustion'! Whatever their faults, current cola drinks certainly do not contain cocaine. Instead, they rely on caffeine to provide the well-known 'lift' associated with cola drinks. From its humble beginnings, Coca-Cola © has achieved dominance among soft drinks. In 1987, the world's population was downing more than 419 million 250 mL drinks of this beverage every day.

If you would like some trivia, the Coca-Cola marketers supplied the following: 'If all the 6.5 ounce [185 mL] bottles of Coke ever produced were loaded onto route trucks filled to capacity and driven, bumper to bumper at 88 km per hour past a point, they would take 3 years and 5 months to pass!' Or try this: 'If all the Coca-Cola ever drunk was placed in cans and stacked next to Mount Everest, 19 million columns would be needed!' And, if you like this sort of stuff: 'If all the Coke ever produced was put into 6.5 ounce [185 mL] bottles and placed end to end, they would wrap around the earth 11,863 times or stretch to the moon 1237 times or go one-third of the distance to Saturn!'

Back to reality: a can of a cola drink has 605 kJ (145 Cals) and contains 10.5 per cent added sugar.

See also Caffeine; Soft drinks.

Cordial

Cordials are made from sugar with added flavourings (natural or artificial) and colourings. They are usually sold in concentrated form with a sugar content of about 35 per cent. Undiluted they contribute 565 kJ (135 Cals) per 100 mL. They have no nutritional value.

Fruit juices

Many fruits are used for juice: orange, apple, pineapple and grape are the most commonly consumed. Apricot, peach, guava, lemon, grapefruit, mango and various tropical fruits are also used for juice.

In some countries, such as Australia, pure fruit juices must contain at least 96 per cent juice. Fruit juice drinks have 25—50 per cent juice and fruit drinks have less than 5—25 per cent juice.

Fruit juices are good sources of vitamins, especially vitamin C and also potassium. Those juices which are orange or red also contribute substantial amounts of carotene.

A negative aspect of fruit juices is that most have lost the fibre which was present in the original fruit. This makes it easy to overconsume the product and take in a large number of kilojoules — a problem for overweight adults and children. Many children who drink juices every time they are thirsty can easily take in enough extra calories to make them overweight. Like many low-fibre foods, juices are deceptively non-filling and, therefore, easily overconsumed. In small quantities they are nutritionally above reproach.

A 250 mL glass of orange juice has 400–505 kJ (95–120 Cals). The same quantity of apple juice has about 485 kJ (115 Cals). Grapefruit is lower at 380 kJ (90 Cals). Most other juices have similar kilojoule values.

Ginger beer

To make a ginger beer 'plant', place 1 teaspoon of yeast, $\frac{1}{2}$ teaspoon of sugar and $\frac{1}{2}$ teaspoon of ginger in 1 cup of water and leave to ferment. For the next week, add $\frac{1}{2}$ teaspoon each of sugar and ginger each day. This mixture is then strained (reserving the sediment) and added to 6 l of water in which 4 cups of sugar have been dissolved. A little lemon juice can also be added. The mixture is then poured into strong bottles, sealed and left in a cool place for a week. Half the sediment is then used to start the 'plant'. A further cup of water is added plus daily doses of sugar and ginger. As the yeast will continue to grow, no further addition of yeast is required. A 250 mL glass of this type of ginger beer will have 710 kJ (170 Cals).

Grenadine

A syrup made from sugar and pomegranate juice. Used in cocktails and desserts.

Lassi

A drink which is very popular throughout India and many Middle Eastern countries. Made from yoghurt mixed with ice water and flavoured with either salt and pepper, sugar or fruit.

Milkshakes

A combination of milk, sugar and fruit or flavouring, sometimes with added icecream. An average commercial milkshake has 1170 kJ (280 Cals). It supplies over 40 per cent of the average person's daily calcium.

Prairie oyster

Used as a 'cure' for a hangover, this drink is made by mixing Worcestershire sauce into tomato juice with a little lemon juice, a dash of olive oil, salt, pepper and paprika. An egg yolk is placed on top. The 'drink' is supposed to be swallowed in one gulp!

Smoothie

A drink made from milk, yoghurt, fruit, honey and ice, blended together until frothy. A smoothie is a good source of calcium and protein and has 1195 kJ (285 Cals).

Soft drinks

see Soft drinks.

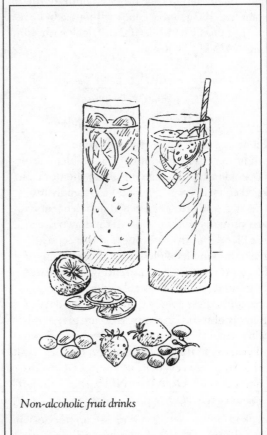

Non-alcoholic fruit drinks

DUCHESS POTATOES

A mixture of mashed potato and egg which is often piped and then browned in a hot oven before serving.

DUCK

The rich flavour of duck makes it a popular food. Compared with chicken, duck has less flesh per kilogram and an average sized duck will serve 3—4 people. Duck also has a higher fat content than other types of poultry, although much of this is concentrated in the skin. Removing the skin leaves a flesh with less than 5 per cent fat content. Duck is a good source of protein, iron and niacin (vitamin B_3) and supplies most of the other vitamins of the B complex. 100 g of roast duck without skin have 800 kJ (190 Cals) while 100 g of duck with skin have 1425 kJ (340 Cals).

DULSE
see Seaweed.

DUMPING SYNDROME

Properly called 'jejunal hyperosmolic syndrome', the symptoms of this problem occur in people who have had surgery to the stomach. Food empties (or is 'dumped') too rapidly into the intestine before it has had sufficient time to mix properly with fluid. Water is drawn from the blood into the intestine and this causes a rapid drop in blood pressure with symptoms of fast pulse, weakness and sweating. It is treated by dividing meals into smaller portions and spreading these evenly throughout the day. Rapidly absorbed carbohydrates are given only with some fat or protein which will slow down their entry to the small intestine.

DUMPLINGS

A light dough formed into balls and steamed or cooked on top of a stew or in a syrup (for dessert dumplings). The dough may contain a variety of different flours, baking powder, eggs, milk, butter and, sometimes, yeast, cheese, herbs or sugar.

DUNDEE CAKE

A light fruit cake enjoyed in Scotland. A 50 g slice has 800 kJ (190 Cals).

DUODENUM

The first part of the small intestine where the acidic contents of the stomach meet the alkaline environment of the small intestine. Digestive juices are secreted into the duodenum to break down proteins, fats and carbohydrates. Pancreatic juice and bile also enter the intestine at the duodenum to begin their job of digestion (see page 94).

DURIAN
see Fruit.

DURUM WHEAT

A high protein 'hard' wheat used for making pasta. Durum wheat also makes strong crusty bread. No good for making a light sponge cake.

DUXELLES

Mushrooms which have been finely chopped and sauteed in butter.

DYSPEPSIA

Indigestion due to some gastrointestinal disorder, eating too quickly without proper mastication, emotional upset or a sensitivity to a particular food ingredient. Treatment is to eat small quantities of food at regular intervals, in a calm atmosphere, taking the time to chew each mouthful properly. Antacids are commonly used for dyspepsia but can interfere with the absorption of minerals such as calcium and magnesium. Relaxation techniques practised just before meals can be useful.

DYSPHAGIA

Difficulty in swallowing.

E

EARL GREY TEA

see Tea.

ECTOMORPH

Long thin body type. Rarely become overweight.

ECZEMA

A skin rash which may be caused by sensitivity to some foods, or a chemical substance from a plant, soap, or material. If a food sensitivity is suspected as being the cause, an elimination diet is used (see page 110).

See also Allergies.

EDAM

see Cheese.

EDIBLE FLOWERS

see Flowers, edible.

EDTA

This chemical substance (ethylenediamine tetraacetic acid) is used to trap metal impurities. Acts as a chelating agent (see page 61). Its safety in humans is unknown.

EEL

see Fish.

EGG

The most commonly eaten eggs come from hens, originally descended from the Indian jungle fowl and domesticated by 2000 BC. These birds were taken to China, Europe and the Middle East, and then to the United States by Christopher Columbus. The eggs of quail, ducks, pigeons, pheasants and ostriches are also eaten throughout the world.

Eggs are intended as the source of food for the growing chick and thus contain most of the important nutrients required for growth. Nutritionally, eggs are a good source of protein, vitamins and minerals, containing every vitamin except C. Each egg has approximately 6 g of fat — about the same amount as in 1 bite of a sausage. An egg has approximately 315 kJ (75 Cals).

Eggs have been condemned for their content of dietary cholesterol. In the context of a fatty diet, this may indeed be a problem. However, research has shown quite clearly that it is the level of saturated fat in the diet which is responsible for cholesterol in the blood rather than the level of dietary cholesterol. A few people do respond very sensitively to dietary cholesterol, but most do not. An intake of 4 eggs a week is suitable for everyone; if you do not have high blood cholesterol and you eat a low-fat diet, you can happily eat an egg each day, if you so desire.

When cooked, the white of an egg coagulates and this is used to provide structure to many cooked foods. The air incorporated into beaten eggs (especially the whites), heats up and expands when sponge cakes, souffles and meringues are being cooked, contributing to the lightness of the products. Egg yolks also form a stable emulsion in foods such as sauces and mayonnaise. Egg whites will trap solid particles in stocks, clarifying them in the process. They also prevent the formation of large ice crystals in icecreams.

Eggs should always be cooked at low to moderate temperatures or their protein will become tough and rubbery.

The colour of an eggshell indicates the variety of hen used and has no relationship to the nutritional value. The colour of the yolk reflects the plants or feed given to the hen. Dark green plants or carotenes in the feed produce orange yolks. There is slightly more carotene in the darker yolked eggs and this will be converted to vitamin A in the body. Since eggs are a good source of pre-formed vitamin A, this small extra contribution from the carotene is insignificant.

Free-range eggs are from hens which are permitted to run around outside rather than being kept caged. Although it may be nicer to think of free-range birds, their eggs have not been shown to be nutritionally superior.

EGG NOG
see Drinks.

EGGPLANT
see Vegetables.

EICOSAPENTAENOIC ACID (EPA)

One of the omega 3 fatty acids found predominantly in deep-sea fish (see Omega 3 fatty acids, page 254).

ELASTIN

An insoluble fibrous connective tissue protein present in arteries, skin and tendons. With ageing, the elastic properties of this tissue decrease. In meats, the elastin content decreases with the age of the animal.

ELDERBERRY
see Fruit.

ELECTROLYTES

Minerals in solution in body fluids which regulate the balance of acids and bases. The major electrolytes — sodium, potassium and chloride — influence distribution of water within cells and in the spaces between them. Other electrolytes include magnesium and

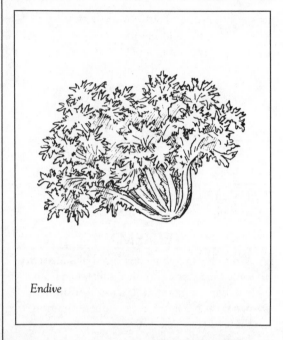

Endive

calcium. Disturbances to the balance of electrolytes occur in severe vomiting, diarrhoea or the heavy sweating common in endurance activities. It is important to realise that after heavy sweating, fluid losses will be proportionally greater than losses of electrolytes such as sodium. Water should always be replaced *before* electrolytes.

ELEPHANT'S APPLE
see Fruit.

ELIMINATION DIET

A diet which omits all foods known to commonly cause allergic reactions or sensitivities. Used in cases of suspected allergy or sensitivity. If the symptoms do not clear up with the elimination diet, it is unlikely that they are related to food. If symptoms do improve, foods with a known content of specific chemical substances (or capsules of the same chemicals) are added and reactions noted. By the gradual process of adding back foods, sensitivities can be discovered. Since there are currently no other reliable tests for food sensitivities, the elimination diet is useful. It is however, very boring, and is not adequate nutritionally. It should not be used without the supervision of a qualified dietitian.

See also Allergies; Dermatitis; Eczema.

EMMENTALER

see Cheese, Emmenthal.

EMULSIFIERS

Substances which keep fats evenly distributed throughout a product. Used in foods such as mayonnaise, sauces, icecream and various desserts, peanut butter, chocolate, coffee whitener, processed cheese, cakes and breads. Commonly used emulsifiers include egg yolk, lecithin, glyceryl monostearate, various stearoyl lactylates and chemical substances such as the sucrose esters of fatty acids. Additive nos. 471–491 are some of the commonly used emulsifiers.

EMULSION

A mixture of tiny droplets of fat and a liquid. Examples in food include mayonnaise, cream, whole milk, butter and salad dressings.

ENCHILADAS

A Mexican dish made from soft cornmeal pancakes (known as tortillas). Usually served wrapped around (or topped with) a spicy sauce containing tomatoes, chilli, cumin, onion and meat, chicken or beans. The dish may be topped with grated cheese, shredded lettuce and hard-boiled egg.

ENDIVE

see Vegetables.

ENDOCRINE GLANDS

Glands without ducts which secrete a variety of hormones to control body processes. Endocrine glands include the pituitary, thyroid, parts of the pancreas, adrenal glands, ovaries, testes and parathyroid gland.

Many of the secretions of these glands work on a feedback basis, so that once production is ample, the glands secrete less. This principle is ignored by some who believe that if a little is good, more must be better.

For example, the pituitary gland secretes a hormone called thyrotropin which, in turn, stimulates the thyroid gland to produce a hormone called thyroxine. This hormone requires iodine for its production and controls the metabolic rate. Many people take extra iodine (usually from kelp) in the hope that this will cause the thyroid to produce more thyroxine and speed up the metabolic rate. In fact, once the thyroxine level increases, the pituitary cuts back on its secretion of thyrotropin, thus preventing more thyroxine being formed, no matter how much extra iodine is supplied. This is called a feedback mechanism and it operates with many of the endocrine functions.

ENDOMORPH

One of the three basic body types originally classified by the American psychologist W. H. Sheldon. The typical endomorph is short and rather round with much of the body fat carried on the abdomen, upper arms and thighs. Weight reduction tends to be difficult for this body type.

ENDORPHINS

Substances released in the brain and related to opium. Larger quantities are produced during endurance exercise and contribute to the familiar 'runner's high'. During childbirth, endorphin production increases, presumably as a natural aid to cope with the pain. It is also thought that the pain relief afforded by acupuncture is related to an increased production of these chemicals.

Some people believe that production of

endorphins increases after eating a hot food such as chilli and this is responsible for the liking for foods which burn the mouth!

ENDOSPERM

The centre part of a grain, seed or nut which stores the protein and carbohydrate needed by the embryo or germ for development. When cereal grains are refined, the endosperm is often separated from the germ and the bran. Until recently, only the endosperm of many cereal grains was used for human consumption. There is now a greater call for wholegrain products which contain the germ and bran as well as the starchy endosperm. In coconut, the endosperm includes both the flesh and the milk. In puffed cereals, it is the endosperm which is heated until its water content expands and the grain 'explodes'.

ENERGY

In nutritional terms, energy refers to the number of kilojoules (or calories) which are released when a food is burned for fuel within the body (see also ATP, page 11). The term energy is popularly used to mean vitality, but this incorporates a psychological aspect in addition to the purely physical use of energy in nutrition. The mixing of the two ideas is confusing and leads many people to believe that energy is good but calories are somehow undesirable. Kilojoules and calories are simply a measure of the quantity of energy which any food can provide. They are also used to describe the quantity of energy needed for particular physical activities, including the basic processes to keep the body alive.

Fats provide the most energy with 37 kJ/g (9 Cals). Alcohol provides 29 kJ/g (7 Cals). Proteins provide 17 kJ/g (4 Cals) and carbohydrates give the lowest energy with 16 kJ/g (4 Cals).

The energy from foods is available to the body for its metabolism, growth (in children) and physical activity. Any energy not used for these purposes is converted into body fat and stored for possible later use. Thus a food which provides a lot of energy (such as chocolate) is not necessarily desirable for those whose lifestyle does not include sufficient physical activity to use up its energy. Few people feel the urge to run out and jump the fence just because they have taken in a heap of energy in a chocolate bar! In fact, the energy for muscular activity depends largely on what you ate the previous day.

In noting how much energy any food provides, it is also necessary to look at the quantity of the nutrients likely to be consumed. Unfortunately, fats still fare badly, since they can be hidden in large quantities in so many foods. Alcohol can also be consumed in large doses. Sugar too slips down so easily that it is easy to take in far more than the body's energy requirements. In small quantities, however, sugar would not provide excessive amounts of energy. The carbohydrate foods which most people fear as being fattening (such as bread and potatoes), usually provide a relatively small quantity of energy in the diet, since it is difficult to eat too much of such filling foods.

See also Carbohydrates.

E NUMBERS

Numbers officially assigned to food additives. The 'E' signifies they are used, by agreement, in European Economic Community (EEC) countries. Other countries, such as Australia, use the same numbers but call them 'additive numbers'.

See also Additives, food.

ENTRECOTE STEAK

A boneless sirloin steak taken from the back of the animal.

ENZYMES

Proteins which occur naturally in all living

organisms and enable chemical reactions to occur. Within the intestine, foods are digested by the action of enzymes. Within foods themselves, it is the action of enzymes which causes them to go bad.

Enzymes are destroyed by heat. This is an important reason why cooked foods last longer than raw ones. It is also the reason why pineapple must be cooked before being put into a gelatine-containing product. Pineapple (and figs and pawpaw) contain an enzyme which breaks down proteins. If raw pineapple comes into contact with gelatine, it breaks down the gelatine so that it cannot set. If the pineapple is cooked, its enzyme will be killed and gelatine can carry out its normal function.

The enzyme papain is extracted from pawpaw and used to break down meat protein to make tough cuts more tender.

Some people take extra enzymes in the belief that they will be of some advantage. This is useless since the enzymes are protein and will simply be digested in the acid environment of the stomach.

See also Lipases; Proteases; Lactase; Amylases; Digestion.

EPA

see Timnodonic acid.
See also Omega 3 fatty acids.

EPILEPSY

Epilepsy itself is not related to diet. Those who maintain that taking extra magnesium will cure epilepsy have no scientifically valid evidence for such claims.

However, epilepsy is related to nutrition in that many of the drugs used to control the condition alter vitamin requirements. Since many of these drugs are taken over a long time, attention to vitamin needs is important. Anti-convulsants may increase the need for folic acid, vitamin D and vitamin B_6 (pyridoxine). A qualified pharmacist should be able to advise on particular drugs.

ERGOCALCIFEROL

One type of vitamin D, known as D_2.

ERGOSTEROL

A substance in plant foods which changes to vitamin D_2 when exposed to ultraviolet light.

ERUCIC ACID

A monounsaturated fat found in rapeseed oil (see page 252). Erucic acid can only be oxidised very slowly and can be harmful to the heart. Recently developed varieties of rapeseed have very little erucic acid.

ERYTHROCYTES

Red blood cells.

ERYTHROSINE

see Colourings.

ESCAROLE

see Vegetables, Endive.

ESKIMO DIET

The Eskimos have a diet which is high in fat. Yet they have low levels of diseases such as heart disease, diabetes and rheumatism. Medical researchers now believe that Eskimos are protected against the problems caused by a high-fat diet because they eat so much fish (around 450 g per person per day). The particular types of fat in fish (see page 120) are polyunsaturated but are different from the polyunsaturated fats found in vegetable oils (see Omega 3 fatty acids and Seal meat.

ESPAGNOLE SAUCE
see Sauces, Brown.

ETHANOL
Another name for ethyl alcohol which is formed from the fermentation of sugars (see Alcohol).

ETHYLENE
A chemical produced naturally by fruit during the ripening process. Fruits such as oranges may be ripened artificially using ethylene. Other fruits, such as bananas, produce a lot of ethylene and can be used to ripen other fruits. This is the reason why an unripe avocado will ripen quickly if placed in a paper bag with a banana.

EUGENOL
The constituent of clove oil which provides its characteristic smell.

EVENING PRIMROSE OIL
A seed oil from the evening primrose plant which has a very high percentage of the polyunsaturated fatty acid, linoleic acid. Also rich in gamma linolenic acid. As a 'new' product, evening primrose oil has been claimed to have many benefits ranging from prevention of pre-menstrual tension (PMT) and hyperactivity, to curing skin disorders. In controlled tests, evening primrose oil has been shown to have no more benefit than a placebo for either PMT or hyperactivity.

EXERCISE
Exercise is a most important factor in weight control. When physical activity is curtailed, the appetite control mechanism does not seem to work properly. Exercise also burns up kilojoules of energy and increases the amount of lean muscle tissue. Since muscle uses up more energy, even when at rest, those who exercise regularly burn up more kilojoules.

It is often quoted that one must walk for several hours to burn up the equivalent number of kilojoules in a piece of chocolate cake, or some such food. This argument ignores the fact that exercise increases the body's metabolic rate for some hours after the walk (or whatever) finishes. It also ignores the benefits of having more lean muscle tissue in place of body fat.

During exercise, the muscles use glycogen and fat as their sources of fuel. Proteins are rarely used. Anaerobic exercise uses only glycogen; aerobic exercise uses a mix of the two. The most limiting factor in exercise is the amount of glycogen stored in muscles. This can be increased by substituting foods high in carbohydrate for those containing fats. The ideal carbohydrate foods include wholemeal bread, wholegrain cereals, rice, pasta, potatoes, other vegetables, legumes and fruit. These foods will also supply the extra vitamins required for carbohydrates to be used by the body.

The fuel for exercise can be either carbohydrate present in the blood, muscle glycogen or fats. With light exercise associated with everyday activities, the fuel used is about 75 per cent fatty acids and 25 per cent carbohydrate (from the blood sugar and the glycogen in muscles). As the exercise intensity increases, carbohydrates (from glycogen) supply a greater percentage of the fuel mixture. For moderate-intensity exercise (heavy work or most sports), fats and carbohydrate contribute almost equal amounts of energy. For the high-intensity activities (competitive sport), the major fuel used is carbohydrate.

See also Carbohydrates; Fats; Glycogen.

EXTRACTION RATE
When grains are ground into flour, the germ and the bran are usually separated from the endosperm of the grain. The extraction rate refers to the weight of flour produced from a given weight of grain — in other words, it

relates to the amount of the grain which ends up in the flour. The higher the extraction rate, the greater the percentage of the grain used and the higher the nutrient content. In Australia, most flour has an extraction rate of 76 per cent, giving even white flour a high nutritional value.

EXTRINSIC FACTOR

An old term for vitamin B_{12}.

EXTRUDED FOODS

Foods (usually grains or mixtures of broken grains) are subjected to increasing temperature and pressure so that their water content becomes very hot steam. The mixture is then forced through small holes. As the pressure drops, the steam evaporates, the material expands and the protein and starch form a gel-like solid substance. This procedure is used to produce some snack foods and breakfast cereals. The extrusion process causes loss of vitamins and some destruction of protein components.

FAECAL SOFTENERS

Substances which absorb water in the large intestine and help give bulk to the faeces. Examples include unprocessed bran, psyllium husk (see page 284), sterculia gum (see page 329) or the small seeds of the plantago species.

See also Laxatives.

FAECES

Waste material excreted from the bowel. With most Western diets, the daily faeces weigh about 80–160 g a day. With a vegetarian diet, this increases to 225 g a day. Some high-fibre African diets give rise to a daily faecal weight of 470 g. The faeces consist largely of bacteria (see dietary fibre, page 92), plus some undigested fibre (largely lignin), bile salts, dead body cells from the intestine and water.

FAGGOTS

A type of sausage made from a mixture of chopped liver, kidneys, sweetbreads and heart,

mixed with oatmeal and eggs, encased in fat and baked.

FAINTING

A nutritional basis for fainting may occur in certain types of anaemia, especially iron-deficiency anaemia. Fainting may also occur if blood volume drops, for example, during dehydration.

FALAFEL
see Felafel.

FAN YONG
see Tea.

FARM CHEESE
see Cheese.

FAST FOODS

The term 'fast foods' is not used simply to denote foods which are fast to prepare, serve and eat, or fresh fruit would be the ultimate fast food. Fast foods are generally cooked items which are available with minimal waiting time. In most cases, the foods need little chewing, have little dietary fibre and so are fast to eat.

Potato chips, hamburgers, pies, sausage rolls, fried chicken and pizza, are generally regarded as fast food. Most are very high in fat and it is the smell of the hot fat which is partially responsible for attracting customers to fast food outlets.

It is difficult to damn fast foods on the basis of any lack of protein, or even a lack of minerals and vitamins. Their nutritional problems lie in their high fat and kilojoule content, and their lack of dietary fibre, as well as vitamins A and C. In theory, it is quite possible to have a range of healthier fast foods than those usually offered.

The fat and kilojoule content of some fast foods are as follows:

FOOD	FAT (g)	(kJ)	CALORIES
Big Mac	31	2400	575
French fries — regular	13	855	205
— large	20	1375	330
Cheeseburger	16	1350	325
Apple pie	17	1120	265
Thickshake	12	1700	405
Standard hamburger	18	1630	390
Fried chicken snack box	34	2385	570
Chicken dinner box	51	3605	860
3 pieces of chicken	43	2515	600
coleslaw, $\frac{1}{3}$ medium tub	5	550	130
corn, each cob	3	960	230
pizza supreme, thin, $\frac{1}{2}$ regular	17	1815	435
pizza supreme, thick, $\frac{1}{2}$ regular	17	2035	485
barbecued chicken			
$\frac{1}{4}$ bird, breast	12	900	215
$\frac{1}{4}$ bird, thigh	18	1100	265
meat pie, each	24	1645	395
sausage roll, each	23	1565	375
fish in batter, 1 piece	23	1555	370
hot chips, av. serve	35	2540	605

FASTING

Fasting entails restricting food and liquids (other than water), usually voluntarily. Some people claim spiritual regeneration through fasting but most people who fast believe that it will clean out toxins from the body. Many also believe fasting is a good way to lose weight.

There is no evidence that fasting results in a loss of toxic substances from the body. Nor is fasting effective for permanent weight control.

The body does not distinguish between fasting and starving — the difference is only one of intent. As far as the body is concerned, a lack of food entering the digestive tract is a signal to reduce its rate of metabolism.

During fasting, the glycogen supplies in the muscles are initially used as fuel for physical activity. Since every gram of glycogen is stored with 3 g of water, the depletion of glycogen results in an apparent loss of weight. Most of this consists of glycogen and water.

To keep the blood sugar level normal during fasting, the body first draws on its glycogen stores in the liver (muscle glycogen can undergo only minimal conversion to blood glucose). The liver glycogen stores last a few hours, after which lean muscle tissue is broken down in the process of gluconeogenesis (see page 164). Thus even a short fast results in a loss of muscle while longer fasts cause extreme muscle wasting. This loss of lean tissue is unavoidable as fat cannot be turned into glucose to maintain blood sugar levels.

For weight reduction, fasting is not a good idea since it is inevitable that lean tissue will be lost in addition to fat. In the absence of carbohydrate, fats are also incompletely burned and ketones are produced (see page 197).

There are many devotees of fasting who believe that almost any illness will disappear more quickly if the subject fasts. The slowing down of metabolism during fasting makes this unlikely.

See also Balanced diet; Diets, slimming.

FAT CELLS

These are the cells which hold body fat. It is now known that fat cells can develop at any age when energy intake exceeds energy expenditure. The greatest proliferation occurs in infancy and at puberty. Fat cells can also disappear but only when weight is lost slowly. Fast weight loss merely empties the cells.

FATIGUE

Tiredness may result from a lack of iron, a lack of food, poor diet or various vitamin deficiencies. Most fatigue, however, is due to a lack of sleep or boredom. Those who are chronically tired, in spite of adequate sleep, should have their blood iron levels checked. Overweight people are also likely to experience greater fatigue from the effort of carrying their excess weight.

FATS
See following pages.

FAVA BEANS
see Legumes.

FAVISM

An anaemia caused by a toxin in broad beans (also known as fava beans) which destroys red blood cells in genetically susceptible people. It may result from eating raw broad beans (the toxin is killed by heat) or inhaling the pollen of the broad-bean plant.

FEIJAO BEAN
see Legumes, Aduki beans.

FEIJOA
see Fruit.

FEINGOLD DIET

Dr Benjamin Feingold gave his name to this diet which he used to treat hyperactive children. The diet excluded all foods with artificial colourings or flavourings, and also restricted certain fruits and vegetables with a high content of salicylates. Feingold only ever claimed that 50 per cent of his subjects improved with his diet. His critics maintained that the diagnosis of hyperactivity invalidated his theory. Those working with hyperactive children today have found that Feingold had only part of the answer in that some hyperactive children do have food sensitivities but that these may be due to a range of substances, including certain colourings as well as some chemicals occurring quite naturally in foods.

FELAFEL

Small Middle Eastern balls made from ground chickpeas, garlic, onion and spices. Usually served with flatbread and tahini (sesame paste).

FENELAR

Norwegian smoked mutton. The leg of mutton is dry-salted with salt, sodium nitrite and sugar and left for several days. After this the mutton is put into a sweetened brine solution and then smoked.

FENITROTHION

A pesticide used to control pests in crops such as wheat. Wheat bran may have high levels of fenitrothion as the pesticide residues lodge in the outside bran layers. If moderate quantities of bran are consumed (1–2 tablespoons a day), the intake of fenitrothion will be low. Those who abuse unprocessed bran by taking 1 cup or more several times a day may take in high levels of the pesticide residue.

FENNEL
see Herbs; Vegetables.

FENNEL SEEDS
see Spices.

FENUGREEK
see Spices.

FATS

More properly known as lipids, fats are organic substances which are insoluble in water. In most Western diets, fats contribute about 40 per cent of the kilojoules — a level which is now considered to be too high.

Fats come in both animal and vegetable foods. They help to make foods palatable, carry some fat soluble vitamins (A, D, E and K) and also contain some fatty acids which are essential for humans. However, the fat soluble vitamins and fatty acids are not found in obviously fatty foods, but occur in small quantities in foods such as fish, lean meat, eggs, oats, seeds, nuts, vegetables and fruits.

Fats in foods contribute more than twice as many kilojoules as either proteins or carbohydrates. This means that it is very easy to overdo kilojoule needs when eating fatty foods. It is also very easy to eat a lot of fatty foods without realising it since fats are so well hidden in many foods.

Excessive amounts of fats contribute to high levels of cholesterol and triglycerides in the blood. This, in turn, increases risks of coronary heart disease, high blood pressure, diabetes and gallstones. A high-fat diet is also a risk factor for cancer of the bowel and for hormone-dependent cancers of the breast and uterus in women, and the prostate gland in men.

Fat content of foods

FOOD	FAT (g)
Meats	
large T-bone steak, including fat	48
small steak, lean, 100 g	10
mince steak, 150 g	24
pork chop with crackling	54
pork loin chop with no visible fat	4
2 lamb loin chops, lean and fat	45
roast leg of lamb, no fat, av. serve	8
veal chops, 2	4
veal steak, crumbed and fried	40
2 sausages, grilled	40
bacon, 2 pieces,	30
meat pie or sausage roll	24
hamburger	30
chicken or turkey breast, av. serve, no fat	3
barbecued chicken, $\frac{1}{4}$	15
chicken — fast food dinner box	51
salami, 60 g	23
egg, 1	6

Seafood	
fish, with batter, av. piece	23
fish, grilled, av. fillet	2
— for butter sauce, add up to	30
oysters, 1 dozen natural	2
prawns, 4 king size, barbecued	2
prawns, 4 king size, battered	18
salmon, canned, 100 g	8
tuna, canned, 100 g	4
Dairy products	
milk, 250 mL	9
skim, 250 mL	0
cream, av. serve	12
cheese, amount on sandwich	8
cottage cheese, $\frac{1}{2}$ cup	4
icecream, rich, 2 scoops	16
— regular, av. serve	7
butter, each tablespoon	16
Fats	
oil, 1 tablespoon	20
mayonnaise, 1 tablespoon	18
margarine, 1 tablespoon	16

Fruits and vegetables

most fruits and vegetables	0
hot potato chips, av. serve	35
roast potato, av. piece	5
avocado, half	20
potato crisps, small packet	10

Breads

bread, 2 slices	1
croissant	14
savoury biscuits, 4	4

Sweets and snacks

apple pie, small piece without cream	18
cheesecake, av. serve	45
chocolate cake, av. piece	35
doughnut	13
sweet biscuits, 2 plain	5
peanuts, 25 g	12
muesli bar	6
chocolate, 100 g bar	31
Mars bar, 70 g size	14

Body fat

Excessive amounts of any type of fat in the diet are stored in the body in fat depots. Excess proteins and carbohydrates can also be converted to body fat. In theory, body fat is a store of energy for leaner times; in practice, in Western societies, the leaner times rarely arrive and excess body fat stores cause health problems. Some fat depots are needed, for example, around the kidneys, to cover and protect joints and as an energy store for lactation.

Saturated fat

Monounsaturated fat

Polyunsaturated fat

Normal body fat levels are higher in women than in men. Female hormones cause extra fat deposits on breasts, thighs, hips and buttocks. If a woman's fat levels fall suddenly, oestrogen levels drop and menstruation ceases. The level of body fat at which this occurs will depend on the individual, but if menstruation ceases, the body fat level is too low for that particular woman. When oestrogen levels fall, calcium retention in bones is also impaired.

Excess body fat is a much greater health risk when it accumulates on the upper body (the 'apple' distribution) than on the lower body (the 'pear' distribution).

Body fat will be used as a source of energy when fewer kilojoules are being ingested than are being used for the body's basic metabolism and physical activity. 1 kg of body fat represents a store of 32,340 kJ (7700 Cals).

The most effective way to lose excess body fat is to eat a little less and to use up more energy in physical activity. It is a mistake to cut food intake back too far since this only slows down the body's rate of metabolism.

Body fat does not accumulate overnight and it will not disappear that way either. Most slimming diets 'work' by removing water and glycogen, rather than by encouraging loss of fat. This type of diet is useless.

See also Diets, slimming.

Types of fats

Fats are described according to the chemical structure of their fatty acids as being saturated, monounsaturated or polyunsaturated. Most foods contain a mixture of each type. The fat in oats, for example, consists of 18 per cent saturated fatty acids, 39 per cent monounsaturated and 43 per cent polyunsaturated. All types of fat contribute the same 37 kJ (9 Cals) per gram and all have the same potential to increase body weight.

Saturated fatty acids

These fats occur in animal and vegetable foods, although the popular misconception is that

119

saturated fats = animal fats. Saturated fats certainly occur in fatty meats and some dairy products. They also occur in palm and coconut oils and chocolate, and find their way into biscuits, cakes, pastries, most fast foods, ready prepared meals, margarine and some types of confectionery.

Saturated fatty acids are a special risk factor for heart disease since they increase the undesirable LDL cholesterol (see page 73) and decrease the protective HDL cholesterol.

Monounsaturated fatty acids

These fats dominate the fatty acids present in olives and olive oil, avocados, peanuts and peanut oil. They also occur in eggs, chicken, some fish (salmon, mackerel, sardines, tuna), macadamias and hazelnuts.

For many years, monounsaturated fatty acids were largely ignored. They were thought to have a rather neutral effect on blood cholesterol levels. More recent research has shown that monounsaturated fatty acids are much more useful than was previously thought because they reduce the undesirable LDL cholesterol but actually raise the protective HDL variety. In addition, populations who have eaten a high proportion of these fats for thousands of years, have very low incidence of both heart disease and cancer. They are thus the fats of choice.

Polyunsaturated fatty acids

Large quantities of these fatty acids are found in vegetable oils and polyunsaturated margarines. Many nuts and seeds are also rich in polyunsaturates, although large quantities of these foods are less likely to be consumed. Most fish contain very little fat but most of what they do have is polyunsaturated.

For further explanation of the different types of polyunsaturated fats, see 'fatty acids' below. See also Cholesterol and Triglycerides.

Essential fatty acids

Fats consist of fatty acids and glycerol. Some of the fatty acids are essential to the body and must be supplied from the diet. These include linoleic acid, linolenic acid and, possibly, arachidonic acid (see also individual entries). They are a vital part of cell membranes, have some ability to control the different types of fats in the blood and are also involved in making prostaglandins, hormone-like substances which, in turn, control many of the body's processes (see page 281).

The fatty acids which are essential are all polyunsaturated. However, not all polyunsaturated fatty acids are essential. There are about 14 fatty acids which occur commonly in foods, and several others which are present only in minute quantities. Large quantities of any fatty acids are undesirable.

Trans fatty acids

These fatty acids are characterised chemically by having their hydrogen atoms on opposite sides of a double carbon bond. Those with their hydrogens on the same side are known as cis fatty acids.

Molecules of trans fatty acids are able to pack more closely together and act more like saturated than polyunsaturated fatty acids.

Some of the fats in meat, milk and cheese are trans fatty acids. More of these fats enter the diet, however, from the hydrogenation of vegetable oils in the manufacture of margarines. In countries such as the United Kingdom, where fish fats are hydrogenated to make edible cooking oils, more trans fatty acids come from these than from margarines made from vegetable sources.

There has been some concern that trans fatty acids may be involved in heart disease or may bring about a deficiency of essential fatty acids. Further research is required to clarify this issue in human nutrition.

See also Carbohydrates; Exercise; Glycogen.

FERMENTATION

A process carried out by micro-organisms and used in making products such as cheese, beer and breads. Asians ferment soya beans to produce soy sauce, tofu, tempeh, miso and various fermented bean products. The fermentation has an added advantage of producing vitamin B_{12} — which can otherwise be missing from totally vegetarian diets.

In the large intestine, fermentation of dietary fibre by bacteria occurs. During this process, the bacteria multiply by the million and their spent bodies then make up about three-quarters of the faecal matter excreted. Acids produced during the fermentation are also valuable as a source of energy and to regulate peristaltic movements of the bowel. They may also be valuable anti-cancer agents.

FERRITIN

A protein which carries iron from its stores to the red cells in the blood. A measure of the ferritin level in the blood gives a good indication of the stores of iron. Normal serum ferritin level is 2–70 mcg/100 mL. Low levels indicate that iron supplementation may be necessary.

FERTILISERS

Natural or manufactured chemical elements needed by plants for growth. Fertilisers are used to bolster poor soil and may include compost or specific nutrients known to be required by the plant. Nitrogen, phosphorus, potassium, magnesium, calcium and sulphur are often used, as are iron, copper, or various trace minerals.

The addition of fertilisers to soils does not change the nutrient content of the products grown in the soil to any great extent. Plants either receive the nutrients they need — and grow — or they fail to meet their nutritional requirements and do not grow and reproduce. The common idea that eating plants grown with fertilisers means that vitamin supplements will be required is not valid.

FETA
see Cheese.

FETTUCINE
see Pasta.

FIBRE
see Dietary fibre.

FIDDLEHEAD FERN
see Vegetables.

FIELD MUSHROOMS
see Vegetables, Mushrooms.

FIG
see Fruit.

FILBERTS
see Nuts, Hazelnuts.

FILO PASTRY
see Pastry.

FINGERNAILS

Fingernails consist of proteins, with sulphur-containing amino acids predominating. If you are very poorly nourished, your fingernails will be affected. But if your fingernails break or split easily, it does not necessarily indicate you are poorly nourished. It is more likely that your fingernails have been in contact with various chemicals which they do not like. These may include some detergents and soap powders, cleaning agents or even the lining of some gloves. Fingernail damage due to poor nutrition usually shows up as ridges across the nails (if they run the length of the nail, they have no significance) and spoon-shaped nails. These features accompany severe malnutrition due either to a lack of food or a wasting disease. White spots on the fingernails are popularly believed to represent a zinc deficiency. There is no scientific backing for this at present and most white spots are the result of banging the fingernails against some object.

FINNAN HADDIE
see Fish.

FIOCHETTI

Pasta shaped like small bows.

FISH
See following pages.

FISH FATS
see Omega 3 fatty acids.

FISH ROE
see Caviar.

FIT FOR LIFE

A popular diet program which maintains that the body works in cycles: from 4 am to noon is the 'elimination cycle'; from noon to 8 pm is the 'appropriation cycle'; from 8 pm to 4 am is the 'assimilation cycle'.

During the elimination cycle, only fruits are to be eaten. This is supposed to help the body rid itself of wastes and food debris. The appropriation cycle is a time when foods can be eaten although proteins and carbohydrates are not supposed to be eaten together. The assimilation cycle is a time for abstinence from food so that the body can absorb and use food.

Although very popular, the Fit for Life Diet is not recommended by qualified nutritionists and dietitians as it has no basis in fact. It sounds plausible but bears little relationship to the facts of digestion. The claim that the secret of weight loss lies in removing 'toxic wastes and excesses' from the body is not correct.

The outcome of the diet will depend on the exact foods consumed, but the program is unlikely to produce a well-balanced diet. Since dairy products are forbidden, calcium intake is low. Sesame seeds are recommended as a source

of calcium, but the lack of absorption of the mineral from the seeds (due to the presence of oxalic acid) is ignored. Other minerals, such as iron and zinc, are also likely to be below recommended levels.

FIVE CORNER FRUIT
see Fruit, Carambola.

FLAGEOLETS
see Legumes.

FLAKY PASTRY
see Pastry.

FLATHEAD
see Fish.

FLATULENCE

Gases in the intestine which arise largely from the fermentation of undigested food and fibre in the colon.

Oxygen and nitrogen are both swallowed in inspired air but are absorbed from the stomach and small intestine. Carbon dioxide is produced during the digestion of foods and also in the large intestine. Hydrogen is also produced within the colon as bacteria ferment certain sugars. Some of this hydrogen is expired from the lungs.

Most of the gases in the intestine are odourless and consist of hydrogen, carbon dioxide, methane and nitrogen. Faecal odour is due to compounds such as skatole, indole, hydrogen sulphide and methyl sulphides.

The more dietary fibre consumed, the more gas produced. It is only in recent years, and in some societies, that this is considered socially unacceptable. It is a major reason why some people are unwilling to consume sufficient dietary fibre to overcome problems such as constipation.

Beans (legumes) and vegetables from the cruciferous family (cabbage, cauliflower, broccoli and Brussels sprouts), are potent sources of intestinal gas. Leaving the husks on legumes has been found to result in less flatus since the husk may bind minerals such as iron or manganese which are required for the formation of flatus.

Sorbitol, a sugar substitute, may cause problems for the half of the population who are intolerant to it (see page 321). It is found in some carbohydrate-modified products and also in some medicinal syrups, including multivitamins and cough mixtures.

FISH

Fish come in many sizes from some tiny fish which are eaten bones and all (such as whitebait) to enormous creatures weighing many kilograms.

Their flesh varies, but all fish have a common feature in being very low in saturated fats. Some, such as trout, salmon or tuna have higher levels of omega 3 fatty acids (see page 254), making them very useful foods.

All fish are rich in protein and several of the B vitamins, especially niacin. They also contain valuable minerals. For those concerned about body fat levels, fish (appropriately prepared) is low in kilojoules and is ideally suited to those needing to lose weight.

Some fish are called by different names in various countries. The fish in some regions are also quite different from those in others. This section can only touch on the types of fish which you may come across.

Albacore
A large fish with fine eating flesh. Blue-finned tuna is sometimes called albacore.

Anchovy
A small fish related to the herring. Often eaten salted or canned, anchovies contribute calcium from their bones but also a high salt content. This is not significant if very small quantities are eaten only occasionally. Anchovies are usually eaten whole and their bones provide some calcium. 100 g of anchovies have 235 kJ (35 Cals).

Argentine
A variety of silver-coloured fish found in the North Atlantic and the Mediterranean. Often confused with smelts, although the two species are different.

Bacalao
A type of cod which is salted and dried. Before cooking bacalao, soak it overnight in water.

Barracuda
see Pike.

Barramundi
A large fish which inhabits waters of northern and western Australia. The barramundi has a dark bluish-grey surface colour and pink eyes which glow at night. Its firm white flesh is eagerly sought as a table fish. Excellent when grilled, barbecued or poached. Like most fish, it is high in nutritional value and low in fat and kilojoules.

Blackfish
An estuarine fish caught in Eastern Australia. Blackfish live in shallow weedy flat areas and feed largely on weed. They are more often caught for sport than for eating. Their reputation as a poor table fish stems from their strong flavour if they are not bled soon after being caught. Many people enjoy their moist white flesh. Like most fish, blackfish have a low fat and kilojoule content.

Bloater

Rather fatty fish eaten in the United Kingdom. The fish are left whole in salt for about 12 hours, washed, threaded onto metal skewers and smoked. They are a good source of protein, iron, vitamin D and most of the B complex vitamins. 100 g of grilled bloater have 1045 kJ (250 Cals).

Blue eye

see Fish, Trevalla.

Blue grenadier

A long silver fish without scales caught off the southern coast of New South Wales. Its moist soft flesh, few bones and mild flavour make it a good fish to use in fish pâtés or baked in a fish casserole. A low-fat fish with plenty of protein and nutrients. Low in kilojoules.

Boarfish

A fish which tastes better than it looks. It has large eyes and a long snout. The adult male fish has yellow spots on its reddish-brown skin. A good meaty fish, usually sold in fillets.

Bombay duck

Not a duck! The bummaloe fish is about the size of a herring and is caught in large numbers near Bombay and salted and dried. Its distinctive smell belies its delicious flavour. It is generally baked until crisp and then crumbled over curry.

Bonito

Tuna fish caught in the Atlantic and Pacific Oceans and in the Mediterranean. Bonito is usually sold cut into steaks or cutlets. It is also used for sashimi.

Bream

A fish which has long been considered one of the finest table fish. Found mainly in rivers, estuaries and around the coast. Those caught in rivers tend to be darker in colour than those caught close to the coast. Sold as either fillets or whole fish, they can be grilled, barbecued, fried or cooked in the microwave. Very low in fat (usually 1–2 per cent) and low in kilojoules, but high in protein and other important nutrients.

Carp

Carp are caught and welcomed as a table fish in Europe but the fish known as 'European carp' in Australia is bony with a strong muddy flavour. Introduced in 1876 to Australian rivers, these carp have wiped out many indigenous fish and are considered a pest. Goldfish (kept as pets) are a variety of carp.

Catfish

Fresh or saltwater catfish are edible. They are commonly sold as fillets and eaten in Europe and parts of the United States.

Chinook salmon

see Salmon.

Cod

There are a number of fish in the cod family, most having a soft white flesh which is due to their habit of resting on the ocean floor rather than being very active (active muscle tends to be darker in colour). Generally considered to be good eating with moist, large flakes.

The hapuka cod (also known as the New Zealand groper) is a large fish and 50–90 kg specimens are often caught. The Queensland groper is the largest cod in Australia and may reach a weight of 300 kg. Those up to a weight of 30 kg are considered palatable.

Pacific, Greenland and polar cod are consumed in the northern hemisphere.

Cod flesh is high in protein and contributes small quantities of many of the B complex vitamins. Fat content is low (usually less than 1 per cent). A 150 g fillet of fish has 460 kJ (110 Cals).

Coral trout

Also known as leopard cod, this pink-red fish is found off the coast of Queensland, Northern Territory and Western Australia. It is an excellent table fish with firm, white, sweet flesh. It is ideally suited to grilling, microwaving or wrapping in foil and barbecuing.

Dhu fish

A fish found only off the coast of Western Australia and considered one of the best eating fish in the world. Very similar to the pearl perch caught off the eastern coast of Australia. Its flesh is moist and has a delicate flavour which needs only simple cooking such as grilling, baking in foil or pan-frying.

Dorado

A large golden-coloured fish of the northern hemisphere. A good table fish, usually sold as fillets or steaks which can be grilled, pan-fried or baked.

Eel

A long fish with fins which extend around the end of the tail. Those which live in saltwater have no scales and are long and slender. Freshwater eels do have scales and are predators. They are born in the sea and go down to the sea to breed. The young then swim upstream until they too are ready to spawn and return to the sea. After breeding, they die.

Freshwater eels range from 1−1.8 m in length and are considered good eating. Smoked eel is regarded as a delicacy.

A number of different varieties of eel are eaten throughout the world. Their flesh is popular, partly because it has no bones. The conger eel is caught off the coast of Europe, Africa and in the Mediterranean. It can be stuffed and baked, smoked or used in seafood casseroles. To smoke eels, they are gutted, headed and left in brine. After this process, they are dry-salted, washed, dipped in boiling water and hung up to smoke. The flesh becomes tender and is served in thin slices.

Nutritionally, the fat content of eel flesh varies from almost none in the young elvers to more than 20 per cent. An 'average' eel has 11 g of fat per 100 g. They are an excellent source of vitamin A and a good source of protein and niacin. They also supply iron and calcium and a selection of vitamins. 100 g of young eel have 320 kJ (76 Cals) while the mature eels have 710 kJ (170 Cals) per 100 g.

File fish

see Leatherjacket.

Finnan haddie

To prepare this Scottish dish, haddock are gutted, split down the backbone and placed in a brine solution. After the salting period, they are threaded onto metal spears and smoked. No dyes are added. Finnan haddie are then steamed or boiled briefly before eating.

Flathead

Over 30 species of flathead occur in Australian waters. They range in length from 30−60 cm, have a firm, dry texture, and make good table fish, either whole or as fillets.

Flounder

A flat fish which often buries itself in sand leaving only its eyes visible. When young, flounder are not flat but have a regular symmetrical shape with an eye on each side of the head. When they are only about 1 cm long, one eye begins to move towards the top of the head and then crosses to lie alongside the other eye. At the same time, the pigment on the fish changes so that the side which has 'lost' the eye becomes white. The side surface which contains the eyes then becomes the 'top' of the fish. In effect, flounder actually swim on their sides, similar to plaice.

In spite of all this body changing, flounder make an excellent table fish with sweet firm flesh. They can be grilled or pan-fried. Flounder, like most white table fish have very little fat (about 2 per cent) and just 375 kJ (90 Cals) per 100 g.

Garfish

The extremely long lower jaw of this fish is usually tipped with bright orange or red.

Garfish live in relatively warm sea water and are herbivores. They swim in shoals close to the surface and are usually caught by netting. They are not very fleshy fish (they grow only to about 45 cm in length and are very thin) but are sweet and highly prized for the table. They are cooked whole, usually pan-fried or baked, allowing 2−4 per serve.

Gemfish

A deep-sea fish caught off the south-eastern coast of Australia during the winter months. These fish were once called 'hake' but are quite different from the true hake. The fish are large and are good eating. With their large flakes, they are also popular as smoked fish. Suitable for grilling, microwaving, pan-frying, baking or wrapping in foil and barbecuing.

Goldfish

see Carp.

Grayling

A silver-coloured fish of the northern hemisphere with a scent a little like the herb thyme. An excellent table fish.

Grouper

A common Mediterranean fish, found especially off the North African coast. Large-mouthed heavy-bodied fish which tend to spend most of their lives in one area. Large groupers can grow as large as 225 kg. Normally sold as steaks which can be wrapped in foil and grilled or baked, or pan-fried. The flesh tends to be a little dry if simply grilled. In Australia, the Queensland groper, a member of the cod family, is similar to the grouper. When young it is an excellent eating fish but becomes rather bland when it reaches very large sizes.

Gurnard

A spiny fish with red 'plates'. From the Sea Robin family. Caught in the northern hemisphere, especially in Mediterranean areas. Some small gurnard are occasionally caught in Australian waters. Can be wrapped in foil and baked. Tend to dry out if grilled.

Haddock

A member of the cod family, haddock is one of the most important commercial fish from the North Atlantic. The fish are bottom-dwellers and feed on smaller sea creatures. They have three dorsal and two anal fins and can be identified by a dark spot on each shoulder and a dark line running along their sides. They grow to about 10 or 11 kg and their firm flake makes them a useful fish to eat fresh or smoked.

Haddock are extremely low in fat, having less than 1 per cent. They are a good source of protein and niacin and provide small quantities of other vitamins and minerals. A 150 g piece of haddock has 460 kJ (110 Cals). Smoked haddock is high in salt.

Hake

A large fish of the cod family, although they are sometimes not classed as such because of skeletal differences. They have large sharp teeth to suit their carnivorous lifestyle, a long, notched dorsal fin (plus a smaller forward dorsal fin) and a long notched anal fin. They are widespread in the Atlantic ocean and are also caught in the eastern Pacific, especially near New Zealand. Their flesh freezes well and is widely used in processed fish products. Hake can be baked, wrapped in foil or steamed. They do not have enough moistness and flavour to be grilled.

Halibut

The largest of the flatfish with both eyes on one side of the body. They are caught in the North Atlantic. The Pacific halibut is a smaller fish. Like most white table fish, the halibut has a low fat content (2 per cent) and is a good source of protein and niacin. A 150 g fillet of halibut has 580 kJ (140 Cals). Can be grilled, pan-fried, microwaved or baked.

Herring

One of the most abundant types of fish in the North Atlantic, herrings are eaten fresh, canned, pickled and smoked. Herrings are high in protein and have a wide range of vitamins, including the fat-soluble vitamins A, D and E. They have varying fat levels depending on the time of year and the amount of plankton available in the water in which they live. Fat levels range from 5 g per 100 g in late winter, to 20 g per 100 g in summer. Within their fat, herrings also have a high percentage of the valuable omega 3 fatty acids. 100 g of herring have 840−990 kJ (200−235 Cals).

Jewfish

In Australia, the jewfish is also known as mulloway and is regarded as one of the finest eating fish. It is a silvery colour and has pale pink flesh, large flakes and firm texture. It is sometimes confused with teraglin, but the latter has a yellow mouth and concave tail (the jewfish's tail is convex).

The Australian jewfish is found on deep offshore reefs but also near coastal beaches and in the mouths of estuaries. It grows to a very large size and is sold as cutlets or fillets. This fish needs to be cooked by pan-frying or wrapping in foil as the flesh can be dry if grilled. The use of marinades during grilling can overcome the problem.

In the United States, the name jewfish is given to a member of the groper family. This jewfish is also very large (up to 320 kg), and is a dull olive brown with faint spots and bands. The adult fish are solitary and stay in the one area for long periods.

To add to the confusion over jewfish, the giant sea bass is sometimes called a jewfish. It grows to a size in excess of 200 kg.

John Dory

The distinguishing dark blotches on the side of this fish are supposed to represent the imprint of St Peter's thumb, left when he took some money from the fish's mouth in the Sea of Galilee. Unfortunately for the story, John Dory does not live in that area. The fish grow to a length of about 40 cm and are regarded as one of the finest of all table fish. They are caught along the coast of Europe, Africa and Australia. Fillets are usually free of bones.

Kingfish

A popular fish with gamefish anglers because of their fighting abilities. In spite of their high level of activity, kingfish are a good table fish and their flesh is particularly suitable for sashimi. Best if pan-fried, cooked in foil, microwaved or grilled with a marinade as the flesh can become dry with straight grilling.

Kippers

Kippers are prepared from top quality herrings which are split, gutted and soaked in a brine solution containing a yellow dye. The fish are then hung on sticks for an hour before being smoked. They are commonly eaten in Scotland and can be fried, baked or grilled. Some of their salt can be reduced by soaking briefly in water before cooking. Like herrings, kippers are high in protein and niacin, and provide some of the fat-soluble vitamins A, D and E, as well as small quantities of other vitamins and minerals. 100 g of baked kippers (weighed with bones) have 460 kJ (110 Cals) and 6 g of fat, mostly polyunsaturated and including the omega 3 fatty acids (see page 254).

Leatherjacket

Also known as file fishes, these rather ugly-looking fish have a tough skin (hence the name), a strong dominant dorsal spine and a rather knobbly-looking head. Their flesh is mild and quite good eating although some of the tropical leatherjackets have a bitter taste. The skin is removed before cooking.

Ling

A member of the cod family, also known as a sea turbot, the ling is a large fish which looks a little like an eel. Both deep and shallow water varieties are found. They are a good table fish, having almost no bones and a firm, white, moist flesh with a rather large flake. They are mostly sold as fillets and can be grilled, pan-fried or microwaved.

Mackerel

The true mackerel are caught in the Atlantic and Mediterranean. A related species, Spanish mackerel, are common around the northern part of the Australian continent. They are mainly found off shore and rarely enter estuaries. In spawning season they leap out of the water, presenting a spectacular display. There is no known explanation for this activity, but it has been observed that the mackerel leave the area soon after. They are good eating fish and are usually sold as cutlets which can be grilled, wrapped in foil and baked, or cooked in wine.

Matjes herrings

Young herrings caught in the spring before they have accumulated too much fat. They are lightly salted and kept for a few days before eating.

Mirror Dory

This fish has a deep body, a large mouth, and a silver scale-free skin. It looks like John Dory but does not have the characteristic dark marks. Fillets do have bones but also a good flavour. Can be grilled, pan-fried, microwaved or wrapped in foil for baking or barbecuing.

Moon fish

Also known as opah or sunfish, this large, plump oval-bodied fish has beautiful pink colourings. It is excellent for sashimi and is highly prized in Japan. Available worldwide, it can be grilled, microwaved, pan-fried or foil-wrapped and barbecued.

Morwong

These fish make up a large part of the commercial catch in Australia. They are usually sold under the name sea bream, but in Tasmania, they are often called perch. They can be cooked in any way and are good for baking, stuffing or rolling around a filling, as the flesh does not break up too easily.

Mullet

The ancient Romans considered mullet a delicacy and paid large prices for these medium sized fish which are caught in freshwater in many countries. Usually caught by netting, sea mullet are caught in estuaries around the Australian coast. Their flesh is excellent when fresh. Sold as whole fish or fillets, mullet has a slightly earthy smell — something they pick up from swimming in mud.

Mullet have a slightly higher oil content than many other fish, and can be baked, grilled, pan-fried, microwaved or barbecued. They are excellent when smoked. Nutritionally, mullet are a good source of the omega 3 fish fats (see page 254).

Mulloway

see Jewfish.

New Zealand groper

see Cod.

Opah

see Moon fish.

Pedah

A partly dried red-coloured fish eaten in Thailand.

Perch

Sea perch come in many shapes, colours and sizes. The red emperor (known as snapper in the United States), is a bottom-dwelling pink-red coloured fish which is particularly abundant along the Great Barrier Reef. The striped sea perch is another bright pink fish with bright yellow fins. Most of the sea perch have firm white flesh and are considered to be good table fish.

There are a number of freshwater perch, also known as bass. They are not fished commercially but make very good eating. The Australian Murray cod is also a perch and grows to about 45 kg. It is considered a fine eating fish with a mild flavour.

Pike

Also called barracuda or sennit, pike are small silvery-green fish with a pointed head and large teeth. They are caught around the Australian coast and are sold whole. Prepare them by grilling, microwaving, pan-frying or baking.

Freshwater pike are caught in Europe. They are traditionally stuffed and baked.

Pilchard

Often sold as sardines, the term 'sardine' is used for a young pilchard. Used fresh, smoked or canned. They are an excellent source of niacin, a good source of iron and contain small quantities of many other vitamins and minerals. 100 g of canned pilchards have 525 kJ (125 Cals) and 5 g of fat.

Plaice

A flat fish, rather like flounder, caught in the North Sea. A good eating fish, available all year round and sold as fillets or whole fish. Cook by grilling, microwaving, wrapping in foil or baking. Similar nutritional content to flounder with 2 per cent fat. A 150 g fillet has 565 kJ (135 Cals).

Pollack

A fish caught all year round in the northern hemisphere. Its flesh is firm and white but generally considered to be slightly inferior to hake or cod. Best used in fish soups, casseroles or steamed.

Rollmops

Herring fillets which are rolled (sometimes around pickled vegetables), secured with wooden skewers and left in a spiced brine for several days, or months. They are not cooked and are popular in Scandinavian countries. Raw herring contains a factor which destroys thiamin. Eating an occasional rollmop will do no harm but a constant diet of raw herrings can lead to a thiamin deficiency.

Salmon

These magnificent fish live in the cold waters of North America and northern Europe. They generally mature in the sea, returning to coastal rivers to spawn. Their flesh ranges from pink to deep red and they are considered one of the finest flavoured fish. Some of the major varieties include the humpback (or pink salmon), chum, chinook, coho and sockeye (often considered the finest). Salmon is available fresh in many parts of the northern hemisphere. It can be poached, wrapped in foil and baked or grilled, and is served hot and cold. Salmon is a good source of omega 3 fatty acids, and also protein, niacin and other B complex vitamins. A 130 g poached salmon steak has 880 kJ (210 Cals). It is also available canned or smoked. 100 g of canned salmon have 545 kJ (130 Cals). If the bones of canned salmon are eaten, it is also a good source of calcium.

To smoke salmon, the fish are headed and gutted and either dry-salted or left in a mixture of saltpetre (sodium nitrite) with some brown sugar and rum. They are then washed in cold water, left to dry and smoked. Smoked salmon is high in salt but low in fat. A 50 g serve has 295 kJ (70 Cals).

Salmon trout

In between salmon and trout in size, these fish return from the sea to spawn in the rivers. The flesh is pale pink, delicately flavoured and delicious poached and served cold. The ocean trout being farmed off the coast of Tasmania have a particularly good tasting moist flesh. They are raised in freshwater and gradually acclimatised to salt. They are then placed in large netted pens in the ocean and fed to produce rapid growth and tender flesh. These fish are highly nutritious and have a fat content which sometimes reaches 20 per cent. They are a good source of omega 3 fatty acids (see page 254).

Sardine

A small Mediterranean fish of the same family as pilchards and anchovies. It migrates to cooler waters in the summer and is caught in large numbers off the coast of France and Portugal. To eat fresh, bend the head back and gently pull it away with the backbone. Either stuff the small fish, coat with flour and pan-fry or grill with a bit of olive oil. In canned sardines, the bones soften and can be eaten, providing a rich source of calcium. 100 g of sardines canned in oil have 900 kJ (215 Cals). They are high in protein, iron, zinc, calcium (100 g have about 70 per cent of the daily requirements), vitamin D, niacin and omega 3 fatty acids. A nutritious little package indeed!

Sea bream

see Morwong.

Sea turbot

see Ling.

Sennit

see Pike.

Shark

Although sharks evoke emotional reactions, their flesh is quite good eating. Since they have no bones (cartilage replaces bone in their skeleton), they are ideal for children and others who have trouble detecting fish bones. The flesh is firm and does not break up if cooked in a casserole, soup or stew. They can also be baked or microwaved. Often sold as boneless fillets.

Silver warehou

Once known as the snotty-nosed trevally, the silver warehou has assumed a sleek new name to match its beautiful silver skin. Its flesh is almost a pinkish colour, mild flavoured and there are few bones. Generally sold as fillets.

Skate

The wings or flaps and the outer body of the skate (related to rays and sharks) are sold. To prepare: place the skate flaps in boiling water and simmer for 2−3 minutes. Peel away the skin and the flesh can be pan-fried.

Snapper

This fish was named by Captain Cook and is caught all year round off the coast of Australia. The fish is distinguished by a bump on the top of its head. Young snapper are called cockney bream; slightly older ones are red bream; the next age group are known as squire, and finally the large fish are snapper. One of the finest table fish and suitable for pan-frying, grilling, microwaving or baking.

Sole

A flat fish, lemon sole is available in Australia. In Europe the varieties include lemon sole (available in winter) and Dover sole (sold all year round). A good eating fish, very similar to flounder. Sold as whole fish or fillets and delicious grilled, baked, pan-fried, microwaved or wrapped in foil and baked.

Sprat

An oily fish related to the herring, caught in cold northern European waters. Available fresh or smoked and can be barbecued, grilled, or baked. During winter, sprats are plump and at their best for eating. Smoked sprats are a popular European delicacy. They are a good source of iron, protein and vitamins.

Sunfish

see Moonfish.

Swordfish

These deep-water fish are caught using long line fishing. They are popular for game fishing. Their flesh is good eating and is usually sold as steaks or cutlets. They are also popular for sashimi. Swordfish tend to dry easily if grilled so baking, fast grilling, pan-frying, microwaving or wrapping in foil and baking, are the best methods of cooking.

Teraglin

This fish comes from the same family as the jewfish but is much smaller in size, has finer scales, a yellow mouth and a concave tail. Its flesh is pale pink and soft. It is sold in fillets or cutlets and can be baked, wrapped in foil and baked, pan-fried or microwaved. It may be dry if grilled.

Trevalla

Also known as blue eye or big eye, the deep sea trevalla is caught by long line fishing. Its moist flesh with large flakes makes it very good eating. It is usually sold in steaks or cutlets and can be grilled, pan-fried, microwaved or baked.

Trevally

These fish belong to the same family as the yellowtail kingfish and jack mackerel. They are a deep-bodied fish, usually a greenish colour on the top and silver underneath. They swim in schools fairly close to the surface. Fillets or whole fish can be baked, barbecued (wrapped in foil), pan-fried or grilled.

Trout

Brown, rainbow, lake or brook trout live in cold water streams, lakes and dams. Their soft, pinkish flesh is delicious. Smoked trout are also a delicacy. It is usual to cook trout whole (preferably by the side of the stream where you have caught them!). They can be pan-fried, grilled, or stuffed and baked. Their fat content varies according to the species and the time of the year. They are one of the fattier fish and have a high content of omega 3 fatty acids. A 500 g trout has an average of 1870 kJ (445 Cals).

Tuna

Large ocean fishes, among the fastest moving fish and a favourite for game fishing. Common species include southern bluefin (the largest tuna caught in Australian waters and having a superb flavour), yellowfin, albacore (white fleshed fish) and northern bluefin (different from the northern hemisphere variety of the same name). Until recently, most tuna was canned, but it has now become a popular table fish. It also makes superb sashimi. When cooking tuna, great care must be taken not to

dry out its flesh. Try pan-frying (don't overcook), wrap tuna fillets in foil and bake, or simply serve it raw.

Turbot

A flat fish caught on the Atlantic coast of Europe, the Mediterranean and the Black Sea. It is excellent when poached and can also be pan-fried.

Wahoo

A large slim game fish found throughout the world but especially in the tropics. The wahoo is a member of the tuna family, has a crescent-shaped tail and is a grey-blue colour with vertical bar markings. It may grow to 55 kg.

Whitebait

These tiny silver herrings or sprats are eaten when they are only 4—5 cm long. They are usually fried in a light batter and eaten whole, including the head. This makes them an excellent source of calcium and if you ate 100 g of whitebait, you would satisfy your entire daily needs for calcium. Since they are usually expensive, a more typical 50 g serve is still valuable and also supplies iron, protein and vitamins. In themselves, whitebait are not high in kilojoules, but since they are almost always served fried, a 50 g serve picks up sufficient oil to have 1115 kJ (265 Cals).

Whiting

Australian whiting are sweet-fleshed fish caught in sandy waters of bays and estuaries. They have very delicate flesh (and fine bones) and many people consider them the finest table fish available. The King George whiting from South Australia and Tasmania is the largest and may weigh 500 g—4 kg.

In Europe, whiting is found off the coasts from the Baltic to the Mediterranean. In the United States, a silver hake is sometimes called a whiting.

Whiting is like most white table fish and is very low in fat (less than 1 per cent). A 150 g fillet has 585 kJ (140 Cals).

FLAVOUR

The flavours of foods come through the senses of taste, smell and touch, and depend on the presence of nerve endings in the mouth and nose. In the mouth, most flavours are detected through the taste buds. The nasal olfactory nerve endings are stimulated by sniffing the food or by swallowing it. Some food flavours are apparent in the raw food; others depend on cooking or certain food combinations to achieve their distinction.

Apart from an inborn liking for sugar and a dislike for bitterness, the human palate is taught which flavours it likes or should reject.

FLAVOURINGS

Flavours are made up of a complex mixture of chemical substances. Flavour chemists study the key elements that provide particular flavours so that they can reproduce them artificially. At other times, flavourings are extracted totally from a particular food.

See also Artificial flavourings.

FLAXSEED
see Linseed.

FLOUNDER
see Fish.

FLOUR

Finely ground product of various grains, seeds or roots. Wheat flour is the most commonly used type in Western countries and produces the best breads and cakes. White flour has the bran and germ removed; wholemeal flour is made by grinding the whole of the wheat grain.

In the milling of wheat, the grain is broken open and the germ and bran layers removed. Through several stages of rolling and sifting, the endosperm is separated and ground to form flour. The final flour product is about 75 per cent of the original grain. It contains 90–95 per cent of the grain's original protein, 50 per cent of the thiamin (vitamin B_1) and around 50 per cent of most of the minerals. White flour products are then bleached to remove any traces of yellow pigments. This is purely a cosmetic process.

Self-raising flour contains bicarbonate of soda (see page 36) and an acid phosphate.

Cake flour is milled from wheats with a lower gluten (protein) content. It has a small particle size to produce fine, tender cakes.

Bread flour has a larger particle size and a high content of gluten (one of the wheat proteins). The gluten is insoluble but can absorb a lot of water to form a strong protein matrix which contributes to the volume and structure of the loaf.

FLOWERS, EDIBLE

Since many flowers are poisonous, it is important to be sure of correct identification before eating flowers. Those which are safe to eat can be used in salads, drinks, breads, rice or as a garnish.

Edible flowers include the flowers of the following:

apple	honeysuckle
borage	jasmine
carnation	lavender
chrysanthemum	lemon
daisy	lilac
dandelion	marigold
day lily	nasturtium
elderberry	pansy
geranium	rose
gladiolus	tulip
hibiscus	violet
hollyhock	

The most commonly eaten flower is probably the nasturtium. It is added to butter or used in salads.

FLUID

About 60 per cent of the body consists of water with about two-thirds of it inside the cells and the rest outside the cells. This fluid balance is maintained by hormonal control of the levels of sodium and potassium.

Fluid comes into the body from food and drinks. It leaves via sweat (visible and invisible), from the lungs (in expired air), the kidneys (via the urine) and the bowel (via the faeces). Fluid levels are regulated by the kidneys, the brain, the heart, various glands and some hormones. Dehydration occurs when the fluid levels in the body fall.

FLUID RETENTION

More properly known as oedema, fluid retention occurs for many reasons. Kidney disease is a common cause. Heart failure and liver diseases may also cause it. Low blood volume (for example, after sweating, vomiting or diarrhoea) will also cause fluid to be retained in the tissues. Once the blood volume drops, fluid will flow out of the blood vessels into the surrounding tissues. A further series of changes cause even more water to flow into the tissues.

Temporary fluid retention occurs if salty foods are eaten. Hormonal changes just before menstruation can also cause a temporary retention of extra fluid in the body. This retention is caused by an increased retention of sodium. The way to get rid of this fluid retention is to drink more water. This may sound paradoxical, but the extra water will flush out the retained sodium which in turn is retaining the water.

Diuretics work to reduce fluid by causing greater excretion of the sodium which is the basic cause of the problem. Unfortunately, diuretics also cause losses of other important minerals (see page 96).

FLUORESCENT LIGHT

These lights can destroy some vitamins in foods if the foods are in a glass container. For example, the riboflavin in bottled milk is destroyed if it is kept in a refrigerated cabinet with flourescent lighting. Cardboard packaging avoids this.

FLUORIDE

Whether fluoride is needed by humans is hotly debated. There is no doubt that small additional quantities strengthen tooth enamel and have played an important role in reducing dental caries. Fluoride may also help slow the bone loss which occurs in osteoporosis.

Too much fluoride is toxic, initially showing up as mottling of the teeth where water levels are greater than 3−5 parts per million (ppm). If the water level rises to 10 ppm, there is a loss of appetite and the bones of the spine and pelvis can become too dense.

See also Teeth.

FOETAL ALCOHOL SYNDROME

A set of symptoms apparent in babies born to mothers who consumed excessive alcohol during their pregnancy. Babies with this condition have growth retardation before and after they are born, mental deficiency, structural abnormalities of the face, head, joints and heart, and delayed development of co-ordination. Researchers have pinpointed these defects on alcohol consumption by the mother and have found that even good nutrition cannot undo the effects of alcohol in pregnancy. Most of the initial research focused on the babies of mothers who were heavy drinkers. More recent research suggests that even as little as two drinks a day may increase the risk of damage to the baby. Until a safe intake of alcohol during pregnancy can be established, it is wise for pregnant women to avoid alcohol throughout pregnancy.

See also Pregnancy.

FOIE GRAS

A rich pâté made from the livers of geese who are fed large quantities of fat. The top rating foie gras comes from Alsace-Lorraine and the

Perigord region of France. Pâté de foie gras is a paste containing goose livers, veal and truffles.

FOLACIN
see Vitamins.

FOLIC ACID
see Vitamins, Folacin.

FONDUE

A Swiss cheese dish made by melting cheese in white wine. The mixture is placed into an earthenware chafing dish and cubes of bread are placed on a long fork and dipped into the fondue pot. Traditionally, anyone who drops their bread into the fondue must kiss everyone present.

Fondue is also made with beef. For this dish, oil is heated in a metal chafing dish and small pieces of fillet steak are placed on the end of long forks and held in the oil until cooked. A variety of sauces are used to flavour the cooked meat morsels.

FOOD ACIDS
see Additives, food.

FOOD ADDITIVES
see Additives, food.

FOOD ALLERGIES
see Allergies.

FOOD GROUPS

A method of arranging foods into categories according to the nutritional contribution they make. Many Western countries have 4 major food groups:
- Breads, grains and cereals
- Fruits and vegetables
- Protein foods such as meat, fish, poultry, eggs, legumes, nuts
- Dairy products such as milk, cheese or yoghurt

Some, such as Australia, add a fifth group for fats and oils. Others split the fruits and vegetables into separate groups.

See also Balanced diet.

FOOD LABELS
see Labels, food.

FOOD POISONING

Illness resulting from eating food which is contaminated by bacteria or their toxins, natural toxicants in foods, mycotoxins produced by fungi, excessive levels of pesticides or additives. Some nutrients which are essential may also be toxic if taken in very large doses.

Symptoms of food poisoning include vomiting, diarrhoea, stomach cramps, fever, physiological shock, and in extreme cases, death.

All substances in, or added to foods, are potentially toxic. In fact, there are no safe substances, only safe quantities.

The major causes of food poisoning are outlined below:

Natural toxins

Some early Arctic explorers died because they ate polar bear liver. The extremely high levels of natural vitamin A in this food were quite toxic. Other naturally occurring toxins are found in plants, fungi or seafoods (usually from contaminated waters).
- *Oxalic acid* (found in rhubarb leaves, spinach, celery tops and tea) would kill you if you consumed enough of it. A kilogram of rhubarb leaves is deadly. In smaller doses, oxalic acid forms chemical complexes with minerals such as calcium.
- *Solanine*, which occurs in potato skins, especially in those which are green, is a common cause of food poisoning. Normal potatoes contain 3−6 mg of solanine in an average-sized potato. A green-skinned potato has more than 20 mg. If all the green skin is removed from a potato which has been exposed to light, the rest of the potato is fine.

- Cabbage, Brussels sprouts, cauliflower, turnips and broccoli contain *goitrins*, which can prevent the thyroid gland making full use of iodine. This is only a problem if excessive quantities of these vegetables are consumed.
- Mustard seed contains chemical substances called *nitriles* and *thiocyanates* which can also interfere with the thyroid gland. Again, it is only in extremely large quantities that these become a problem.
- Lima beans and cassava contain highly toxic *cyanide* compounds. In populations where very large quantities of cassava are consumed (750 g/day), blindness and degenerative diseases of the nerves occur due to cyanide poisoning.
- Heavy metals such as *mercury* and *cadmium* occur in some seafoods and can cause serious food poisoning. This is only a problem with seafoods which come from contaminated waters. Many samples of kelp and other seaweeds are so high in arsenic that they are not permitted to be sold in some areas. Strangely enough, kelp is usually used by those seeking 'natural' food substances. It is quite 'naturally' toxic.
- Comfrey contains *alkaloids* which can cause liver cancer.
- Icthyosarcotoxin is found in the flesh of some fish from tropical waters. It is not destroyed by cooking. It causes extreme illness and even death.
- *Furanoterpenes* occur in moulds which grow on sweet potatoes. All moulds should be removed from vegetables and grains.
- *Caffeine* in tea, coffee, chocolate and cola products is quite toxic in excess (see page 50).
- Fungi, including some varieties of mushrooms, contain *toxic* substances which cause delirium, fever, vomiting, and death.

Some foods containing natural toxicants also have other factors which are protective against the toxicity. For example, a high content of zinc in molluscs can protect against the toxicity of cadmium. In general, however, naturally-occurring toxins deserve some of the attention which is given to man-made toxins.

Bacterial toxins

In some countries, bacterial food poisoning is a notifiable disease. It is more common during summer and can occur in foods which look and taste perfectly normal.

Most bacteria are not harmful, but a few are. They can multiply rapidly in foods, given the right conditions. Sometimes it is the sheer number of the bacteria themselves which cause food poisoning; in other cases, the bacteria themselves are harmless but the toxins they produce do the damage. The distinction between whether it is the bacteria themselves or their toxins which are harmful is important, as the bacteria will be killed by heating the food, but their toxins may not be. Reheating food does not always guarantee safety.

The major bacteria which cause harm are *salmonella*. The most common ones which produce toxins to cause food poisoning are staphylococci, clostridium welchii and clostridium botulinum.

Salmonella live and grow in the intestines of humans, household pets and birds, and are transmitted by excreta, flies, cockroaches and other pests. Strict standards of hygiene, especially washing hands after using the toilet, are important to control these bacteria. Cooking will destroy salmonella, but if cooked foods come into contact with raw foods, they may be recontaminated. For example, cooking a chicken will kill any salmonella, but if a knife used to cut raw chicken is used on cooked chicken, without being washed, the salmonella will begin to grow.

Staphylococci are bacteria which live in cuts, pimples, under fingernails, in the nose and, sometimes, just on the skin. Coughing, sneezing and handling food spread the bacteria. Staphylococci produce a toxin which

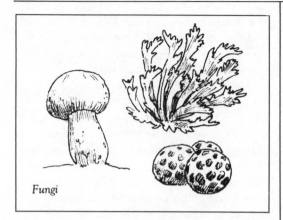
Fungi

contaminates the food, but does not make it look or smell any different. The toxin is not destroyed by heating. Foods which are commonly a cause of this type of food poisoning include potato salad, custard tarts, cold meats, meat pies and cream cakes (especially those left sitting in the cake shop window).

The *clostridium welchii bacteria* abound in the faeces of humans and animals. They present a special hazard in large cuts of meat. Cooking will kill the bacteria on the surface but those deep inside may survive. After the meat is cooked, these survivors begin to multiply, especially if the meat is left at room temperature. This type of food poisoning is common in institutions. It can be prevented by eating meat while it is hot or refrigerating immediately after cooking.

Botulism is a rare and very serious form of food poisoning (see page 41).

The term *ciguatera* came from the name used by Spanish settlers in the Caribbean to describe poisoning from a sea snail known as cigua. The term is now used to describe food poisoning from a toxin produced by a bacterium present in decaying coral reefs such as those affected by crown-of-thorns starfish. Small fish feed on the algae and are in turn eaten by larger bottom-feeding fish such as the Spanish mackerel, coral trout and red emperor. The toxin is highly poisonous and 1−30 hrs after eating the

infected fish causes diarrhoea, abdominal pain, nausea, chills, weakness, tingling, numbness and a hot sensation after eating cold foods. Some of the symptoms, such as chills and tingling, may persist for months or years. Death may occasionally occur.

To protect against food poisoning:
- Personal hygiene is important
- Those with cuts and respiratory infections should avoid handling food to be consumed by others
- Hot foods should be kept piping hot
- Foods to be served cold should be refrigerated immediately after cooking
- Utensils and equipment used for raw foods should be washed well before using for cooked foods
- Pet food should be stored away from human food

FOOD SENSITIVITIES
see Allergies.

FORTIFICATION

The process of adding nutrients to a food. For example, most breakfast cereals are fortified with vitamins to make up for the losses due to processing.

F-PLAN

A popular slimming diet written by the English writer Audrey Eyton, featuring high-fibre foods. The F-Plan swept through many countries, providing a reasonably well-balanced diet. The rationale for the diet was that a high fibre intake would decrease the number of kilojoules absorbed. This is not strictly correct since the bacterial fermentation of fibre in the large intestine does provide kilojoules. Nevertheless, the diet was well received since it represented a much better eating pattern than was evident in most popular diets.

FRANKFURT
see Sausages.

FREE RADICALS

Highly reactive molecules which try to stabilise themselves by taking an electron from another molecule. The polyunsaturated fatty acids in the membranes around cells are vulnerable to attack by free radicals. This leads to a destruction of the tissue.

Radiation, light, iron and copper, cigarettes, urban pollution and the presence of oxygen in the tissues, can all start free radical reactions.

Antioxidants such as vitamins C, A and E, are scavengers of substances which start these reactions.

Free radicals are thought to play a role in degenerative diseases including heart disease, cancer and inflammatory conditions. They are also thought to be involved in ageing. At this stage, without a complete understanding of how free radicals work, large doses of antioxidants are not recommended. However, there can be no harm, and possibly much good may stem, from eating foods which supply natural antioxidants such as fruits, vegetables and wholegrain products (see also Ageing and diet; Vitamin E).

FREE-RANGE EGGS
see Eggs.

FREEZE-DRIED FOODS
see Dehydration.

FREEZING OF FOODS

The most satisfactory method of preserving many foods, freezing stops chemical activity in the cells of foods. It is suitable for a wide selection of foods, including many vegetables (except salad vegetables), fruits, breads, meats, fish and cooked dishes.

The water crystals which form during the freezing process also rupture some cells in the food so that once the food is thawed, it has a different (usually softer) texture than before. Foods with a very high water content (such as lettuce, tomatoes, cucumber and some fruits), will have so many ice crystals that their structure will be damaged severely during freezing. Other fruits, such as watermelon, strawberries or grapes, can be eaten frozen but are mushy if thawed.

When freezing meats, the spaces between the muscle cells freeze first and then draw water out of the cells by osmosis (see page 256). This causes the dry patches of 'freezer burn' sometimes seen on frozen meat. The faster foods are frozen, the smaller the ice crystals which form and the less damage there is to cell structure.

Freezing greatly reduces spoilage of foods but it cannot eliminate it completely. Frozen foods do have a limited life. All foods to be frozen should be wrapped to exclude air and lessen drying out.

Vegetables must be blanched before freezing. This involves a short heating period to kill enzymes which would otherwise make the vegetables go bad.

Losses of vitamins are much less with freezing than with most other means of keeping food. In many cases frozen foods will have a higher vitamin content than their fresh counterparts. With vegetables, for example, the practice of blanching and freezing takes place almost as soon as the vegetables are picked. Further vitamin losses are less than would be involved in the marketing and home storage of the vegetables.

When frozen foods thaw, some water soluble vitamins will be lost in the juices which inevitably drip out. For vegetables, this is not a problem, since they are cooked from the frozen state. For meats, some of the B vitamins will be lost.

FRENCH BEANS
see Vegetables, Beans.

FRONTIGNAN
see Wine, Varieties.

FRUCTOSE

The sugar in fruits and honey with small amounts found in some vegetables. Fructose (also called fruit sugar or levulose) is also one of the two sugars which make up sucrose (regular sugar). Unlike glucose, fructose does not stimulate the production of insulin. However, it does contribute just as many kilojoules as any other sugar and so is not a suitable product for many diabetics. For other people, there is absolutely no advantage in paying high prices for fructose instead of regular sugar.

Fructose is slightly sweeter than sugar in cold foods. This may give a slight advantage if it means that a smaller quantity of the sugar will be used.

Fructose can decrease the rate at which alcohol is absorbed into the blood, but only to a small extent. Although it is sometimes sold as an instant cure for heavy drinking, the amount of fructose which has to be taken to achieve a significant effect will usually cause stomach cramps and vomiting. Which is worse — the alcohol or the cure?

See also Carbohydrates; Sucrose.

FRUIT

See following pages.

FRUIT JUICES

see Drinks, Non-alcoholic.

FRYING

Cooking with some type of fat. Pan-frying uses only a small amount of fat; deep-frying, as the term suggests, uses a large quantity. With pan-frying, the fat prevents the food from sticking, seals the surface of the food to prevent flavour loss and itself contributes flavour. Iron pots should not be used for frying as the iron can accelerate the breakdown of fats, causing them to become rancid.

Fried food has a high fat content, the exact amount of fat or oil absorbed depending on the food. Foods such as potatoes soak up a lot of fat and twice-fried chips (a common practice in many take-away food shops), have almost twice as much fat as chips which have been fried only once. Small, thin chips will also take up a lot more fat than large chips, since the smaller products have a greater surface area to absorb the fat.

Whatever the type of fat used in frying, the resulting product will have a similar calorie and total fat level. The different types of fats used will have other benefits or disadvantages.

See also Fats.

FUDGE

A candy made by boiling sugar syrup to 132°C (270°F), adding chocolate and milk (or cream) and beating the mixture vigorously as it cools to produce a smooth, non-grainy texture. Corn syrup in the mixture produces very fine crystals which help give a smooth texture. The composition of the final product varies according to the ingredients, but, on average, 100 g fudge contains about 1680 kJ (400 Cals) and has about 13 g of fat.

FUJI FRUIT

see Fruit.

FUL MEDAMES

see Legumes.

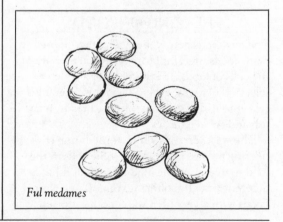

Ful medames

FRUIT

Fruits consist of fleshy ovaries surrounding the seed which will produce a new plant. Technically, fruits include some foods which we call vegetables (such as tomatoes, cucumbers and beans) and some we refer to as nuts (such as almonds, pecans and walnuts). In practice, we restrict fruits to sweet-fleshed products.

Fruits are sweet because of the sugars they contain, the major one being fructose or fruit sugar. They are also good sources of vitamins and contain some dietary fibre and a selection of minerals. Only a few fruits, such as bananas and custard apples, contain the complex carbohydrates found in grains, cereals and vegetables. In general, the vitamins in fruits are well-preserved while the fruit is undamaged and retains its skin. Once cut or exposed to oxygen in the atmosphere enzymes bring about chemical changes which alter the taste and destroy the nutritional value of the fruits.

Many fruits grow in tropical areas while others thrive in colder climates. Modern methods of transportation and refrigeration now ensure that a wide variety of fruits are available. There are many other fruits available in particular parts of the world; a complete list would take up an entire book.

Acerola
Also known as the Barbados or West Indian cherry, the tart red fruits are one of the richest known sources of vitamin C. 100 g of the fruit have 1680 mg vitamin C (which is 56 times the average daily requirement) and 135 kJ (32 Cals). It can be eaten raw or used in jams and jellies. If not completely ripe, it has a rather resinous flavour.

Akee
A fruit about the size of a peach. When ripe, the skin is yellow and splits open to reveal shiny black seeds and a white edible flesh (the seeds are poisonous). Originally brought to the West Indies from West Africa by William Bligh (of *The Bounty*), the akee is usually cooked and eaten with salted fish, rice, or in small pastries.

Alligator pear
see Avocado.

Apple
A member of the 'pome' family (meaning that they have a compartmentalised core), apples come in over 7000 varieties, and have been eaten for thousands of years. About 100 varieties are grown commercially with approximately one-quarter of the world crop being used to make apple cider.

Nutritionally, apples are a source of the soluble dietary fibre, pectin. They also supply small quantities of minerals and vitamins. It is likely that the saying 'an apple a day keeps the doctor away' originated because of their dietary fibre content. An average-sized apple (140 g) has 285 kJ (68 Cals).

Apricot
A stone fruit which is a member of the rose family, *Prunus*. Originally grown in China, apricots are now used throughout the world, either fresh, canned or dried.

Apricots are a good source of dietary fibre

and potassium and also supply some carotene which is converted into vitamin A in the body. Dried apricots are an excellent source of dietary fibre and a good source of iron. Two or three apricots (100 g) have 170 kJ (40 Cals).

Apricot kernels contain substances called cyanogenetic glycosides which release cyanide and are poisonous. With some varieties of apricots, eating 25 kernels could be lethal. Claims that apricot kernels can cure cancer are incorrect; even if the poisonous substances could kill cancer cells, they also kill healthy cells and, ultimately, the person.

Avocado

The fruit of a tree which originated in Central and South America. Also known as alligator pear, different varieties of avocado have a green or black skin which may be wrinkled or smooth.

The avocado is unusual among fruits and vegetables in that it contains fat. However, the avocado does not have any cholesterol — no vegetable food does. Nor is it likely to increase levels of cholesterol in the blood since most of its fat is in the form of monounsaturated fatty acids which can help lower blood cholesterol levels. The high fat level does mean that the avocado has a higher level of kilojoules than other fruits and vegetables.

The avocado is a good source of vitamins E, folate and B_6, has useful quantities of vitamin C and potassium, and supplies some riboflavin and niacin (B vitamins). It also has small quantities of other vitamins and minerals. Half an average avocado has 820 kJ (196 Cals).

Azarole

A member of the rose family, the azarole or medlar originated in Iran and Southeast Europe. It now grows wild in many countries and is highly prized in Italy, France, Spain and Algeria. The fruits come in clusters and are 1–1.5 cm in diameter. The fruit of the medlar can be distinguished from its relatives the apple

and pear, because it is open at one end, revealing its carpels. The fruit ripens in late autumn. It is brown, apple-shaped and its leathery skin is quite hard. As it begins to rot and turns a brown colour, the flesh becomes buttery and delicious. The rotting process is known as 'bletting' and can be carried out artificially by placing the medlars on a bed of hay for up to 2 months.

The fruit of the medlar is eaten raw, sometimes mixed with a little cream, or is made into jellies or preserves. It is high in dietary fibre and contains small quantities of minerals and vitamins. 100 g of the flesh have 175 kJ (42 Cals).

Babaco

The babaco, sometimes called 'the fruit of the gods', looks a little like a seedless, pale-orange version of its relative, the pawpaw. It originated in Equador and has a delicate flavour which is said to resemble a mixture of passionfruit, pineapple and strawberry. The babaco is an excellent source of vitamin C and is low in kilojoules. 100 g have 85 kJ (20 Cals).

Banana

One of the most useful fruits which probably originated in China as a more bitter product with many black seeds. There is a legend that it was a variety of banana known as Adam's Apple which was the forbidden fruit offered to Adam by Eve.

In some parts of the world, green bananas are baked whole and eaten as a vegetable. When the skin is yellow, the banana is ripe, much of its starch has been converted to sugar, and it tastes quite sweet. They can be eaten raw, cooked or dried.

The most commonly grown variety of banana is the cavendish. Other varieties include lady's fingers, a sweet-tasting banana which grows well in slightly cooler areas, and sugar bananas, small, plump, thin-skinned fruits which grow in smaller bunches.

Nutritionally, bananas are a good source of

dietary fibre, vitamin C and potassium, and have small quantities of other minerals and vitamins. They are also one of the few fruits which contain complex carbohydrate, with the sugar banana having more than the regular cavendish variety.

Contrary to popular belief, bananas are unlikely to be fattening. An average-sized banana has 375 kJ (90 Cals).

Banana passionfruit

A slender, yellow-coloured fruit with a soft skin and flesh which looks and tastes like passionfruit with a hint of banana flavour. Nutritionally, it is similar to the passionfruit and is a good source of dietary fibre.

Barbados cherry

see Acerola.

Barbary fig

see Prickly pear.

Barberry

The bright red fruit of the barberry bush. Has a rather acidic taste which goes well with meats. Used in jellies, pickles and jams.

Bell apple

Another name for a passionfruit with a yellow skin, rather like a banana passionfruit.

Bergamot

An orange cultivated in Calabria for its oil. The bitterness of bergamot oranges is used in some liqueurs such as Curacao.

Berries

Berries are made up of small aggregates of several small fruits with each segment being a fruit with a stony layer surrounding the seed. Blueberries, cranberries, red and blackcurrants are all true berries; blackberries and raspberries are multiple fruits; strawberries are not technically berries at all. See also individual fruits.

Bilberry

A European berry (also known as the whortleberry) with a blue-purple colour and a slightly astringent flavour. The staple food of grouse, they are mainly used for jams, jellies and tarts. Bilberries go well with game meats.

Blackberry

A member of the rose family, blackberries (also called brambles) are not really a true berry but are aggregates of several small fruits. The blackberry bush is a prickly climber which often grows wild, and is regarded as a nuisance. The flavour and nutritional value of the fruit, however, are hard to fault. The hard green fruit ripens and swells in early autumn to a dark purple-coloured delicacy which can be eaten raw or stewed. Blackberries are a good source of dietary fibre, vitamins C and E and provide small quantities of many other vitamins and minerals. Half a punnet of blackberries (125 g) has 150 kJ (35 Cals).

Blackcurrant

A European berry which also grows in northern Asia, the richly coloured blackcurrants have a slightly tough skin, a somewhat acid taste and a distinctive aroma. They should not be confused with dried currants. Usually preferred cooked or made into jams, jellies or syrups, blackcurrants are also used in the French liqueur cassis.

Blackcurrants are an excellent source of vitamin C, a good source of dietary fibre, and provide some iron as well as other minerals and vitamins. 100 g have 120 kJ (28 Cals).

Blood orange

An orange from Malta with sweet, juicy reddish-coloured flesh. Its nutritional value is similar to other oranges.

Blueberry

A true berry, blueberries are a member of the heather family and grow wild in Northern Europe and North America. Once the berries ripen to a blue colour, they should be left on the bush for a few days to produce a much sweeter flavour. They can be eaten raw or in pies, cakes or muffins. They are a good source of vitamin C and provide small quantities of dietary fibre, minerals and vitamins. Half a punnet (100 g) of blueberries has 235 kJ (55 Cals).

Boysenberry

A hybrid berry developed from a raspberry and loganberry and first grown in California in the 1930s. Grown mainly in the United States, New Zealand and Australia, the berries are large and plump and turn dark red when ripe in late summer. The fruit is an excellent source of dietary fibre and provides a range of minerals and vitamins. Half a punnet (100 g) has 210 kJ (50 Cals).

Bramble

see Blackberry.

Breadfruit

The breadfruit is a member of the mulberry family and comes from Asia where it is used as a vegetable or, when fully ripe, as a fruit. Covered with a thick, rough green skin, the flesh of the large fruits (weighing 1–2 kg) is yellow when ripe and is usually served mashed with milk and sugar or with a sweet sauce. The seeds can be roasted and eaten like chestnuts. As a vegetable, the flesh can be baked and used in much the same way as potatoes, either mashed, baked, fried or diced into a salad. Captain Cook was taken with the breadfruit trees growing in Tahiti. Eleven years later Bligh left on his ill-fated trip on *The Bounty* to collect 1000 potted breadfruit trees. The mutiny on board *The Bounty* prevented the breadfruit reaching their destination.

Breadfruit is an excellent source of vitamin C, a good source of complex carbohydrate, and provides some dietary fibre as well as small quantities of vitamins and minerals. 100 g (raw weight) have 420 kJ (100 Cals).

Bullock's heart

West Indian name for custard apple.

Cactus berry

see Prickly pear.

Canteloupe

see Rockmelon, Melons.

Cape gooseberry

Also known as golden berry and Chinese lantern, this is a small round yellow fruit with a delightfully fresh flavour. It is reminiscent of a mixture of passionfruit, tomato and cherry. The fruit originated in South America and was later cultivated around the Cape of Good Hope (hence its name).

Carambola

A popular fruit in Indonesia, carambola is also grown in China, South America and Australia. The fruit is juicy with a sweet, pleasant flavour and can still be sweet enough to eat when green. The star-shape of slices of the fruit look attractive and the fruit is also used in preserves, pickles and chutneys.

Nutritionally, it is an excellent source of vitamin C and provides some dietary fibre plus small quantities of vitamins and minerals. 100 g have 230 kJ (55 Cals).

Carambola is also known as star fruit or five corner fruit.

Casaba melon

A gold-yellow-coloured melon with a mild flavour and very little aroma. Like all melons, it is a good source of vitamin C and provides small quantities of other vitamins and minerals plus some dietary fibre. 100 g of casaba have 105 kJ (25 Cals).

See also Melons.

Cherimoya

A large, creamy-coloured fruit with a green skin covering its bumpy shape, weighing anything from half to several kilograms. Native to tropical America but also grown in Australia, Israel and the West Indies. Very similar to the custard apple. The pulpy flesh has a fragrant, sweet, slightly acidic flavour, sometimes described as a cross between a strawberry and a pineapple. The fruit ripens in autumn and early winter and is best eaten when fully ripe, at which time the carpels separate a little. In some varieties, the skin blackens when ripe. The black seeds are not edible but can be crushed and used as an insecticide.

Nutritionally, the cherimoya is an excellent source of vitamin C and dietary fibre and supplies small quantities of many minerals and vitamins. It also contains a small quantity of complex carbohydrate. 100 g of the fruit have 315 kJ (75 Cals).

Cherry

The cherry is a member of the rose family and there are many varieties which have been cultivated since many centuries BC. The fruits can vary in colour from yellow to red to a dark purple and may have varying degrees of sweetness. There are three major types grown: those with sweet fruits, those with sour fruits, and an in-between group.

Cherries are eaten raw, stewed, in jams, in chutneys, served with meats (especially game meats or pork), and are used to make the cherry liqueur, kirsch.

Nutritionally, cherries contribute some vitamin C, dietary fibre, potassium and other minerals and vitamins. 100 g cherries have 225 kJ (54 Cals).

Chinese gooseberry

see Kiwi fruit.

Chinese lantern

see Cape gooseberry.

Chocolate pudding fruit

see Sapote.

Citrange

A variety of orange originating from a cross between a sweet orange and a trifoliate orange. The fruits are 2.5—10 cm in diameter and have a skin which is yellow or reddish-orange. The skin contains an oil which tastes unpleasant but the flesh is juicy and slightly acid tasting.

Citron

A variety of lemon used only for its very thick peel which is candied and used as confectionery.

Citrus fruits

Lemons, limes, oranges, tangerines, grapefruit and citron belong to the citrus group of fruits. They are used for their flesh, juice and rind. All are rich in vitamin C and pectin (a form of dietary fibre) with the skin and pith containing much higher quantities of these than the flesh.

Citrus fruits are native to Southeast Asia. They were first cultivated in India, China and other Asian countries. They are now grown throughout the world, with particular types being specialities of certain areas.

After picking, there is little increase in the sweetness of citrus fruits; they should therefore be left to ripen on the tree.

For more information, see individual varieties.

Cloudberry

A berry which grows in areas close to the Arctic circle. The sweet juicy yellow and red berries have a flavour which is similar to apples.

Crabapple

A small wild apple which probably originated in Northern China. The raw fruits are too sour to eat but are used to make jellies, pickles, a sour juice and a drink known as lamb's wool (made by roasting and mashing crabapples, mixing with ale, pressing through a strainer and seasoning with a little nutmeg before serving hot). 100 g crabapples have 315 kJ (75 Cals).

Cranberry

A crimson berry of the heather family. Popular in the United States and used in Scandinavia where it grows wild and provides one of the few available good sources of vitamin C. Cranberries are acidic and are usually cooked with sugar. Often served as a preserve, especially with turkey. The fruits contribute dietary fibre and small quantities of minerals and vitamins. 100 g contain 210 kJ (50 Cals).

Cumquat

Originally grown in China, now flourishing in Japan, Malaysia and Australia. The cumquat (sometimes called kumquat) looks like a miniature orange and is often grown as a decorative tub plant. The skin is quite edible and the whole fruit is often pickled, made into marmalade or cooked to serve with foods as diverse as icecream or curries. Like all citrus fruits, cumquats are an excellent source of vitamin C. They are also a good source of dietary fibre and have smaller quantities of many vitamins and minerals. 100 g cumquats have 270 kJ (65 Cals).

Custard apple

A close relative of the cherimoya, although the flesh is a little more granular. Uses and nutritional characteristics are similar to cherimoya.

Damson

see Plum.

Date

The fruit of the date palm, native to India but grown widely in North Africa since 3000 BC. Also grown in Iraq, Iran, Saudi Arabi, Egypt and in any place where the temperature is high and the humidity low. A bunch of dates may contain more than 1000 dates. Can be eaten fresh, semi-dry or dried. The very dry dates used in Arab countries are often ground into a powder. The fresh fruit has a flesh which is a dull yellow-brown colour with a soft buttery flavour. The fruit darkens as it dries.

Dates are a good source of dietary fibre and provide some iron and other minerals and vitamins. They are high in sugars. The exact kilojoule count depends on the extent to which they have been dried; an average figure for pitted semi-dry dates is 1045 kJ (250 Cals) per 100 g. Fresh dates have approximately 840 kJ (200 Cals) per 100 g.

Durian

A large fruit weighing 2−5 kg and cultivated throughout Asia. Under the thick heavy skin is a creamy flesh whose distinctive odour is offensive and bears no relationship to the highly prized flavour. Can be eaten raw, cooked in rice dishes, fermented or used in cakes or icecream.

Nutritionally, durian is an excellent source of vitamin C and provides small quantities of other vitamins and minerals. 100 g of the fruit have 520 kJ (124 Cals).

Elderberry

A member of the honeysuckle family, elderberries are ripe when they turn a deep purplish-black. Major uses are in syrups, pickles or jams. The flowers of the elder are sometimes used for making wine.

Nutritionally, elderberries are an excellent source of vitamins and dietary fibre, and also provide carotene (converted to vitamin A), iron and potassium. 100 g have 315 kJ (75 Cals).

Elephant's apple

A Javanese fruit about the size of an apple but with a grey skin covering a woody shell. The flesh is used for making jams or jellies. The fruit also produces a gum, a little like gum arabic. The gum is an excellent source of dietary fibre.

Feijoa

A fruit about the size of a passionfruit, with a green skin and creamy flesh. Also called the pineapple guava. Its flavour is like a scented pear with a hint of pineapple. Grown in New Zealand, the whole fruit, apart from its skin, is edible. Can be eaten raw, stewed or in jellies.

Fig

The fig tree is a member of the mulberry family and probably originated in Asia many thousands of years ago. Figs are pollinated by a certain kind of wasp. The pear-shaped ripe fruit has a skin with colours of green, purple and brown. When ripe, the skin starts to split. The flesh is delicately but richly flavoured and sweet when ripe. Because they do not keep well, most figs are dried.

FRUIT

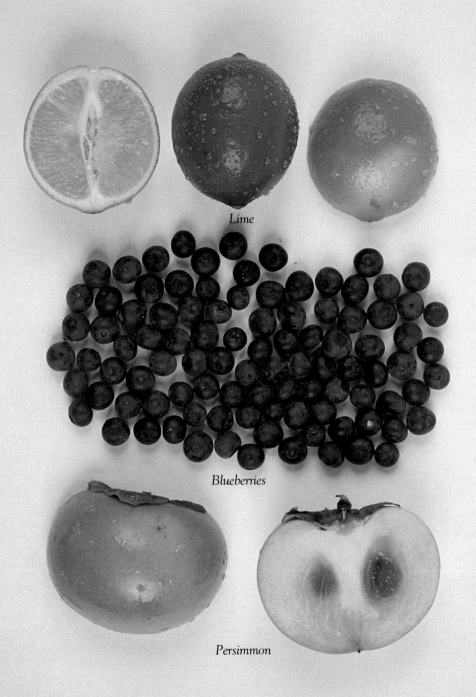

Lime

Blueberries

Persimmon

FRUIT

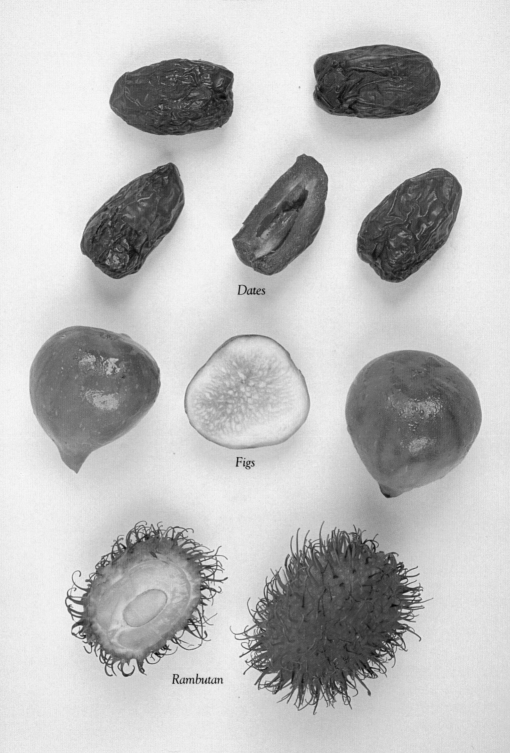

Dates

Figs

Rambutan

Nutritionally, figs are a good source of dietary fibre and provide small amounts of many minerals and vitamins. When dried, these nutrients become more concentrated, and dried figs are especially valuable for their high fibre content. A 100 g fresh fig has 170 kJ (40 Cals) while 100 g of dried figs have 900 kJ (215 Cals).

Five corner fruit

see Carambola.

Fuji fruit

Related to the persimmon, the fuji fruit has a slightly more delicate flavour and is edible even when slightly underripe. Similar nutritional value to persimmon (see page 153).

Golden berry

see Cape gooseberry.

Gooseberry

A hairy covered berry with a ripe fruit which can be green, white, yellow or red. Originally from North Africa, the gooseberry bush grows wild in many parts of Europe. Gooseberries were once very popular in England and 'gooseberry clubs' were established in many villages with the aim of producing giant gooseberries.

Gooseberries can be made into jams, jellies, pies and other desserts. In France, they are used to make a sauce to serve with mackerel. Gooseberry wine, made from yellow gooseberries, is said to resemble champagne.

They are an excellent source of vitamin C and a good source of dietary fibre. Gooseberries also supply small quantities of many vitamins and minerals. 100 g have 70 kJ (17 Cals).

Gramma

An orange-coloured fruit which looks like a large pumpkin. Stewed and used in jams and pies.

Granadilla

see Passionfruit.

Grape

One of the oldest plants in cultivation, the grape originally grew wild in western Asia, southern Europe and parts of northern Africa. Some varieties come from America. Many varieties of grapes are now grown throughout Europe, Australia, New Zealand, South Africa and the United States, and are used for eating as table grapes, wine making or dried as sultanas or raisins. In the United States, sultanas are known as 'seedless raisins'.

Grapes have either black or green skins. Black grapes are used for eating, for making raisins and for red or white Wines. Green grapes are used as a table grape, for sultanas or for making white wines. See under Wine, Varieties, for varieties of grapes used to make different wines.

In addition to their role in making wines, grapes go well with cheese platters, can be used with meats, fish or poultry, or made into desserts. For a healthy snack, bunches of sultana grapes can also be frozen.

Grapes contribute dietary fibre and some potassium. They have more sugar (in the form of equal amounts of glucose and fructose) than other fruits. Contrary to popular belief, black grapes have little iron. Because they are easy to eat, those aiming to lose weight are sometimes advised to give grapes a miss. While this is unnecessary, it is important for the overweight not to eat the large quantities of grapes which some people find possible. A small bunch of grapes (125 g) has 340 kJ (80 Cals).

Grapefruit

Also called pomelo or shaddock, this fruit originated in the West Indies but was not extensively cultivated until it was taken to Florida in 1823 by the chief surgeon of Napoleon's army. By the late nineteenth and early twentieth centuries, grapefruit were extensively cultivated in this area and rapidly spread to Central America, Israel, Greece, Spain, parts of Asia and South Africa.

There is some dispute as to whether the pomelo and the shaddock are the same fruit. The term shaddock was originally given to the fruits with a pink flesh (the pink is from a higher content of carotene). The pomelo may have yellow, pink or red flesh, a thick rind which peels easily away from the fruit and it is easily segmented. The confusion has arisen because the fruit known as a pomelo was taken to the West Indies by a Captain Shaddock.

Grapefruit can be made into marmalade, squeezed for their juice, added to salads or used in desserts. Their major use is as a breakfast food, served plain or sprinkled with sugar.

Like other citrus fruits, the grapefruit is an excellent source of vitamin C and a good source of dietary fibre. It also has small quantities of a range of minerals and vitamins. Half a grapefruit (120 g edible portion) has 135 kJ (32 Cals).

Guava

A common tropical fruit and one of the richest sources of vitamin C, the guava is part of the myrtle and eucalyptus family. Guavas are native to tropical parts of America and also grow in the south of France, India and Algeria.

The highly scented fruit is botanically a berry and may be yellow, red, green or white. The pulpy flesh contains hard seeds and is usually pink or red but may be white or yellow. The cherry guava is small and reddish-purple at the outside of the flesh, lighter (even white) at the centre.

Guavas are used for their juice or to make jellies, pastes, relishes and sauces. In Central America, guavas are also used in stuffings.

Nutritionally, guavas are rich in vitamin C (almost 5 times as much as in oranges) and have a high content of dietary fibre. They also supply carotene (converted to vitamin A in the body) and small quantities of many minerals and vitamins. An average-sized guava (115 g edible flesh) has 115 kJ (27 Cals).

Honeydew melon

A variety of winter melon with a hard smooth white rind and sweet green flesh. Served raw, with ham as an entree, in salads, with other fruits or in drinks or desserts. The fruit is an excellent source of vitamin C and also supplies some calcium and small quantities of other minerals and vitamins.

See also Melons.

Huckleberry

A blue or red berry which grows on the north-west coast of the United States. Generally considered to have slightly more flavour than the blueberry. Similar nutritional value to the blueberry.

Indian fig

see Prickly pear.

Jackfruit

Native to India and Malaysia, the jackfruit is now widely grown in tropical areas in Asia, America, Africa and Australia. The fruits are large, weighing over 20 kg, have a hard, rough, yellowish-brown rind and take 6–8 months to ripen. The yellow flesh has a pungent odour and is very juicy. The seeds (white or brown) can be roasted and eaten. The flesh can be eaten underripe as a vegetable or, when ripe, as a fruit. Jackfruit fritters are sold along the roadside in some parts of Asia.

The fruit is a source of dietary fibre, carotene, potassium and iron. It also has small quantities of other minerals and vitamins. Jackfruit has a higher sugar content than many fruits and 100 g have 335 kJ (80 Cals).

Jambo

Also known as the rose apple, Brazilian cherry, the Santo Domingo apricot, pitanga or lillipilli, this fruit is a member of the myrtle family and grows in eastern Asia and South America. A variety which grows in Australia is known as the lillipilli; its fruits are somewhat inferior to those of the Asian jambos.

The fruits are about 4 cm in diameter and look a little like an apple with pale yellow-pink colouring rather like that of the apricot. The flesh is the same colour as the skin, has a slight rose scent and, in some varieties, has a slightly resinous flavour. When completely ripe the flavour is more agreeable and can be used in salads, pies or other desserts. The seeds should be removed before eating. A jelly can be made from the unripe fruit.

The fruits are a good source of vitamin C and also supply carotene. 100 g have 140 kJ (33 Cals).

Jujube

Also known as the Chinese date, the origins of this small fruit are not known. Records show that it was used in China in the third century BC, while some believe it is native to the Mediterranean area. It grows wild in Syria and is also found in Arabia, Asia, southern Europe and Russia. The fruit is first green, then turns red and finally goes brown when it is ripe. The flesh is white and the stone is inedible. The fruit is often left to dry until it is crisp and sweet. It can be eaten raw or made into desserts, jellies or pastes. The dried jujubes are eaten like dates.

Jujubes are rich in vitamin C and contain dietary fibre and a range of minerals and vitamins. 100 g of the fruit have 195 kJ (47 Cals).

Kaki or kakee

A brilliantly coloured Chinese persimmon, grown for many centuries in China and Japan. Now grown in Mediterranean countries.

See also Persimmon.

Kiwi fruit

Previously known as the Chinese gooseberry, this fruit underwent a change of name with a clever marketing exercise by New Zealand. The fruit has no relationship to the gooseberry, apart from having a slightly hairy skin.

True to its original name, the fruit is a native climbing deciduous shrub of China. It has only been cultivated by Europeans this century and is now grown in New Zealand, Australia, Israel, France, Italy, Spain and the United States.

The green-coloured juicy flesh of the fruit contains tiny seeds which add to the attractive appearance of slices of the fruit. The brown skin is quite edible. The fruit is eaten raw, used in, or to decorate, desserts, and can also be made into a kiwi fruit wine. Kiwi fruits also go well with poultry, meats and salads.

Kiwi fruit are an excellent source of vitamin C, a good source of dietary fibre and provide small quantities of many vitamins and minerals. One kiwi fruit (80 g edible portion) supplies 2.5 days' needs for vitamin C and 170 kJ (40 Cals).

Kumquat

see Cumquat.

Lemon

A member of the citrus family, the lemon is thought to have originated in India, Burma or south China. It was not popularised until about the fourteenth or fifteenth century when the Arabs took it to North Africa. From here the Crusaders took the lemon to Britain. It is now grown in the Mediterranean regions, Israel, North America and Australia. In tropical areas it is replaced by the lime. In some of these areas, the lemon tree flowers and fruits throughout the year.

Lemons are used in both sweet and savoury dishes and in drinks. The peel (or zest) is also finely chopped for use in marmalade, and to give flavour to desserts and cakes.

Like all citrus fruits, lemons are an excellent source of vitamin C. They also supply dietary fibre and small quantities of many minerals and vitamins. The pectin in lemons is important in the jelling of jam and provides an important type of dietary fibre. A lemon (100 g) has 95 kJ (22 Cals).

Lillipilli

see Jambo.

Lime

Limes are thought to have originated in tropical Asia and were extensively cultivated in the West Indies. The Arabs took the fruit to Persia and India and it is now grown in most tropical areas, where it has replaced the lemon. Limes can be used in the same way as lemons — to flavour drinks, seafood dishes, meats, chicken, desserts, cakes, biscuits, marmalade and confectionery. Limes received great publicity when they were used by Dr James Lind, well-known Scottish physician, to prevent scurvy in sailors, who then became known as 'limeys'.

Lime juice has the ability to break down the protein in raw fish and is used extensively in this way in the marinaded raw-fish dishes of Pacific Islands.

The nutritional value of limes is almost identical to that of lemons, being an excellent source of vitamin C. 100 g of lime contain 90 kJ (21 Cals).

Loganberry

A member of the rose family, the loganberry was named after its Californian producer, James Logan, in 1881. It is a hybrid of the American blackberry and a raspberry.

Like most berries, loganberries are high in dietary fibre and vitamin C. Half a punnet of the berries (100 g) has 230 kJ (55 Cals).

Longan

A native of India, the longan, sometimes spelled lungan, comes from the same family as the lychee and has been cultivated in China for thousands of years. It also grows well in sub-tropical climates. The fruit is similar to that of a lychee with a light brown shell covering the pale yellow flesh. It can be eaten fresh or cooked in a sugar syrup or canned.

The longan has a high content of vitamin C and supplies potassium and dietary fibre as well as small quantities of vitamins and minerals. 100 g of the fruit (the flesh of 4–5 longans) have 250 kJ (60 Cals).

Loquat

A native of China and a relative of the apple and pear, the loquat was introduced to Japan and then brought to India. It was cultivated in Europe for its foliage rather than its fruit but is now grown in California, Australia and around the Mediterranean. It fruits best in warm climates.

Loquats have yellow or slightly orange-coloured skins and come in clusters of about 10 small (4 cm-long) slightly pear-shaped fruits. Their flesh is white or soft yellow, slightly acid and perfumed. Different varieties have one or two small or large seeds. They ripen in spring and early summer.

The fruits can be eaten fresh, served with a sweet syrup or a little lemon juice or made into a jelly. They contribute some dietary fibre and small quantities of other nutrients. 4 loquats have only 55 kJ (13 Cals).

Lychee

Also spelled litchee, lichi or lichee, this delicately flavoured fruit is a member of the same family as the longan. The evergreen tree originated in China where it has been cultivated for thousands of years. It is now also grown in Australia, New Zealand, South Africa, Hawaii, Florida and certain parts of the Mediterranean.

The ripe fruits are about the size of a small plum and have a reddish brown or purple, rough 'shell' surrounding the translucent jelly-like white flesh. The hard brown seed is inedible. The flesh is sweet and delicately flavoured with a slight acidity. It is considered the perfect ending to a Chinese meal.

Canned lychees are widely available but do not compare with the flavour of the fresh fruit.

Lychees are an excellent source of vitamin C and also provide dietary fibre and small quantities of minerals and vitamins. 4 fresh lychees have 185 kJ (44 Cals).

See also Rambutan.

Mammee

The mammee is also known as mamey, a mammee apple or Santo Domingo apricot and is native to South America, Africa and the West Indies. It is now popular in the Bahamas.

Its fruit is brown and globular-shaped with a rough leathery skin. Its pink-orange flesh is described as having a delicious flavour somewhere between that of an apricot and a raspberry. Christopher Columbus thought it 'the size of a lemon with the flavour of a peach'. The inner skin is bitter and should be removed. The flesh can then be eaten raw or used in pies and desserts.

The mammee fruit is large (usually about 800 g) and provides some vitamin C as well as small quantities of other vitamins and minerals. 100 g of the flesh have 210 kJ (50 Cals).

Mandarin

Related to the tangerine and mandarin orange, mandarins are a member of the citrus family and originally came from China. There is little difference between mandarins and tangerines, the latter name being used for fruits with a very deep orange or reddish colour.

Widely grown, especially in South Africa, Australia, southern Europe, the United States and parts of France. The fruits are slightly smaller than an orange with a loose skin which comes away from the fruit easily. They are eaten raw, added to drinks, desserts or used in marmalade.

Like other citrus fruits, mandarins are an excellent source of vitamin C and also provide carotene and dietary fibre. A fruit with 120 g edible portion has 190 kJ (45 Cals).

Mandarin orange

A variety of mandarin which is a hybrid of a mandarin and an orange. It is widely grown in China and is often canned for use in desserts, salads or drinks.

Mango

Native to India, the mango is an important fruit which comes from the same family as the cashew and the pistachio. To Indians, the mango is an important tree and Buddha is supposed to have done much of his meditating in a mango grove. India is still the world's largest grower of mangoes although they are also grown in South America, Southeast Asia, Australia, Spain, Israel, South Africa, Hawaii and the Philippines.

The are many varieties of mango and those whose fruit is especially prized have short fibres and a rich-tasting deep orange flesh. The fruits are green initially and become yellow, orange or pink-tinged when ripe.

Ripe mangoes are eaten raw or used in drinks, desserts or chutneys. Green mangoes are also eaten raw in Asia and are made into pickles or chutneys to serve with curry.

The flesh of the mango is an excellent source of vitamin C and carotene (converted to vitamin A in the body). They also supply potassium and small quantities of other minerals and vitamins. 100 g of mango flesh have 245 kJ (58 Cals).

Mangosteen

A native tree of Asia and tropical Africa, the mangosteen is now grown in the West Indies and parts of tropical Australia. The fruit (about 6 cm in diameter) is considered delicious, and has a dark red-purple rind covering about 6 segments, each with a seed surrounded by a white jelly-like flesh.

The fruits should not be picked until ripe but then need to be eaten without too much delay. Nutritionally, the mangosteen contains small quantities of many minerals and vitamins. 100 g of the flesh have 230 kJ (55 Cals).

Medlar

see Azarole.

Melon pear

see Pepino.

Melons

Melons were originally native to Asia but were widely cultivated in the Nile Valley in ancient times. They were not introduced to Europe until the fifteenth century. Today, various varieties of melon are grown throughout the world, especially in Asia, Australia, Italy and France.

Some of the most commonly grown varieties include:

- Canteloupe (also called the rockmelon) — has orange flesh
- Honeydew (another variety of winter melon) — has a hard white smooth skin and green flesh and keeps much longer than other melons
- Ogen melon — a small round orange melon with green ribs
- Casaba (or winter melon) — is oval in shape and has pale green or yellow flesh with less flavour than most other melons
- Musk melon — a round melon with a network of ribs on the skin and flesh which is green, orange or pink-orange
- Watermelon — one of the most popular melons

There are also hairy melons and bitter melons which are used as vegetables in Asian cookery (see Vegetables, Melons). The watermelon comes from a different family (see page 158).

Melons should be allowed to ripen on the vine to develop maximum sweetness. When ripe, the melon will easily detach from the stem which joins it to the vine.

Melons are usually eaten raw, either as an appetiser, for breakfast or for dessert. With watermelon, the white flesh (between the green rind and the pink flesh) can be steamed or pickled.

The nutritional value varies according to the particular melon. Most are excellent sources of vitamin C and provide some dietary fibre as well as small quantities of minerals and vitamins. Rockmelons, especially those with darker orange flesh, are also a good source of carotene. Watermelons are not rich in any particular nutrient. In kilojoules, 200 g of rockmelon flesh have 185 kJ (44 Cals); 200 g of honeydew melon have 245 kJ (58 Cals); 200 g of ogen melon (generally the whole melon) have 220 kJ (52 Cals); 200 g of watermelon have 200 kJ (47 Cals).

Mirabelle

A small golden plum which looks a little like an apricot. Also known as a golden gage (see page 154). Usually eaten raw or made into jams, the mirabelle also forms the basis of the flavouring of a French spirit. In nutritional value, the mirabelle resembles other plums (see page 154).

Monstera

From Mexico we have this plant with its distinctive fruit which is also called the Mexican breadfruit or the Swiss cheese plant. The plant is widely grown in Australia although there is little commercial marketing of the fruit. The monstera fruit takes almost a year to mature and looks like a long green cone covered in hexagonal scales. When ripe, the scales fall away from the bottom of the fruit revealing the white flesh. Unripe fruits cause a burning around the mouth and throat and should be avoided. The best method of ripening is to pick the fruit when the bottom half begins to wrinkle, wrap it in paper and leave for a few days. When unwrapped, the scales should fall off.

The flavour is sometimes described as resembling fruit salad. Those who do not like it cite other references for its slightly pungent aroma and flavour. The fruit is eaten raw or used in icecreams and desserts, or in drinks.

Morello

A dark fleshed cherry which is prized among its species. Eaten raw or used in jams or preserves.

See also Cherry.

Mulberry

A member of the same family as the fig and

breadfruit, the mulberry originated either in Persia or Nepal. Valued for its leaves (which are eaten by silkworms to produce fine silk), the white mulberry is rarely used for human food. Black mulberry leaves do not produce the same quality of silk but have more flavoursome berries. Widely grown throughout Europe, India, Iran, Turkey, Japan, China and Australia.

The unripe fruits are a light green and become deep purple when ripe. They are sweet and yet slightly tart and their juice stains fingers and clothes. Stains can be removed by rubbing with an unripe berry.

Mulberries can be eaten raw or made into sauces (excellent with game meats or lamb) or used in jams, jellies and desserts. Home-made mulberry wine was once popular.

Nutritionally, mulberries are a good source of dietary fibre and potassium and provide some vitamin C. 100 g have 120 kJ (28 Cals).

Musk melon

Also known as the netted melon, the musk melon has a green skin overlaid with lighter coloured rib work or 'netting'.

See also Melons.

Naseberry

see Sapodilla.

Nashi fruit

Originally grown in Northern Asia, the nashi fruit is a pear but looks like a greeny-brown skinned apple. Crisp and very juicy, it is served in thin slices.

Nectarine

A variety of peach, the nectarine may have been cultivated in China along with the peach. The smooth-skinned fruit was introduced into Europe and Britain in the sixteenth century and took its name from 'nectar', the drink of the gods. It is grown in New Zealand, Australia, the United States and in Britain.

The flesh varies from white to yellow to red. Australian nectarines are usually the small, white-fleshed variety while those from New

Zealand are much larger, have yellow flesh and are less likely to bruise.

The fruits are usually eaten raw or stewed and may be served with poultry or meats. They are good sources of dietary fibre and provide small quantities of minerals and vitamins. 100 g of nectarine flesh have 185 kJ (44 Cals).

Ogen melon

see Melons.

Olive

see page 249.

Orange

Probably originally from India or China, oranges are the most popular of the citrus fruits. The modern sweet orange was first grown around the Mediterranean and is now grown throughout the world, especially in Australia, California, Florida, Israel, Spain, Italy, North and South Africa and Brazil.

The bitter (or Seville) orange is not pleasant to eat but makes wonderful marmalade (see page 220). The Bergamot orange is grown mainly for the fragrance of its peel which is used in various perfumes and toilet preparations as well as in some liqueurs. The Navel orange is a popular eating orange with no pips.

Oranges are eaten as fruit or used for their juice. They can also be used in salads, desserts, with meats, fish or poultry, and in drinks, including the liqueurs Curacao and Van der Hum. Orange flower water, or Neroli, is produced in Italy and is used to flavour desserts.

Oranges have long been known as an excellent source of vitamin C, one orange containing about 2.5 days' supply. They are also good sources of dietary fibre and supply some calcium, carotene and potassium. An average-sized orange (150 g of flesh) has 245 kJ (58 Cals).

Orange juice was once squeezed in the home kitchen. Today most orange juice is commercially prepared. Some sugar is added and, in Australia, 4 per cent sugar may be added to a product labelled as 'pure orange juice'. Nutritionally, orange juice is an excellent product. However, it is also a product which is easy to overconsume. Many children drink orange juice whenever they feel thirsty and may take in far more calories from this source than they realise. A 250 mL carton or glass of juice has 500 kJ (120 Cals) — about the same as in 2 slices of bread. For those who drink 4—5 glasses of juice — in addition to their regular meals and snacks — it is easy to become overweight.

Passionfruit

Also known as bell apple or granadilla, passionfruit grow on a climbing vine which originated in South America. Different varieties now flourish in Australia, New Zealand, Kenya, South Africa and Malaysia. The name passionfruit relates to the beautiful flowers of the vine which Spanish priests used when attempting to convert South Americans to their faith. The three styles of the flower represented the nails used in the Crucifixion, the ovary of the flower was the sponge soaked in vinegar which Jesus called for, the stamens represented his wounds, the filaments his crown of thorns and the petals his apostles. The flower became known as the passion flower and its fruit, the passionfruit.

The passionfruit has a hard, green-brown skin which darkens to a deep purple (or it may be yellow or green in some varieties) and becomes wrinkly. Inside the skin, the edible black seeds are in a yellow-orange pulp which is sweet and slightly acidic. Both seeds and pulp are eaten together. The richly scented aroma of the passionfruit is unforgettable.

Passionfruit can be eaten straight or used in drinks, desserts or spreads. The classic pavlova is always decorated with passionfruit which seems to marry well with the sweetness of the dish.

Dietary fibre is found in seeds so it is not surprising that the passionfruit is an excellent source of fibre — having the highest fibre content of any commonly eaten fruit. It is also a source of vitamin C and niacin. The flesh of two passionfruit (approximately 50 g) contributes 100 kJ (24 Cals).

Pawpaw

Also called papaw, or papaya, the pawpaw tree originated in tropical America but is now grown in Australia, the West Indies, Hawaii, many Pacific islands and Malaysia. Its fruits may be 10—50 cm in diameter and may weigh 500 g—8 or 9 kg. The fruits from female trees are round or oval; those from hermaphrodite trees tend to be long and narrow.

The skin of the fruits usually turns yellow as the fruit ripens, although some varieties remain green. The flesh may be yellow, orange or pink. It is sweet and succulent and is eaten raw or in fruit salads or desserts. In some areas, green pawpaw flesh is used in pickles, chutneys and curried dishes.

Pawpaw leaves and fruit contain an enzyme called papain which breaks down some of the fibres in meat, tenderising it. This is the principle behind the Pacific Island custom of wrapping meat in pawpaw leaves for cooking. Papain is also used in some chewing gums and indigestion mixtures.

Pawpaw is a most nutritious fruit being a rich source of vitamin C (a 150 g portion has 3 days' supply), a good source of carotene and dietary fibre, and supplies small quantities of many minerals and vitamins. 150 g have 185 kJ (44 Cals).

Peach

Peaches have been cultivated in their country of origin, China, since at least 550 BC. They are regarded as a symbol of immortality and a token of friendship. Peaches have also been enjoyed in Persia since the first century BC, and were welcomed into Britain in Anglo-Saxon times. They are now grown in Italy, the United States, China, Japan, New Zealand, Australia, Israel, Spain and Mediterranean countries.

The downy skin of the fruit may be white, pale green or yellow, often with a flush of pink. The juicy flesh may cling to the stone or be easily freed and is white or yellow. The best flavoured peach is a matter of personal taste.

Peaches are eaten raw, canned (usually the yellow varieties), used in drinks and desserts. They may also accompany meats or poultry.

They have some vitamin C and dietary fibre as well as small quantities of various vitamins and minerals. Yellow peaches are also a source of carotene. An average peach (85 g of flesh) has 120 kJ (28 Cals).

Peaches are also dried and this concentrates their nutritional value. Dried peaches are a good source of dietary fibre, carotene and iron. 100 g have 880 kJ (210 Cals).

Pear

A member of the rose family, pears are native to Europe and western Asia and have been used for at least 4000 years. Many varieties of pears have been cultivated and major growing areas include France, Belgium, Germany, Australia, the United States, Great Britain and China.

Pears may have the typical pear shape or be more rounded like an apple. Their skins may be green, brown or yellow, but the flesh is always white. They continue to ripen after being picked and are ready to eat when there is a slight give near the stalk. If soft to the touch, they will be overripe. Many people waste pears, fearing that their firmness indicates that they are not ready to eat.

Pears are eaten raw, stewed, canned, made into relishes and chutneys, used in desserts and drinks. Pear juice has become a cheap way of providing a minimum fruit juice content in many processed fruit juice products. They can also be dried.

Pears are not rich in any vitamins or minerals, but they are a very good source of

dietary fibre. Their kilojoule value varies. A 150 g pear has 190—300 kJ (45—72 Cals).

Pepino

Also known as the melon pear, this fruit originally grew in Peru and Chile. It is now grown in Florida, New Zealand and Australia. The fruit has pale yellow flesh, is very juicy and has a delicate flavour half-way between that of a melon and a pear. Its smooth, shiny skin is also pale yellow, streaked with purple. It is eaten raw or in fruit salads or desserts. Unripe fruits are crisper and have little flavour.

The pepino is an excellent source of vitamin C and provides small quantities of other vitamins, minerals and dietary fibre. 100 g have 95 kJ (22 Cals).

Persimmon

Native to North America, China, Japan, western Asia and the region of the Himalayas, the persimmon kakee is a delightful sweet fruit when ripe. When unripe, its high tannic acid content gives it an unpleasant astringency.

The fruit of the most common variety is about the size of a tomato and has a bright orange-red thin skin covering its deep orange flesh. It is ripe when its flesh develops almost a jelly-like consistency. Some smaller varieties (such as the date palm) are only 1—2 cm in diameter and turn from yellow to purple-black when ripe. Others, such as the American persimmon, are 3—4 cm in diameter and are yellow, dark red or plum-coloured when ripe. Unripe persimmon skin often has a bloom on it.

The fruits are eaten raw or in sauces (excellent with game or pork). They are a good source of vitamin C, carotene and dietary fibre. An average persimmon (85 g) has 230 kJ (55 Cals).

See also Kaki or Kakee.

Pineapple

Native to Brazil, the pineapple is now grown in most of the tropical areas of the world.

Christopher Columbus first took the fruit to Spain. It is now grown commercially in Hawaii, Australia, Brazil, the West Indies, Mexico, South Africa and the Canary Islands.

The rough skin of the fruit ripens from a green colour to yellow, yellow-green, orange or red. The flesh is yellow and very juicy.

Like pawpaw, pineapple contains an enzyme which can tenderise meats. It also breaks down the structure of the protein in gelatin and prevents jellies from setting. Cooking the pineapple kills the enzyme, so cooked or canned pineapple can be set into jellies.

Pineapple is eaten raw, in salads, desserts and drinks, grilled or fried or used with meats, fish, chicken, in kebabs or various cooked dishes. It is a good source of vitamin C and provides dietary fibre and a little calcium, as well as other minerals and vitamins. 100 g of pineapple have 160 kJ (38 Cals)

Pineapple guava
see Feijoa.

Pitanga
see Jambo.

Plantain
A direct relation of the banana, the plantain is used as a vegetable when underripe. Once the skin blackens and the fruit is ripe, it is sweet enough to eat raw. The plantain is a good source of dietary fibre, potassium, carotene and vitamin C. 100 g of plantain have 500 kJ (120 Cals).

Plum
A member of the rose family, there are more than 200 varieties of plums and their original ancestry is unknown. Some varieties of plum are known as 'gages'. These are distinguished from plums by their sweet flavour and scent. The golden gage (also known as a mirabelle, see page 150), and the green gage, are considered tops for flavour. Damsons are considered to be excellent cooking plums and

are used in pies and desserts. The blood plums are some of the largest and best eating plums. The Australian green bush plum is one of the world's richest known sources of vitamin C. Until recently, it was known only to Aboriginal people.

Plums with a firm flesh and small stone can also be dried as prunes. With some of their water removed, prunes become an excellent source of dietary fibre and a more concentrated source of minerals such as iron.

Plums may have purple, yellow or green edible skins while their flesh may be deep-red, pink, yellow or green. They provide dietary fibre and small quantities of minerals and vitamins, the exception being the green bush plum which has large quantities of vitamin C. 100 g of plums have 135 kJ (32 Cals).

Pomegranate
Literally a 'grain apple', the pomegranate comes from the Mediterranean region and is also cultivated in India, Spain (Granada is supposed to have been named after it) and Egypt. The pomegranate has always been associated with religious ceremonies and fertility. It is found in temple carvings in Rhodes, in Chinese paintings, and is mentioned many times in the Bible. Its refreshing juice and the fact that it keeps well (its skin becomes leathery and hard but preserves the fruit beautifully) have also established its popularity in the Middle East.

The skin of the fruit is quite beautiful with colours ranging from yellow to red to a red-purple. The inside of the fruit is divided by pithy walls and each compartment contains pink flesh surrounding crisp edible seeds. The small kernels inside the seeds are usually not swallowed but are quite edible. When fully ripe, the skin splits.

Pomegranate seeds are used in both sweet and savoury dishes, for example, in rice dishes or salads, cooked with chicken, or made into jelly. The juice is perhaps more widely used as a drink or an ingredient in desserts, soups or savoury dishes. Pomegranate juice was once used in making grenadine syrup but is usually replaced by artificial flavours nowadays.

The pomegranate is a very good source of dietary fibre, and provides vitamin C, some iron and small quantities of minerals and vitamins. The edible portion of an average-sized fruit (400 g) has 630 kJ (150 Cals). 100 mL of pomegranate juice has 190 kJ (45 Cals).

Pomelo

see Grapefruit.

Prickly pear

Also known as cactus berry, Indian fig or Barbary fig, the prickly pear is one of the many edible fruits of cactus plants. The prickly pear originated in South America and was brought back to Europe by Christopher Columbus. The plant was introduced to Australia in the early days of the colony to nurture the cochineal insect which feeds on its leaves. The insect itself was introduced to produce the red dye needed for military uniforms. The prickly pear spread and became a pest until it was brought under control by a moth which eats it. Fortunately the moth has not, in turn, become a pest.

The fruit has a yellow, orange or red skin when ripe and has fine bristles which are very difficult to remove from the skin. The flesh is white, pink, yellow, orange or red; the seeds are edible. Delicious raw. If cooked, the seeds become hard and are difficult to remove unless the fruit is sieved. It can also be used for jam.

The fruit is high in dietary fibre and is a good source of vitamin C. It also contains some calcium and small quantities of other minerals and vitamins. An average fruit (110 g) has 145 kJ (35 Cals).

Prune

A partially dried plum usually from a variety with a small seed. The dark rich plums of Agen in France are said to produce the best quality prunes.

Prunes are an excellent source of dietary fibre and a good source of iron, potassium and carotene. 100 g of prunes (10–12 prunes) have 670 kJ (160 Cals).

Quandong

The fruit of a native peach tree which grows in Australia. The fruit changes from green to bright red when ripe and is excellent eaten fresh or dried. It also makes superb jam. The seeds can easily be parted from the flesh and are usually roasted and eaten like a nut.

Quince

Another member of the rose family, the quince has been used for so long that its origins are somewhat obscure. It probably originated in the area between Iran and the Caspian Sea. In ancient times it was dedicated to both Venus and Aphrodite as a symbol of love and fertility. It is grown in Greece, Spain (where it is called the marmelo), Israel, parts of South America, Turkey, the United States and Australia (less popular now than formerly).

The hard, yellow-skinned fruits are covered with a down. The yellow flesh is hard and quite acidic with a pleasant aroma. The fruit is usually stewed, baked or even roasted, and the hard flesh turns pink and soft. Its flavour marries well with meats and chicken. It is also used in pies and desserts. With its very high pectin content, it makes marvellous marmalades and jellies. Clear, dark-pink quince jelly is served with bread and butter or with chicken or lamb.

Quinces are rich in vitamin C and dietary fibre (especially pectin) and contain small quantities of various vitamins and minerals. 100 g of quince have 200 kJ (48 Cals).

Raisin

A dried black grape. In the United States, sultanas are called raisins while the sultana is called a seedless raisin. Raisins are high in potassium, dietary fibre and contribute some iron. 100 g of raisins have 1025 kJ (245 Cals).

Rambutan

Also known as the hairy lychee, this strange-looking fruit comes from Malaysia and is related to the lychee. It is bright red or orange when ripe and the rather tough skin has long, soft black spines. When the skin is split, a fruit resembling the soft white colour of a lychee is revealed.

The fruit is eaten raw and used with salads. It is an excellent source of vitamin C and provides dietary fibre. The flesh of 4 rambutans (60 g) has 170 kJ (40 Cals).

See also Lychee.

Raspberry

A member of the rose family, the raspberry is native throughout much of Europe, including Scandinavia and the United Kingdom. It grows well in Tasmania and New Zealand. Raspberries need a cool climate and an acidic soil. European varieties do not grow well in the United States and American varieties have been developed with yellow, purple or black berries.

The fruits are considered one of the best tasting of all fruits. They are eaten raw, stewed with sugar, made into desserts or sauces to serve with desserts or with game meats, pork, veal or poultry. Raspberry vinegar, raspberry wine and raspberry juice are also popular.

Nutritionally, raspberries are an excellent source of vitamin C and a good source of dietary fibre. They also contain some iron and small quantities of various vitamins and minerals. Half a punnet (100 g) of raspberries has 105 kJ (25 Cals).

Red currant

These somewhat acidic fruits grow wild throughout Europe, parts of Asia and even as far afield as Siberia. One variety, the white currant, is less acidic.

The red currant is actually a many-seeded berry. It is used in sauces or jellies served with meats or poultry, and in desserts, including several popular Scandinavian dishes. The unripe fruits are sometimes cooked and need less sugar to sweeten them than the riper fruits.

Red currants are an excellent source of vitamin C and dietary fibre and also supply some iron, other minerals and vitamins. 100 g of berries have 90 kJ (21 Cals).

Rhubarb

Botanically, rhubarb is a vegetable rather than a fruit, although it is generally used as a fruit. Native to Siberia, the Himalayas and eastern parts of Asia, rhubarb has been cultivated for thousands of years. Initially, however, rhubarb was grown for the pharmaceutical properties of its root as a laxative and astringent. It was not until the eighteenth century in Britain, that rhubarb was used as a fruit.

Rhubarb needs to be cooked before eating. The leaves should not be eaten as they have a very high content of oxalic acid and are quite toxic. The rhubarb stalks are usually stewed with sugar and then used in pies, desserts, jams or pickles. Rhubarb wine can also be made.

Rhubarb contains only small quantities of minerals and vitamins plus some dietary fibre. 100 g have 80 kJ (19 Cals); if sugar is added, each tablespoon of sugar will contribute a further 335 kJ (80 Cals).

Rockmelon

Also known as the canteloupe, this melon has a ridged skin and a sweet orange flesh. The melon was originally developed at Cantalupo, a former papal garden near Rome. Related to the musk melon, it is an excellent source of vitamin C.

See also Melons.

Rose apple

see Jambo.

Rose hip

Roses grow wild in areas as diverse as Alaska, Mexico, India, the Philippines, northern parts of Europe and Ethiopia. Their fruits, or hips, come in various sizes and different intensities of flavour. They are generally orange or red and all are edible, although their seeds are not as they irritate the throat.

Rose hips are used in desserts and to make jellies or jams. They are rich in vitamin C.

Rosella

A tropical fruit which grows in Australia, Hawaii, the West Indies and parts of Asia and consists of the fleshy calyx surrounding the petals of a yellow flower. The fruits are usually stewed, made into jams, jellies or used in drinks. Rosellas have much more calcium than most fruits (215 mg/100 g). They also contribute some vitamin C, dietary fibre and iron. 100 g of rosellas have 210 kJ (50 Cals).

Rowan

Also called mountain ash, the rowan produces edible red berries which are very high in pectin (a valuable form of dietary fibre). It is native to Europe and western Asia. Since the rowan fruits are rather bitter and have so much pectin, they are usually used to make jellies or sauces to serve with rich meats or game.

Sapodilla

Also known as the Santo Domingo Apricot or the Naseberry, the sapodilla is a native of Central America and the West Indies, and is mainly grown for its sap which is used as a basis of chewing gum (see page 68). In tropical countries, it is also cultivated for its round, brown, tough-skinned berries whose yellow-brown, juicy, sweet flesh is edible when fully ripe. The hook-shaped black seeds should not be swallowed. The flesh is eaten raw or used in fruit salads, with savoury salads, as a topping for pancakes or breads.

The sapodilla fruits are a source of vitamin C and dietary fibre. 100 g of the flesh have 335 kJ (80 Cals).

Sapote

Native to Central America, the sapote comes in several different varieties including the black sapote (also called the chocolate pudding fruit), the green sapote (which grows in cooler climates) and the white sapote. The colour of the fruits varies from the normal reddish-brown flesh to the richly chocolate coloured flesh of the black sapote (rather like a chocolate coloured persimmon). The fruit can be eaten raw, stewed or made into jams.

Nutritionally, the sapote is a good source of vitamin C and supplies potassium, carotene (converted to vitamin A) and dietary fibre. 100 g of the fruit have 565 kJ (135 Cals).

Shaddock

see Grapefruit.

Soursop

A tropical American fruit with a sour-smelling skin, related to cherimoya and custard apples. The green-skinned fruit has rows of soft spines and often weighs several kilograms. The fruit is eaten raw or stewed with sugar. Its texture is off-putting to some people, so it is often pureed and served with icecream or made into jellies or drinks.

Nutritionally, the soursop is a good source of vitamin C and provides small quantities of other vitamins and minerals. 100 g have 280 kJ (66 Cals).

Star apple

A relative of the sapodilla, this fruit grows in the West Indies, Central America, Africa, parts of Asia and Australia. The fruit resembles an apple with flattened ends and has a skin which may be yellow, pink or a dark purple; the flesh is white with a dry layer under the skin. The skin contains a type of latex and is unpleasant but the flesh is sweet and jelly-like.

Star fruit

see Carambola.

Strawberry

Commercially grown strawberries are rather different from the original wild strawberries which grow throughout Europe and in parts of North and South America. The cultivated strawberry has been grown since the fourteenth century and was much in demand in England by the seventeenth and eighteenth centuries.

The best-tasting strawberries are allowed to mature on the plant until the skin is shiny. They are eaten raw, used in desserts, drinks, sauces, jams or to garnish almost any dish.

Nutritionally, the strawberry is rich in vitamin C and contains some dietary fibre and a selection of vitamins and minerals. Low in calories: half a punnet (100 g) has 80 kJ (19 Cals).

Swiss cheese plant

see Monstera.

Tamarillo

Also known as the tree tomato, this fruit is native to South America but is mainly grown in New Zealand and Australia. The fruits have a dark red or yellow skin and a firm orange or reddish flesh with many edible dark-purple seeds. The flavour is sometimes said to resemble a cross between a tomato and a Cape gooseberry. Its flesh can be scooped out and eaten raw or it can be used in fruit salads or jams.

The tamarillo is a good source of dietary fibre, vitamin C and carotene and has small quantities of many minerals and vitamins. An average-sized fruit (95 g) has 80 kJ (19 Cals).

Tamarind

A native of Africa and Asia, the tamarind is a member of the pea family. Its leaves, bark, flowers, seed pods and seeds are used. The mature pods are 10–15 cm long and are a rich brown colour when ripe. The acidic seeds are used to season curries and meat, fish or rice dishes or to make chutney, especially in India. The pods contain pulp which is also eaten raw or dried and cooked with sugar. Tamarind juice is also used as a refreshing drink.

Tamarind is high in dietary fibre and potassium and is a source of iron, calcium, and thiamin (vitamin B_1). One tablespoon of the pulp has 210 kJ (50 Cals).

Tangelo

A cross between two different varieties of mandarin. Grown in New Zealand.
See also Mandarin.

Tangerine

A citrus fruit which is also known as a mandarin. The term tangerine is usually used for deep orange or orange-red fruits.
See also Mandarin.

Ugli

A hybrid of a tangerine and a grapefruit, with similar uses and value to either of these fruits.

Watermelon

A melon believed to have originated in southern Italy although some maintain it is native to India or tropical Africa. Now grown in the United States, Australia, Israel, Asia and southern Europe, melons may weigh 2–25 kg. The flesh may be pale pink or bright red and has a white rim near the rind. The white flesh has much less sugar and flavour than the pink flesh but is steamed, candied or made into pickles. The seeds contain an edible oil. Contrary to popular belief, they are not toxic.
See also Melons.

Wax jambu

Also known as the waxy rose apple or the Java rose apple, this tropical fruit is native to Malaysia. The tree has dark glossy leaves, white flowers and produces small pear-shaped fruit about 3–4 cm in diameter. The skin of the fruits is white and red and its pulp is pale and watery in texture, with or without seeds.

The fruits are a good source of vitamin C and provide small quantities of other vitamins, minerals and dietary fibre. 100 g have 70 kJ (17 Cals).

Whortleberry

see Bilberry.

Winter melon

see Vegetables, Melons.

FUNGI

Edible fungi include mushrooms, morels and truffles. Yeasts and moulds are also types of fungi. These organisms live on the decaying parts of other organisms, or on tree roots. In some cases, the fungi takes sugars from the roots and provides minerals such as phosphorus to the soil for the benefit of the tree.

The part of mushrooms and fungi which we eat is the fruiting body which develops for the purposes of making and disseminating spores.

Many types of fungi are eaten throughout the world; others are quite toxic. Those which are enjoyed give distinctive flavours to foods. This is partly due to their high content of an amino acid, glutamic acid, which intensifies flavours. (Monosodium glutamate is the sodium salt of glutamic acid.)

Fungi continue to 'breathe' after being picked and should be used while fresh.

See also Vegetables, Mushrooms; Truffles.

FURANOTERPENES
see Food poisoning.

FUSILLI

Pasta made in the spiral shape of a corkscrew.

G

GADO GADO
see Salads.

GALACTOMANNAN

A gummy type of dietary fibre which is found in legumes. The fibre is water soluble and is made up of polysaccharides of the sugars mannose and galactose. In the stomach, galactomannan absorbs water to form a gel which slows down the rate at which foods are emptied from the stomach. This is of great value to diabetics and anyone with fluctuating blood sugar levels as it means that sugars in foods will take longer to be absorbed into the blood and smaller amounts of insulin will be required.

Galactomannan also prevents some cholesterol being absorbed. Whether it is effective as a bulking agent to help overweight people eat less remains to be seen. Positive results probably depend on the individual and whether he or she stops eating once the stomach feels full.

See also pages 75, 174 and Dietary fibre.

GALACTOSAEMIA

A condition of high levels of galactose (see below) in the blood. It occurs when there is a lack of the enzymes which would normally break down galactose to glucose. In galactosaemia, galactose, and all products which contain lactose, must be omitted from the diet. If not, cataracts and blindness, and occasionally mental retardation, may occur.

GALACTOSE

A simple sugar which is formed when the lactose in milk is digested. Also a constituent of the dietary fibres pectin and galactomannan. Once in the liver, galactose is converted to glucose.

A few people have an inability to metabolise galactose. Such people should avoid milk, fruits and vegetables with a high galactose content.

Galactose content of foods

FRUIT	GALACTOSE (g)
Apple, 1 av., 150g	1.3
Apricot, 2 av.	0.6
canned, 4 halves	0.3
dried, 50 g	0.3
Avocado, $\frac{1}{2}$	0.7
Banana, 1 av.	0.2
Blackberries, 100 g	1.0
Cherries, 120 g, as purchased	0.5
Cranberries, 100 g	1.2
Currants, red, 100 g	0.8
Dates, 50 g	0.4
Figs, fresh, 1	0.5
dried, 2 halves	0.3
Grapefruit, $\frac{1}{2}$ medium	1.5
Grapes, sultana, 120 g	0.4
black, 120 g	0.2
Kiwi fruit, 1 (80 g edible portion)	0.6
Mango, 1 medium (200 g flesh)	3.4
Melon, 150 g slice	0.6
Nectarine, 1 av. 100 g	1.1
Orange, 1 av. 140 g	2.5
Orange juice, 250ml	0.5
Passionfruit, 2 av.	0.3
Peach, 1, 120 g	1.6
canned, $\frac{1}{2}$ cup	0.5
Pear, 1 av. 160 g	1.0
Pineapple, 100 g	0.7
Plums, 2 av. 100 g	2.6
Prunes, 5 av., 80 g	1.4
Raisins, 50 g	0
Raspberries, 100 g	0.9
Rhubarb, 100 g	1.5
Strawberries, 100 g	0.5

VEGETABLES	
Asparagus, 100 g	2.8
Bean sprouts, 50 g	1.4
Beans, 100 g, green	4.1
100 g, green, frozen	5.1
Beans, 120 g baked, canned	1.0
Beans dried, 1 cup cooked	2.7
Beetroot, 100 g	1.1
Broccoli, 100 g	2.7
Brussels sprouts, cooked, 100 g	4.1
Cabbage, raw, 100 g	4.4
Carrots, raw, 100 g	3.4
cooked, 100 g	4.6
Cauliflower, cooked, 100 g	3.2
Celery, 100 g	2.7
Cucumber, 100 g	1.6
Eggplant, 100 g	3.5
Leeks, cooked, 100 g	6.6
Lettuce, 2 leaves, 50 g	1.0
Mushrooms, raw, 100 g	1.1
Onion, raw, 100 g	4.5
Parsnip, cooked, 100 g	2.2
Peas, cooked, 100 g	0.8
Potato, 1 medium, 130 g	2.5
Potato crisps, packet, 30 g	0.7
Pumpkin, raw, 100 g	2.4
Spinach, cooked, 100 g	1.4
Sweetcorn, $\frac{1}{2}$ cup	0.5
Tomato, 1 medium, 120 g	2.0

NUTS	
Chestnuts, 100 g	2.7
Coconut, fresh, 100g	0.8

See also Carbohydrates.

GALANGAL
see Spices.

GALETTE

A flat cake traditionally eaten on Twelfth Night in France. The galette may be sweet or savoury and may have pastry, meringue, potato or a yeast dough as a crust.

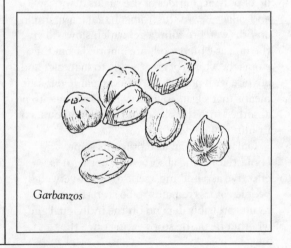

Garbanzos

GALLBLADDER

The organ which concentrates and stores bile from the liver. The presence of food, especially fat, in the upper part of the small intestine, stimulates the gallbladder to contract and squirt its contents through the bile duct into the small intestine.

If the gallbladder becomes inflamed from the presence of gallstones, it may need to be surgically removed. Following surgery, bile passes directly from the liver to the intestine.

GALLIANO
see Drinks, Alcoholic.

GALLSTONES

Gallstones consist of cholesterol, bile pigments and mineral salts. They form when the liver makes bile which is supersaturated with cholesterol and contains abnormally low levels of bile salts and lecithin. Under normal circumstances, these latter substances keep cholesterol in solution. Gallstones are known to occur more commonly in overweight people, particularly women. However, they can occur in thin people if too high a proportion of the diet consists of fat. Polyunsaturated fats seem to be just as bad (some studies have found them to be worse) as any other fat in the formation of gallstones.

Gallstones may rest undisturbed in the gallbladder, but if they move to the bile duct and block it, severe pain results.

Sometimes small gallstones will spontaneously pass into the intestine and will be excreted. In most cases, they must be surgically removed or broken up using laser surgery. If gallstones inflame the gallbladder, or become lodged in the bile duct, fats should be restricted. This is usually no problem as the thought of eating fats nauseates the patient.

GAME
The flesh of any wild animal or bird. Game is sometimes divided into 3 categories:
- Small birds — such as quail
- Winged larger birds — such as wild duck, geese, pheasant, partridge, or ground game — such as rabbit, hare
- Big game — such as venison, wild boar, kangaroo

The larger the game, the stronger the flavour tends to be. Big game often needs to be marinaded and cooked carefully to keep the flesh tender.

Wild animals have nutritional advantages over domesticated animals in that they are much leaner. Left to find their own food, most animals do not become overly fat. The small amount of fat in game is structural fat and is largely polyunsaturated.

Game meats have as much protein, minerals and vitamins as domesticated meats. With their lower fat content, they have fewer kilojoules.

GAMMA LINOLENIC ACID

A polyunsaturated fatty acid with 18 carbon atoms and 3 double bonds. Formed during the metabolism of linoleic acid, and does not occur to any extent in the diet. The few food sources include breast milk and oils made from borage, blackcurrant and evening primrose.

GAMMELOST
see Cheese.

GARAM MASALA
see Spices.

GARBANZOS
see Legumes.

GARFISH
see Fish.

GARLAND CHRYSANTHEMUM
see Vegetables.

GARLIC

see Herbs.

GAS

see Flatulence.

GASTRIC JUICE

The secretions released into the stomach by cells in the stomach walls. Gastric juice is highly acidic (pH about 1.0) and contains the enzymes pepsin and rennin which begin the digestion of proteins.

See also Digestion.

GASTRIN

A hormone which is produced by the stomach walls when food enters the stomach. Gastrin then regulates the flow of gastric juices.

GASTROINTESTINAL TRACT

The tube which begins at the mouth and includes the oesophagus, the stomach, the small intestine (made up of the duodenum, ileum and jejunum) and the large intestine (the colon and rectum) before ending at the anus. The gastrointestinal tract is about 10 m in length.

See also Digestion.

GATEAU

The French term for a cake. Outside France, the term is often used for a rich concoction of several layers of cake with whipped cream, butter cream or other rich fillings.

GAZPACHO

A Spanish soup made from tomatoes, onion, garlic, cucumber, capsicum and olive oil flavoured with pepper and herbs. Served chilled. An average bowl has 670 kJ (160 Cals).

GEFILTE FISH

A Jewish dish of fishballs made from minced fish, onion, matzo meal, bread, eggs and seasonings.

GELATIN

A protein substance extracted from the collagen in animal hides, connective tissue and bone. Forms a gel or glue and is used to make aspic, jellies, souffles, confectionery and also has some industrial uses as glue.

Unlike most animal proteins, gelatin is deficient in several amino acids. It cannot support life or growth. There is no evidence to support the idea that taking extra gelatin will strengthen fingernails. Gelatin contains virtually no vitamins or minerals. Each tablespoon (7 g) has 100 kJ (24 Cals).

Pineapple, pawpaw and figs contain a protein-splitting enzyme which breaks down the protein in gelatin and prevents it forming a gel. To set these fruits in a jelly, they must be cooked to kill the enzyme and allow the gelatin to set. Gelatin is also added to cream to make it more viscous and stabilise the bubbles when it is whipped.

Meat fibres and bones contain gelatin. This is extracted in making stocks and provides the slightly thick texture to sauces made from reduced stocks. When meats with a high content of connective tissue are subjected to long slow cooking, the collagen is converted to gelatin and becomes tender.

GELATO

A flavoured iced dessert usually made from sugar, water, fruits or juices and egg whites. True gelato has no cream or egg yolk and, hence, no fat. Commercial gelato may or may not stick to the basic low-fat formula.

GEMFISH

see fish.

GENOISE SPONGE

A sponge cake made by beating eggs and sugar over hot water until thick and then folding in sifted flour and some melted butter. A small slice (50 g) has 670 kJ (160 Cals).

GHEE

Clarified butter, widely used in Indian cooking. To clarify butter, it is heated until a sediment (made up of a small amount of protein and salt from the butter) settles on the bottom. The melted butter is carefully poured off. Ghee is a purer form of butter and can be heated to a higher temperature without burning.

GHERKIN

Small pickled cucumbers. A true gherkin is a particular type of cucumber with a furrowed prickly skin and is 5–6 cm long.

GIBLETS

The neck, heart, liver and gizzards of poultry. Used for making soups and stocks with a good chicken flavour.

GIMLET
see Drinks, Alcoholic.

GIN
see Drinks, Alcoholic.

GINGER
see Spices.

GINGER BEER
see Drinks, Non-alcoholic.

GINSENG

A plant grown in Korea and surrounded by stories of its powers to cure all manner of diseases. The name ginseng comes from the same Greek root as the word 'panacea'.

Top of ginseng's long list of credits is its supposed aphrodisiac qualities. It is also supposed to relieve fatigue, counteract the effects of alcohol, improve hormone production and fertility, and reduce blood fats. Ginseng is also used as a dietary supplement to promote general health and finds its way into tea, drinks, shampoos, soaps and face creams.

The original ginseng legend concerned a woman to whom a god revealed in a dream a secret place on a high mountain. Here she would find a special plant growing. The woman was to nurture the plant for 6 years and then eat an extract from its root which would bring her great health and happiness. From this humble story, the power of ginseng grew. Today it is one of Korea's major exports, and is also grown in the United States and China. Ginseng is so valuable that it is carefully tended for the 5–7 years it takes to mature from seed to plant.

Analysis of ginseng shows that it contains small quantities of steroid hormones. The amounts present in most ginseng preparations are too small to have any significant effect and most of its reputed actions are due to a placebo effect. However, those with high blood pressure are warned against taking any concentrated ginseng products as they could make their condition worse.

GIN SLING
see Drinks, Alcoholic.

GIZZARDS

The hind part of a bird's stomach, located behind the crop and the intestine. Contains small stones which have a mechanical effect in helping to grind food. In some countries, hen's gizzards are boiled to use for soups, stocks or to eat.

GJETOST
see Cheese.

GLIADIN

Part of the protein gluten in wheat. Gliadin proteins are long molecules made up of several thousand atoms which tend to form compact balls. They are important in giving structure to bread doughs.

GLOBE ARTICHOKE
see Vegetables, Artichoke.

GLOBULINS

Proteins which are insoluble in water but will dissolve in salt water. Found in blood (in the serum), in egg white (they provide some of the stability of beaten egg whites) and in milk.

GLOGG
see Drinks, Alcoholic.

GLOSSITIS

An inflammation of the tongue in which it appears red, swollen and inflamed. May arise from deficiencies of several of the B vitamins or iron.

GLUCONEOGENESIS

The process whereby the body produces glucose from proteins, lactic acid, glycerol and pyruvic acid. This process is important to keep the body's blood sugar level normal when no carbohydrate foods are being eaten (as occurs with some slimming diets and with fasting). Gluconeogenesis usually means that lean muscle tissue will be broken down. It is the body's way of protecting vital organs such as the brain which need glucose as a fuel.

See also Blood sugar.

GLUCOSE

Also known as dextrose or grape sugar, glucose is the major sugar in the blood and ultimately provides energy for all body cells. However, we do not need to eat glucose as such. It is formed from the digestion of all other simple and complex carbohydrates and can also be made from proteins in the diet or from muscle protein.

In spite of the advertisements which imply that glucose will provide instant energy, there is absolutely no advantage in eating glucose. The energy for physical activity comes from

glycogen in the muscle cells and this depends on carbohydrates eaten many hours earlier. Eating glucose will put glucose into the stomach from where it will go to the small intestine from where it will pass into the blood. This process is not instant and takes some hours. Glucose is only useful when being given by intravenous drip to by-pass the stomach.

When glucose is absorbed, the pancreas produces insulin, the hormone which is necessary for glucose to enter the cells. Once in the cells, glucose is metabolised to provide energy for use by compounds such as ATP (see page 11).

Glucose is present in some foods. Honey is about one-third glucose and some fruits and vegetables also contain naturally occurring glucose. The highest content of glucose in these products is as follows:

FOOD	GLUCOSE (g)
Mango, av.	11
Grapes, 120 g	8
Cherries, 120 g	7
Banana, av.	7
Orange, 1 medium	4
Onion, 1 medium	2
Apricots, 100 g	2
Strawberries, 100 g	2

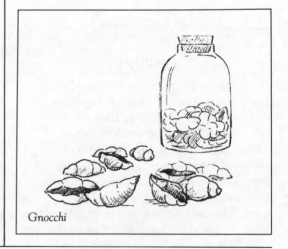

Gnocchi

Mueslis and health-food bars may also contain added glucose. In soft drinks, the added sugar (sucrose) breaks down to glucose and fructose. Prepared fruit juices also contain glucose.

See also Carbohydrates.

GLUCOSE TOLERANCE TEST (GTT)

A test to measure how well one secretes insulin in response to a given load of glucose. Used as one of the diagnostic tests for diabetes mellitus. After fasting overnight, 75 g of glucose are given and the blood glucose levels measured every half hour. Normally, blood glucose level does not rise above 8 mmol/L and returns to 4−5 mmol/L within two hours. In diabetes, there is a greater rise in blood sugar and glucose may spill over from the blood into the urine.

GLUTAMIC ACID

An amino acid which is involved in the formation of a substance which carries nerve impulses in the brain. Not essential in the diet since it can be made from other amino acids. The intense flavour of truffles is due in part to their high content of glutamic acid. The sodium salt of glutamic acid is monosodium glutamate (see page 233).

GLUTEN

The most important protein in wheat, made up of gliadin and glutenin. When mixed with water, gluten becomes sticky and holds wheat flour together to give a firm strength to the structure of dough. Hard wheats have a high gluten content and are used for making pasta and bread. Soft wheats have less gluten and are more suitable for fine crumbed products such as cakes and biscuits.

High gluten flours from hard wheat produce breads of good volume with a well-developed crust and a strong, elastic texture.

Wheat has much more gluten than other grains. Rye has some gluten but tends to make a heavier, less crusty bread. Oats and barley have only small amounts of gluten.

Gluten extracted from wheat is also used to make vegetarian products, sausages and pet foods.

Some people have an inherited sensitivity to gluten (coeliac disease) and must avoid it by having a gluten-free diet. Gluten-free breads, biscuits, cakes, pasta and breakfast cereals are available for these people. Without gluten, breads tend to be heavy and more like a scone in texture than bread.

See also Coeliac Disease.

GLUTENIN

Along with gliadin, glutenin makes up gluten, the protein in wheat.

GLYCEROL

A clear sweet substance which is chemically an alcohol. Widely used as a softening agent in cakes, shortenings, icings and desserts. Glycerol also has many non-food uses in lotions, cosmetics, candles, various drugs, serums and vaccines and in protective coatings and paints.

In nutrition, glycerol attaches itself to fatty acids to make up triglycerides — the major type of fat present in foods. Glycerol forms about 10 per cent of triglycerides (see page 348).

GLYCOGEN

The storage form of carbohydrate in animals, glycogen consists of chains of glucose molecules. Glycogen is stored in liver and muscles. Liver glycogen is used to replenish the blood sugar level. About 80−90 g of glycogen are stored in the liver after meals which contain carbohydrate. This is used up as required during the ensuing period. After 12 hours without food, liver glycogen stores are empty. The blood sugar level is then maintained by breaking down proteins in lean muscle tissue.

Muscle glycogen stores are much larger and are very much influenced by diet and exercise.

Muscle glycogen cannot be broken down to supply glucose to the blood as the enzyme necessary for the conversion is not present in muscles. Glycogen in muscles is solely for the use of muscles. During anaerobic activity (without oxygen, see page 23), glycogen is the only fuel available for muscles. Even in aerobic activity, glycogen is still an important fuel and its supplies are usually the limiting factor for physical endurance.

For athletes, it is extremely important to maintain adequate stores of glycogen in the muscles and liver. Glycogen stores in muscles can be increased by increasing the amount of carbohydrate in the diet (see Carbohydrate loading, page 56). In the short term, any type of carbohydrate (that is, sugars or complex carbohydrates) will increase glycogen stores. However, in the longer term, the best increases have been obtained from complex carbohydrates rather than sugar. For other nutritional reasons, athletes are advised to build up their glycogen stores by eating more grains, breads, cereals, vegetables and fruits rather than simply eating more sugar.

High intensity exercise, such as competitive sport, uses glycogen for fuel. Maximising glycogen stores is therefore important for sportspeople. However, even for those who do not follow such active pursuits, glycogen is an important fuel for physical activity. Slimming diets which 'work' by depleting glycogen stores thus make exercise difficult.

Once glycogen stores fall, fatigue results. This may often be the cause of mistakes and accidents. It thus makes sense to eat a diet which will provide good stores of glycogen.

Once glycogen stores are depleted, re-feeding will increase them beyond their previous level. This is the principle behind carbohydrate loading. The same situation occurs when people come 'off' a slimming diet. With a low carbohydrate diet, the muscle cells will have used their glycogen. As soon as the person begins to eat normally, the muscle cells immediately store up extra glycogen. Since every gram of glycogen is stored with almost 3 times its weight of water, re-feeding someone who has not been eating results in a greater weight gain (see Diets, slimming, page 93).

See also Carbohydrates; Exercise; Fats; Weight reduction.

GNOCCHI

A type of pasta made from a cornmeal/milk mixture or semolina/pureed vegetable mixture. The paste is cooked over a low heat, spread out to set, cut into squares (or other shapes) and simmered in boiling water.

GOAT

The flesh of young goats (kids) is eaten in some parts of the world, especially in Middle Eastern countries. The young flesh is quite tender but older goats tend to be tough and require long slow cooking. The meat is fairly low in fat and high in protein, iron and various other minerals and vitamins. 100 g of goat meat have 755 kJ (180 Cals).

GOAT'S MILK

Goat's milk is an alternative to cow's milk. Nutritionally, the products have a number of similarities and a few differences. These are shown below:

PER 100 g	COW'S MILK	GOAT'S MILK
protein (g)	3.3	3.3
fat (g)	3.8	4.5
carbohydrate (g)	4.7	4.6
sodium (mg)	50	40
potassium (mg)	150	180
calcium (mg)	120	130
phosphorus (mg)	95	110
iron (mg)	0.05	0.04
vitamin A (mcg)	39	40
vitamin D (mcg)	0.03	0.06
vitamin B1 (mg)	0.04	0.04
riboflavin (mg)	0.19	0.15

niacin (mg)	0.08	0.19
vitamin C (mg)	1.5	1.5
vitamin B_6 (mg)	0.04	0.04
vitamin B_{12}		
(mcg)	0.3	trace
folacin (mcg)	5.0	1.0
pantothenic acid		
(mg)	0.35	0.34
biotin (mcg)	2.0	2.0
calories	65	71
kilojoules	275	300

The important differences are that goat's milk has more fat and less vitamin B_{12} and folacin than cow's milk. These differences can be significant for infants being fed goat's milk.

Most children who are allergic to cow's milk protein are also allergic to goat's milk protein. These allergic reactions occur in an immature digestive system which does not break the proteins down to their smallest amino acid units. As the child matures, the problem usually disappears.

A few children who react to cow's milk do not have any problems with goat's milk. For the rest, there is no advantage in switching to goat's milk unless it is more convenient or economical.

Goat's milk is also made into excellent quality yoghurts and cheeses.

GOITRE

An enlargement of the thyroid gland due to a dietary deficiency of iodine.

See also Iodine.

GOITRINS

Compounds which occur naturally in vegetables of the cabbage family, cassava and soya beans, which interfere with the way the thyroid gland uses iodine. In areas of long-term iodine deficiency, eating a very large quantity of cabbage or cauliflower could exacerbate goitre. In practice, you are unlikely to get goitre from eating cauliflower or cabbage but such a practice could make an existing goitre worse.

See also Food poisoning.

GOLDEN BERRY

see Fruit, Cape gooseberry.

GOLDEN SYRUP

A syrup produced during the refining of sugar. The golden colour of the syrup comes from the small amounts of molasses which still remain. Golden syrup has bout 20 per cent water and contains some potassium and a little calcium. It has no vitamins. 100 g of golden syrup have 1230 kJ (295 Cals).

GOLDFISH

see Carp.

GOOSE

The flesh of the goose is sometimes used as a meat but it is the liver of the goose which is particularly prized for making the rich pâté, foie gras. The flesh of goose is high in protein, fat, iron and potassium. Only young birds are tender enough to be eaten. 100 g roast goose have 22 g of fat (about 5 times the level in chicken and turkey) and 1340 kJ (320 Cals).

Colonial goose was an Australian dish made from a boned and stuffed shoulder of hogget and popular in the early days of the colony. The resemblance to a goose was achieved by removing the flat blade bone but leaving the shank attached. When cooked, this bone was meant to look like a goose with its head raised.

GOOSEBERRY

see Fruit.

GORGONZOLA

see Cheese.

GOUDA

see Cheese.

167

GOUGERE

A choux pastry mixture cooked as one large
'puff' and served with a sauce or filling.

GOULASH

A Hungarian stew flavoured with paprika. An
average serve has 1900 kJ (455 Cals).

GOURDS
see Vegetables.

GOUT

A form of arthritis which affects the joints,
especially the joint in the big toe. Crystals of
sodium urate (from uric acid) accumulate in the
joint causing swelling, redness and extreme
pain. Kidney stones may also develop. The uric
acid is derived from purines which are
constituents of nucleoproteins.

Treatment for gout involves weight
reduction (if overweight) plus some restriction
on alcohol, and on foods containing purines
and fats (see also Purines).

Drugs are normally used to treat gout and the
major dietary restrictions these days are
alcoholic drinks and fatty foods.

Alcohol is involved in gout because it causes
the level of lactic acid in the blood to rise.
Lactic acid competes for the same transport
system in the kidneys as uric acid and when
large amounts of alcohol are consumed, the
kidneys cannot excrete uric acid properly. The
uric acid level in the blood rises, causing gout.

See also Uric acid.

GRAINS
See following pages.

GRAMMA
see Fruit.

GRANADILLA
see Fruit, Passionfruit.

GRAND MARNIER
see Drinks, Alcoholic.

GRANOLA

The original granola was a breakfast cereal
devised by Dr John Harvey Kellogg in 1877.
It was made from wheat, oats and cornmeal
baked into biscuits and then ground up.
Modern versions of granola use a mixture of
cereals, vegetable fat (usually palm or coconut
oil), dried fruits, sugar and/or honey and nuts
baked and then broken up. In some countries
the modern product is known as toasted muesli.
It is high in fat and sugar and its only
redeeming nutritional virtue is that it may
contain some dietary fibre.

For a typical granola recipe, $\frac{1}{2}$ cup (60 g) has
16 g of fat and 1220 kJ (290 Cals).

GRANULATED SUGAR

The term used in the United States for general
purpose white sugar.

GRAPE
see Fruit.

GRAPEFRUIT
see Fruit.

GRAPE SEED OIL
see Oils.

GRAPE SUGAR
see Glucose.

GRASSHOPPER
see Drinks, Alcoholic.

GRAVAD LAX

Smoked salmon.

GRAYLING
see Fish.

GREAT NORTHERN BEAN
see Legumes.

GREEK SALAD
see Salads.

GRAINS

The cultivation of cereal grains was a momentous step in human history. It marked a transition from a nomadic way of life to the development of settlements, towns and cities.

Grains were first gathered from wild grasses and either boiled and eaten, or, more commonly, pounded into flour, mixed with water and roasted. Different types of grain crops were grown in various parts of the world, according to the seeds available and climatic conditions.

All grains are valuable from the nutritional point of view. They are rich in complex carbohydrates and provide a good source of different types of dietary fibre as well as contributing most of the world's protein and a large portion of the minerals and vitamins needed. They are relatively easy to grow and transport and can be stored for long periods with their nutritional value intact.

Barley

One of the oldest cultivated cereals, barley is a tough grain which can be grown in both drought and frosty areas. It does less well in acidic soil. Barley originally grew in northern Africa and Southeast Asia, and was once used as the basic unit of the Sumerian measuring system from 4000–2000 BC.

Until the early part of this century, barley was the major grain used in Japan. The barley was 'pearled' (meaning the outer brown layers were removed). Barley was also widely used in China, often ground into a flour with lentils and used to make bread. Today barley is still eaten in the Middle East and also in Tibet. In Middle Eastern countries, it is either ground into a flour and made into flat cakes, or boiled and used like rice. In Tibet, Buddhist monks carry a bag of barley flour to mix with yak's milk and cook into a porridge called tsampa. If cooking facilities are not available, the flour and milk are mixed to a dough, rolled into small balls and eaten raw.

Nutritionally, barley is a useful grain with about 6.5 per cent dietary fibre, much of which is valuable soluble fibre. It contains slightly more of most nutrients than rice. 100 g of raw barley have 1535 kJ (360 Cals) — about the same as most grains.

Buckwheat

Although it is usually included with cereals, buckwheat is not a true cereal but the fruit of a herbaceous plant. It originated in Asia and flourished in China where it was made into a bread. Once introduced to Europe, buckwheat was more commonly made into a porridge or eaten steamed. It grows well on poor soil which will not support grains.

Buckwheat is made into pancakes, pasta and biscuit products and is useful for people who are allergic to wheat.

Nutritionally, it resembles grains with about 8 per cent protein, vitamins of the B group, a selection of minerals and some dietary fibre. 100 g have 1520 kJ (363 Cals).

Bulgur

A product made by grinding wheat which has already been cooked and dried. Its subtle, slightly nutty flavour is popular in Eastern Europe. Because the wheat has already been cooked, bulgur takes little preparation. Simply pour boiling water over the grain, allowing 2 cups of water to 1 cup of bulgur. Cover tightly and leave to stand for about 10 mins until all the water is absorbed. The bulgur can be eaten hot as an accompaniment to poultry or meats (as you would serve rice), or mixed with

169

parsley, cucumber, tomato and dressing and served as a salad.

Corn

Native to Mexico, corn has been the staple food for the Indians of South and Central America for thousands of years (see page 83). Different varieties of corn are now grown for human and animal food. It is used both as a vegetable and a grain and is also important in the United States as a base material for corn syrup, corn oil (more commonly called maize oil, see page 251) and as a base material in making bourbon whisky.

Nutritionally, corn lacks some amino acids (see page 21) but contains adequate quantities of vitamins and minerals and is an important source of complex carbohydrate and dietary fibre. 100 g of cornmeal have 1485 kJ (355 Cals). Sweetcorn has 1655 kJ (395 Cals) in 100 g.

Millet

Millet is mostly regarded as a bird seed, but this hardy grain was once the main cereal in Europe. It began life well before that, however, in Egypt and simultaneously in parts of Africa and Asia. It was a staple grain in China before rice and is still widely used in India, Ethiopia, the Soviet Union and Egypt. Millet has a good content of protein but does not contain the gluten which is needed for a good loaf of bread. It is used for flat breads and is the major ingredient in the national bread of Ethiopia, injera. It is also used in stews and soups, or mixed with various legumes.

Millet contains dietary fibre, various vitamins of the B complex and a selection of minerals. 100 g of millet have 1485 kJ (355 Cals).

Oats

Native to Central Europe, oats were neglected as a grain for some time. They were first used when the legions of the Roman Empire discovered them growing in amongst barley. As oats were well-suited to cool wet areas, they became a staple in Scotland, Ireland and the north of England. Although the consumption of oats has declined dramatically in Scotland, the Scots still love their oatmeal porridge and oat cakes. Oats are also an ingredient in the famous Scottish haggis (see page 303).

Oats have been returned to favour in the Western world since the discovery that the soluble fibre they contain is useful to lower blood cholesterol levels (see Dietary fibre, page 92). They are now being consumed as porridge, muesli or in the form of oat bran (see page 248).

Nutritionally, oats are an excellent product. They contain more fat than most grains and this is high in the essential fatty acids. They also have a much higher protein level than most grains and are a good source of iron, zinc, potassium and other minerals (including manganese), vitamin E and other vitamins. They have a higher level of dietary fibre than most cereals and, like barley, much of this fibre is in the form of valuable gums. 100 g of oats have 1675 kJ (400 Cals). Since an average serve of porridge can be made from 25 g of oats, plus water and milk or low-fat milk if desired, the idea that porridge is a fattening food is quite unfounded. A bowl of porridge has no more kilojoules than a bowl of a light, puffed or popped breakfast cereal. Oats can be quickly cooked in a microwave. By making it in the bowl, there is no need to wash up a dirty porridge saucepan.

Rolled oats are made by flattening the oat. Quick cooking oats are made by cutting the oats into finer flakes. No nutritional value is lost. Oat bran is a finer product again. Unless the oat bran retains some of the endosperm of the oat, it will not have the kind of dietary fibre which is valuable for lowering blood cholesterol.

Rice

Once believed to be native to China, it is now thought that rice originated in India. It has, however, been used as the staple diet in China for at least 5000 years. Rice thrives in warm humid areas and needs copious quantities of water. It is usually grown in paddies which are submerged in water until the grain is ready to ripen. The paddies are then drained and the rice is picked and harvested by machines.

There are many types of rice available. The most commonly eaten is polished white rice in which the bran has been removed by abrasive milling. Unfortunately, this also removes some of the dietary fibre, minerals and vitamins. Parboiled or converted rice is partially cooked with the bran layer still present, then dried and the bran removed. Many of the nutrients pass into the grain. Brown rice includes all the bran and has the highest nutritional value.

Grains of rice may be round or long and narrow (long-grained rice). The more broken grains present in raw rice, the more gluggy the rice will be when cooked. Sticky or glutinous rice is a variety which becomes quite sticky when cooked. It is available as black sticky rice (more of a purple colour) or white. It is used in some parts of Asia, often for sweets. Basmati rice grows in the foothills of the Himalayas and has a slightly aromatic flavour.

Patna rice is a high quality long-grained rice with grains which tend to remain firm and fluffy when cooked. Slightly creamy-coloured. Also known as Carolina rice.

Wild rice is not really a rice at all but a tall aquatic grass which grows in China, Japan and the Great Lakes region of North America. It is difficult to cultivate which is the reason for its high cost.

Brown and parboiled rice are good sources of dietary fibre, minerals and vitamins but all rice supplies some of these. Rice is also a good source of complex carbohydrate. 100 g of raw rice have 1505 kJ (360 Cals). It absorbs water during cooking and a cup of cooked rice (160 g) has 860 kJ (205 Cals). Many people believe rice to be a fattening food. The number of slender Asian people who eat up to a kilogram of raw rice each day shows that this is not the case. It is not grains which contribute kilojoules so much as what is served with them.

Rye

A fairly recent grain in comparison with other grains, rye was taken to Britain by the Saxons in AD 500. Rye made up a large part of the basic dark breads commonly eaten throughout Europe. Today, rye is still eaten in Eastern Europe and in Germany (in pumperknickel bread) and Scandinavia. In parts of the United States which were originally settled by the Dutch, rye breads are also popular. Only small quantities of rye are used in Australia.

Rye flour contains gluten but not as much as wheat flour. In making bread, rye produces a heavy loaf unless mixed with some wheat flour.

Rye is a nutritious grain and supplies dietary fibre as well as many minerals and vitamins. 100 g of rye have 1400 kJ (335 Cals).

Sorghum

The staple grain of Africa and parts of Asia, sorghum is rarely used in most Western countries. Its history is not well known although it is clear that the Egyptians cultivated sorghum in 2200 BC. Sorghum is also called kaffir corn, Guinea corn or African corn. Sorghum can be used in the same way as rice or it can be ground into a flour to use in flat breads and cakes. When young, the sorghum plant contains a high level of prussic acid which is poisonous to cattle (and humans). As the plant matures and is cut and dried, the prussic acid content is dissipated and it can be used for cattle feed.

Sorghum grain is high in protein, iron, niacin and dietary fibre. It also contains a range of other minerals and vitamins. 100 g of raw grain have 1380 kJ (330 Cals).

Triticale

This grain is a hybrid of rye and wheat and was first developed in the 1960s in an effort to produce a rye with a higher gluten content. Triticale is used only to a small extent in breads and some specialised pasta and biscuits. It can be used in place of wheat or rye grains or flour.

Nutritionally, triticale is an excellent product with a good content of protein, iron, potassium and vitamins of the B complex. 100 g of the grain have 1505 kJ (360 Cals).

Wheat

Wheat was first cultivated in western parts of Asia, and has been milled since at least 4000 BC when the Egyptians used stone grinding wheels to break down the grain. They added water and made flat cakes which were baked on hot stones. Today wheat is grown in many parts of the world with the United States, the Soviet Union, Canada, Argentina, Australia and European countries being the largest producers.

Most wheat is used to make bread (see page 43). It is ideally suited to this because of its high content of gluten, a protein which gives structure to bread (see page 165).

Hard wheats have the highest gluten content; soft wheats the lowest. The very hard wheats such as durum wheat are used to make pasta. Hard wheats are also used to make breads while soft wheats are used for cake flour.

Cracked wheat (burghul or bulgur) is also used in many European and Middle Eastern countries. It is sold in parboiled form, is quick to prepare and can be used like rice (see page 171).

Wheat flour is available as wholemeal (or wholewheat in the United States) or white flour. Some countries, including Australia, allow the flour to be bleached (see Flour, page 132) to look white; others find bleaching an unnecessary step and sell a white flour which is cream coloured.

Wheat is also used to make pasta of all shapes and sizes, breakfast cereals (the largest selling cereal in Australia is a wholewheat breakfast biscuit) and a range of baked goods.

Wholegrain wheat is a highly nutritious grain with plenty of vitamins of the B complex, vitamin E, protein, dietary fibre and a range of minerals. 100 g of wheat have 1380 kJ (300 Cals).

White flour still retains a substantial proportion of its nutrients although more than half the dietary fibre is lost. In some countries, white flour has added vitamins or minerals. In Australia, the white flour is considered nutritious enough not to need this fortification.

GREEN BEANS
see Vegetables, Beans.

GREEN GODDESS DRESSING

A mayonnaise dressing flavoured with tarragon vinegar, garlic, anchovies and pepper. Sometimes has added parsley.

GREEN GRAM
see Legumes, Mung beans.

GREEN PEPPER
see Vegetables, Capsicum.

GREENS
see Colourings.

GREEN SALAD
see Salads.

GREEN TEA
see Tea.

GRENACHE
see Wine, Varieties.

GRENADINE
see Drinks, Non-alcoholic.

GRIDDLE CAKES

Flat cakes originally cooked on a hot iron plate. Some griddle cakes are thin, others are made from a thicker batter. They may be sweet or savoury and encompass pikelets (see page 268), Scottish bannocks (see page 33) or blini (see page 39). The basic batter is made from flour, a leavening agent (usually baking powder), milk and eggs.

GRILLING

Called 'broiling' in the United States, food is grilled by placing it close to an intense heat until brown. If necessary, the food is then turned to brown the other side. Meats are cooked on both sides, cheese is grilled until it melts, most fish only need to be grilled on one side. Meats with a large proportion of connective tissue are not suitable for grilling. Since it uses no fat, and permits fat to drip out of products, such as meats, grilling is generally considered a healthy method of cooking. However, there is some loss of niacin (one of the B vitamins) and minerals such as iron in the meat drippings. The longer meat is grilled, the greater the nutrient losses.

GRITS

Coarsely ground grain or beans. Corn grits (also known as hominy) and soya bean grits are the most commonly used.

GROATS

Wholegrain products, especially oats.

GROPER, OR GROUPER
see Fish.

GROUNDNUTS
see Nuts, Peanuts.

GROUSE

Generally considered to be the best-tasting of the game birds. The bird is native to Scotland and there are many varieties in Europe but no true grouse in the United States. The birds are fairly small and one bird may be served to each person. They can be roasted or grilled. Older birds can be cooked in casseroles.

GROWTH, CHILDREN AND NUTRITION
see Children, growth and nutrition.

GRUEL

A thin porridge made by simmering rice, wheat or oats with water. Although often recommended for invalids, gruel has no nutritional advantages over thicker porridges or some more appetising dish incorporating grains.

GRUYERE

see Cheese.

GTT

see Glucose Tolerance Test.

GUACAMOLE

A Mexican dish made from avocado, chilli, garlic, lemon and onion. Often served with corn chips. A quarter of a cup has 460 kJ (110 Cals).

GUAR GUM

A soluble type of dietary fibre derived from the seeds of the cluster bean, a leguminous plant which grows in India. The gum is a creamy white powder obtained by removing the husk and germ from the seed and grinding the remaining endosperm to a white powder.

See also pages 75, 159.

Guar has a great ability to form a gel in water. In small quantities it has been used in icecream, soft-serve icecream products, salad dressings, relishes and in doughs for baked goods. Large quantities have not been used since it is unpalatable and difficult to swallow before it sets into a hard gel in the throat.

Some recent guar gum products have included biscuits and capsules which dissolve in water and can be drunk before becoming too thick.

The reason for using guar has been to improve diabetic control. Guar contains

galactomannan (see page 159), a valuable gelling agent. Attempts have also been made to use guar as a pre-meal substance for overweight people so that they will consume less food. At this stage, guar appears to be a helpful product for diabetics to improve glucose control and, possibly, to help lower cholesterol levels. Its major problem is its unpalatability.

GUAVA

see Fruit.

GUGELHOF

A yeasted cake containing flour, eggs, yeast, butter and rum-soaked dried fruits, the gugelhof was the first of this type of cake and was traditionally made in Alsace. Subsequently, the savarin and baba versions have developed.

GUINEA FOWL

Originally from Africa, guinea fowl have been domesticated in many parts of the world. The flesh is tender (especially that of the hens) and has a gamey flavour a little like pheasant. Usually roasted or cooked in a casserole.

GUMBO

The word gumbo comes from an African word for okra (see page 366). Gumbo is a Creole stew containing the vegetable okra plus tomatoes, onion, smoked ham and either chicken, seafood or meat. The okra gives the gumbo a thick, smooth, almost jelly-like texture.

GUMS

Substances found naturally in certain plants and seaweeds. Used in foods as thickeners and to provide texture to foods such as salad dressings. Gum arabic from the *Acacia senegal* tree prevents sugars crystallising in foods. Gum tragacanth is used for coating sugar cake decorations so that they do not pick up moisture from the atmosphere.

The type of dietary fibre in gums may be

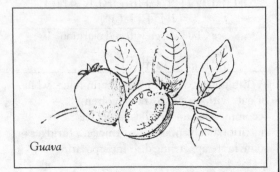
Guava

valuable in the treatment of diabetes and fluctuating blood sugar levels, and also in the prevention and treatment of constipation.

Gums such as those found in oats and legumes, as well as guar gum extracted from the cluster bean, form gels in the stomach. This slows down the rate at which carbohydrates are released for absorption into the blood.

Carbohydrates are normally digested to glucose which is then absorbed into the blood. As the blood glucose level increases, insulin is released from the pancreas. A sudden flow of glucose into the blood results in a sharp increase in insulin production. When gums are present, the glucose enters the blood much more slowly and spreads out the production of insulin. This is of benefit to diabetics and others who cannot tolerate sudden peaks in blood sugar levels.

Further down the intestine, gums are completely digested by bacteria, causing the bacteria to multiply in the process. The bodies of these bacteria then add to the faecal bulk and prevent constipation. During the bacterial fermentation, some acids are also produced which may be of benefit.

The quantity of gums added to foods such as thickened cream or salad dressing, is small. Those wishing to take in more gums are advised to eat oats and legumes.

See also Dietary fibre; Grains, Oats; Guar gum.

GURNARD

see Fish.

HADDOCK

see Fish.

HAEM IRON

The type of iron found in haemoglobin. In foods, haem iron comes from animal muscle and is found in meat, chicken and seafoods. Non-haem iron in vegetables and grains is not as well-absorbed by the body as the haem iron.

See also Iron.

HAEMOCHROMATOSIS

A condition of excessive iron in the liver. Occurs in some African tribes who brew beer in iron pots. The alcohol causes iron to dissolve into the beverage.

See also Siderosis.

HAEMOGLOBIN

A compound in red blood cells consisting of a protein (the globin) and a haem molecule which contains iron. As red blood cells pass through the lungs, oxygen attaches itself to the heme part of haemoglobin and is then transported to the tissues where it is needed for the production of energy.

HAEMORRHOIDS

Commonly called 'piles', haemorrhoids occur in the anus as a result of constipation. They are common in people in Western countries, occurring in almost half the population over 50 in the United States. They are rare in countries where the dietary fibre intake is high.

Haemorrhoids occur when normal cushions

of blood vessels in the anus are subjected to pressure from hard stools. As a result of abdominal straining to pass stools, the blood vessels become engorged with blood and swell. Straining gradually pushes the cushions down through the anal canal until they protrude and may bleed. Haemorrhoids can be prevented by a high-fibre diet and plenty of water so that only soft stools are produced.

HAGGIS
see Sausages.

HAIR

The condition of hair depends partly on diet. In malnutrition, hair is dull, has no lustre and may become very wiry. The normal differences between fine and coarse hair are related to genetics rather than diet. Those who have naturally coarse or wiry hair need not fear they are malnourished. Greying of hair and baldness are also unrelated to nutrition. Rats which are deficient in pantothenic acid (vitamin B_5) do turn grey but this is not the cause of grey hair in humans. In spite of enthusiastic salespeople, taking pantothenic acid supplements will not restore hair colour.

HAKE
see Fish.

HALIBUT
see Fish.

HALOUMI
see Cheese.

HALVA

A sweet made from sugar, water, butter, semolina and nuts or seeds. Indian halva is flavoured with cardamom and saffron, while halva prepared in Mediterranean countries usually contains cinnamon.

Nutritional values for halva will vary with the recipe used. It is a good source of iron and vitamins and also supplies some protein and dietary fibre. In energy, an average value would be 770 kJ (185 Cals) for a 30 g piece.

HAM

Pig meat (from the leg or shoulder) which is preserved by salting, smoking or drying. Sodium nitrite is also added as a preservative and to maintain the pink colour. This slows down the growth of bacteria and so gives longer keeping qualities. Most hams now have a lower level of salt and preservatives and must be kept refrigerated. Leg ham has the best flavour. Many shoulder or sandwich hams are made from pork offcuts.

Hams have been produced for thousands of years throughout Europe and parts of Asia. They are unacceptable to those whose religious beliefs do not allow them to eat pig.

Sugar-cured hams have slightly less salt and a softer texture. They are generally regarded as top quality products.

Nutritionally, hams vary depending on the cut of meat used. Their fat content may be as low as 3–5 per cent, or many times that much. Salt content also varies and reduced salt products are now available. Average sodium content for regular hams in 50 g of ham is around 600 mg. 50 g of an average lean ham would have 275 kJ (65 Cals).

HAMBURGER

A popular fast food which originated as a minced steak patty in the German city of Hamburg and was popularised in the United States. A hamburger consists of a meat patty placed inside a soft bread roll, with ingredients such as tomato sauce, lettuce, tomato, onion, egg, bacon, cheese, mayonnaise or dill pickles added. Australian hamburgers traditionally contain a slice of beetroot. Depending on the ingredients, a hamburger can be a well-balanced meal. Some large hamburgers, however, are high in fat and kilojoules. A Big

FRUIT

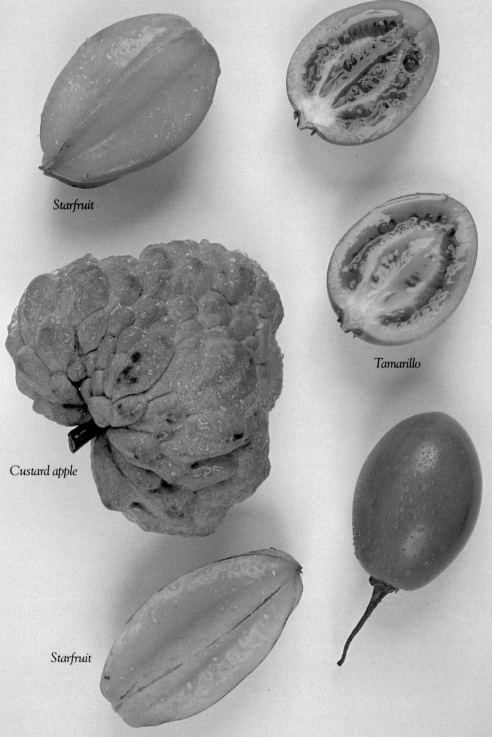

Starfruit

Tamarillo

Custard apple

Starfruit

GRAINS

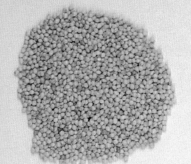

Millet (unhulled)

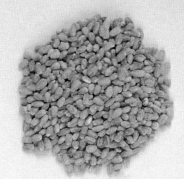

Barley (unpearled)

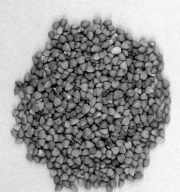

Buckwheat (raw)

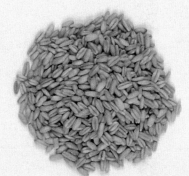

Oats (hulled)

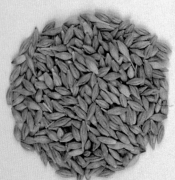

Barley (unhulled)

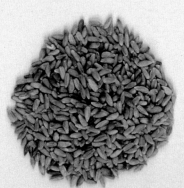

Rye (whole)

Mac has 2405 kJ (570 Cals) and 31 g of fat. A regular hamburger has 1630 kJ (390 Cals) and 18 g of fat.

HARD SAUCE

A combination of butter, sugar and usually some type of alcohol (such as rum or brandy). A lump of this solid 'sauce' is traditionally served with hot plum pudding. Also known as brandy or rum butter. A 60 g serve has 1200 kJ (285 Cals).

HARICOT BEANS
see Legumes.

HARICOT OF MUTTON

A casserole made from pieces of mutton (or lamb), potatoes, onions, turnips and herbs. The ingredients are cut into small pieces and cooked in a moderate oven.

HARVEY WALLBANGER
see Drinks, Alcoholic.

HASH BROWNS

A North American dish made by browning sliced potatoes in oil, butter or some other type of fat. Nutritionally, hash browns are high in fat and kilojoules; the exact amount will vary according to the amount of fat used. An average cup of hash browns has 1490 kJ (355 Cals).

HAVARTI
see Cheese.

HAY FEVER

A condition characterised by runny nose, sore eyes and headache, caused by an allergy to seeds and pollens, typically those in the air when hay is being cut. Some sufferers of hay fever may have a sensitivity to either a natural or added chemical in foods.

See also Allergies.

HAZELNUT
see Nuts.

HAZELNUT OIL
see Oils.

HDL CHOLESTEROL
see Lipoproteins.

HEALTH FOODS

The term used to describe foods which have been subjected to minimal processing. Some use it for products which have been grown without fertilisers or pesticides.

HEART

The heart pumps blood containing oxygen and nutrients to all body tissues. For its size (230–340 g), the heart is a remarkable organ, pumping some 10,000 L of blood each day. The muscular wall of the heart (the myocardium) does so much work that it needs much more blood than any other muscle in the body. This is supplied by the coronary arteries — narrow branching structures with a diameter similar to that of a drinking straw. A blockage in a coronary artery (either from a blood clot or a build-up of fatty deposits) leads to a myocardial infarction, or heart attack (an interruption to the blood supply to the heart wall, or myocardium). When this occurs, an area of the heart muscle is deprived of oxygen and dies. This may result in sudden death, or the area may heal (leaving a scar).

See also Atherosclerosis.

HEARTBURN

This condition has nothing to do with love. It is a sharp burning pain felt immediately behind the sternum (breast bone) and is due to acid from the stomach hitting the wall of the oesophagus. Eating small amounts of food often and thorough chewing bring relief. Avoiding alcohol (especially on an empty stomach), coffee and pepper are the main dietary requirements.

177

HEART DISEASE

Properly known as coronary heart disease or ischaemic heart disease, the term includes conditions which arise when the heart muscle does not receive a full supply of blood. Myocardial infarction, angina pectoris, and sudden death come under the heading of heart disease. Atherosclerosis (fatty deposits in the arteries) and arteriosclerosis (hardening of the arteries) are also classified as heart disease.

See also Atherosclerosis.

HEMICELLULOSES

One of the major types of dietary fibre which occur in breads, grains and vegetables. Chemically, hemicelluloses are made up of polyuronic acids plus sugars such as xylose, galactose, mannose and arabinose.

The hemicelluloses are not digested in the small intestine but can be fermented by bacteria in the large bowel. Different hemicelluloses are fermented to varying degrees; generally about 80 per cent are digested in this process.

They are valuable in the prevention of constipation and may also bind some bile acids and thus remove cholesterol from the body.

See also Dietary fibre.

HEPARIN

An anticoagulant used to thin the blood. Altering the intake of vitamin K in the diet will change the dose of heparin required. For this reason, those for whom heparin has been prescibed, should not alter their usual intake of foods rich in vitamin K, such as green leafy vegetables and liver.

HEPATITIS

Inflammation of the liver, caused by a specific virus. Hepatitis A is known as infectious hepatitis and usually comes from food or water which is contaminated by the virus. The virus lives in the digestive tract. Hepatitis B, or serum hepatitis, can be transmitted by injection or by sexual contact with an infected person. This virus lives in the blood, saliva and semen.

The disease is characterised by fever, headache, nausea, muscle pains and, occasionally, joint pains. Bile pigments are excreted in the urine which appears dark. The liver is enlarged and tender and jaundice may be present.

The diet during hepatitis should be high in protein so that liver cells can regenerate. Plenty of carbohydrates should also be given so that protein is 'spared' for cell regeneration. Fats are usually not well-tolerated and all fried foods and high fat foods should be omitted. Plenty of fluid, but absolutely no alcohol, should be given. Tolerance to fat usually returns slowly.

HERBAL TEA
see Tea, Herbal.

HERBS
See following pages.

HERRING
see Fish.

HESPERIDIN
see Bioflavenoids.

HERBS

The broad category of herbs includes the leaves, stems and seeds of plants containing volatile oils. For many thousands of years, herbs were gathered from the wild. They were first cultivated in monastery gardens for their healing properties and many found their way into the liqueurs which were made by the monks.

The uses of herbs then extended to their preservative qualities and, only in comparatively recent times, have they been used to impart specific flavours to particular foods.

The medicinal value of some herbs is questioned by modern medicine but their ability to enhance the natural flavours of foods is beyond doubt.

Angelica

A variety of herb of the parsley family native to Europe and Syria but now also grown in Europe and Asia. Its stalk is coated with sugar and cut into slivers to use as cake decoration. Its roots can also be eaten. In Iceland (where the plant grows well), it is eaten as a vegetable.

Balm

Once believed to calm the heart, balm is a herb whose leaves add a lemony flavour to dishes such as fish. It is also used as a tea and makes a refreshing drink.

Basil

A herb which is a member of the mint family and native to India. Comes in several forms, the most common being sweet basil (a summer annual) or the more robust bush basil (may survive winter). Widely used in Italian cooking, especially with tomatoes and in pesto (see page 265) and an important ingredient in the cuisine of Thailand. Basil is also used to flavour the liqueur chartreuse.

Nutritionally, basil is a good source of calcium and iron, if used in sufficient quantities. This may occur with the use of pesto. Like most herbs, it has few kilojoules. 100 g of sweet basil leaves have 170 kJ (40 Cals).

Bay leaf

The leaf from the bay laurel tree, native to the Mediterranean region. Dried bay leaves add flavour to soups, stews, casseroles, sauces and the liquid used for poaching meats, fish or vegetables. The leaf is removed before serving. Insufficient quantities are consumed to provide any particular nutritional value.

Bergamot

An American herb with a sweet scent used for tea and added to punch. Also added to salads. A member of the mint family. Insufficient quantities are usually consumed to make a nutritional contribution.

Borage

A Middle Eastern herb with greyish coloured leaves which can be added to salads or cooked as a vegetable. The faint cucumber-like flavour has made borage a popular ingredient in drinks. The blue flowers of the borage plant are also sometimes floated in punch bowls and form an ingredient in the drink marketed as Pimms.

Bouquet garni

A bundle of herbs, tied together and immersed in soups, stews, casseroles and stocks to provide flavour. A traditional bouquet garni consists of parsley stalks, bay leaf and thyme. If dried herbs are used, they are usually tied in a piece of muslin and removed from the dish before serving. Other ingredients such as celery may be added.

Chervil

A herb which looks rather like a lacy version of parsley but has a more tender and delicately flavoured leaf. Native to southern Russia and the Middle East. Classically used in 'omelette aux fines herbes', chervil can also be used in salads, soups and sauces.

Chives

A native of Europe, chives are a member of the onion family. They are finely chopped and added to egg dishes, soups, salads, sandwiches and savoury dishes. Onion and garlic chives are available.

Comfrey

A flowering plant of the borage family. Comfrey roots, when beaten, boiled and mixed with hot water, form a poultice. This has a high content of gums which set hard, making it useful to form a cast around a broken limb. It has no specific healing powers.

A tea can be made from comfrey and some people eat the leaves. Other people use comfrey as a source of vitamin B_{12} — a vitamin found mainly in animal foods. However, the content of B_{12} in comfrey is small and the plant contains alkaloids which are known to cause liver cancer. It is probably best avoided for this reason.

Coriander

One of the oldest known herbs which looks a little like a feathery type of parsley. A member of the carrot family, it is native to the Mediterranean and parts of Asia and is widely used in Indian, Thai, Mexican and Mediterranean cooking. Both the leaves and seeds are used, the latter going into pickles, sauces and curry powders (as a spice).

Dill

A delicate aniseed-flavoured herb, which is a member of the carrot family. Originally cultivated in India, Asia and around the Mediterranean, it is popular in India and Scandinavia. Both its fine, feathery, green foliage and its yellow seeds are used; the former being popular with fish, seafoods and eggs while the seeds are used in pickles.

Fennel

As well as being used as a vegetable, the foliage of fennel is used as a herb to flavour salads, soups, fish dishes and vegetables. It grows around the Mediterranean and was first used by the Egyptians. It is also added to sweets and liqueurs. The flavour is a little like aniseed.

See also Vegetables, Fennel.

Fenugreek

Although commonly regarded as a spice, fenugreek leaves can be added to curries or salads or used as a vegetable.

Garlic

Related to onions and chives, garlic grows from multi-cloved bulbs. Garlic was used by the slaves who built the great pyramids (about 2700 BC) and supposedly gave them the strength for the task. More recently garlic has been reported to reduce levels of cholesterol in the blood — a property attributed to its content of the sulphur-containing substance, allicin (see page 20). Garlic is also supposed to be a natural antiseptic and to cure colds.

The flavour of garlic is generally liked, and is used throughout Asia and in French and Mediterranean cookery. Unfortunately, its odour lingers on the breath and is difficult to remove. Popular suggestions are to chew parsley or fennel seeds. Neither is totally effective.

For most people, the quantity of garlic consumed means its nutritional value is insignificant.

Lemongrass

A grass, native to Southeast Asia and widely used in Asian, especially Thai, cuisine. Its delicate lemon flavour marries well with those of coriander and other spices. Dried lemongrass is sold as sereh powder.

Lemongrass is also used to make tea; it has no caffeine and no known undesirable effects.

Lemon verbena

A lemon-scented plant with small white or mauve flowers which was originally grown in South America. The leaves can be added to drinks, both hot or cold.

Lovage

A tall plant from Mediterranean regions. It can grow up to 2 m in height. The stalk, young leaves and foliage have a celery flavour and can be used in soups or salads.

Marjoram

A herb which is similar to its wild cousin, oregano. Originally grown in Greece, this small herb with purple flowers is now a popular addition to most Mediterranean cuisines. Sweet marjoram is not quite as robust as the regular herb but has a delicious flavour which goes well with salads, stuffings, sauces, meat dishes and eggs.

Mint

There are many varieties of mint — all native to the Mediterranean region. The unique flavour of mints comes from menthol released from tiny oil glands on the hairs on the surfaces of the leaves and stems. Menthol has a cooling effect in the mouth. Apple and pineapple mints are delightful in drinks or salads; spearmint goes well in mint sauce (to serve with roast lamb) or in mashed potatoes or with eggs; peppermint is used medicinally; eau de cologne mint is used in teas or cold drinks.

Oregano

A wild form of marjoram, the term oregano means 'mountain joy'. The herb is widely used in Italian and Greek cooking and goes well with pasta, eggplant, tomatoes, shellfish and meat sauces.

Parsley

A member of the carrot family, parsley is probably the best known of all herbs. The Romans introduced it to Britain and it is now also popular in Middle Eastern cookery, where the large quantities consumed can make a valuable contribution to the diet. Parsley is rich in vitamins A and C, dietary fibre, iron, potassium and calcium. If used only as a garnish, the quantities of these nutrients will not be significant. In a dish such as tabbouli, however, its nutrients will make a very valuable contribution. Flat leaf parsleys are used in Italy and other parts of Europe while the English prefer the curly leafed variety.

Pennyroyal

A variety of mint, pennyroyal is not pleasant to eat but is occasionally used as a tea.

Rosemary

The needles of this evergreen Mediterrranean shrub were originally used in ancient Rome as a medicine. Today its sweet, strong flavour is used in many dishes. It goes particularly well with lamb and is also used with pork or vegetable dishes. Used as the symbol of remembrance, rosemary's scent stays on the fingers for some time after the herb has been touched.

Sage

Originally grown in the Mediterranean countries, the grey-green leaves of sage are popular in meat dishes (especially veal and pork), fish meals, stuffings and soups.

Salad burnet

A small European herb with a cool cucumber-like flavour. Used in drinks and salads and also with fresh fruit.

Savory

Summer and winter varieties of this herb are related. Summer savory is an annual with a more delicate, sweeter flavour. It grows wild around the Mediterranean and is popular in cheeses, scones and in sauces. Winter savory is a small bush which has masses of small white flowers in summer which attract many bees. Its slightly more peppery flavour is appreciated in meat dishes, stews and with vegetables.

Sorrel

see Vegetables.

Tarragon

The variety known as French tarragon is a perennial, a member of the daisy family and native to southern Europe. It is used in meat, fish or poultry dishes and is the characteristic flavour of tarragon vinegar and Bearnaise sauce. Russian tarragon is a larger plant with a coarser leaf and an inferior flavour.

Thyme

There are numerous varieties of this popular herb, originally grown in Mediterranean regions. Its name comes from a Greek word meaning courage. Its oil, thymol, is used as a disinfectant, a mouthwash and in cough lollies. Wild thyme, the original plant, still grows and attracts many bees to its lilac-coloured flowers.

HIATUS HERNIA

A condition in which a small portion of the stomach pushes back through a hole in the diaphragm through which the oesophagus usually passes. This allows acid from the stomach to irritate the oesophagus, causing heartburn and sometimes regurgitation of food or fluid into the mouth. The effect is particularly noticeable with a change of posture. Common in overweight people and sometimes occurs during pregnancy.

The diet for hiatus hernia can contain normal foods but they should be eaten in small portions at more frequent intervals throughout the day. Thorough chewing is important.

HICKORY NUTS
see Nuts.

HIGH BLOOD PRESSURE
see Hypertension.

HIGH-DENSITY LIPOPROTEIN
see Lipoproteins.

HISTAMINE

A substance formed from histidine. Affects smooth muscle, blood pressure and the production of acid in the stomach. Also released in allergic reactions and causes hives, hay fever and rashes. Antihistamines act by reducing the action of histamine and other amines (see page 21).

HISTIDINE

One of the amino acids found in proteins which is essential for normal growth in children.

HOGGET

The meat from an animal in age between lamb and mutton. Hogget is not readily available. It is tougher than lamb but many people consider it has more flavour.

HOISIN SAUCE

A sweet barbecue sauce containing garlic and a little mild chilli.

HOLLANDAISE SAUCE

A rich sauce made from butter, egg yolks and lemon juice. Often served with vegetables such as asparagus, fish and chicken. The sauce must be made in a double boiler with constant whisking until it thickens. Should hollandaise curdle (because of too much heat), it can be 'saved' by taking a clean bowl and gradually whisking the curdled mixture into another mixture of a little fresh lemon juice and one tablespoon of the sauce.

HOMEOPATHY

A system of medicine which assumes that agents which cause disease, when given in very small doses, are able to cure the disease. The system relies heavily on the use of herbs.

HOMINY

A grain product made from corn. Not especially rich in any nutrients. 100 g have 1515 kJ (360 Cals).

HOMOGENISATION

The process of forcing milk at high pressure through very small holes onto a hard surface where the fat globules are broken so small that they disperse throughout the milk rather than rising to the top. There appears to be little effect on the nutritional value of milk after this process.

HONEY

The material produced by bees from the nectar collected from flowers. The flavour of honey depends on the flowers from which the nectar came. In general, darker honeys have a stronger flavour. The wild bush honeys of central and northern Australia are strongly flavoured and contain more solid material than commercial honeys.

The production of honey is marvellous. A bee will fly the equivalent of 6 times around the earth to collect enough nectar to make 1 kg of honey. The bee's saliva contains an enzyme, invertase, which breaks down the sucrose in nectar to glucose and fructose. This process continues in the hive. The glucose and fructose are more soluble than the original sucrose and so a more concentrated solution of honey can be formed.

In the hive, the nectar is concentrated and deposited on the honeycomb wax. Some other substances from the nectar are also broken down to other substances which act as natural antiseptics.

Honey consists of about 20 per cent water, 78 per cent sugars plus some minerals and acids. It has little protein or fat. Nutritionally, honey is not particularly suitable for humans as the quantities of minerals and vitamins it contains are really only significant in the diet of something as small as a bee — nature's intended recipient for honey. 1 tablespoon of honey has 250 kJ (60 Cals).

Most honey sold in shops has been collected from a number of beehives, heated (to destroy any yeasts), blended and filtered to remove any pollen. This processing results in some loss of individual flavours which are apparent in individual samples of honey.

Candied honey is honey which has less moisture than clear honey. Creamed honey is produced by whipping honey.

HONEYCOMB

The hexagonal cells of wax in a beehive which supports the honey.

HONEYDEW

A sweet liquid formed when insects such as aphids suck out sap from plants and then excrete it. The air causes some of the honeydew's water to evaporate leaving a concentrated form of the original sap. Bees and ants then take the ready-made concentrated sugar for their own use. The production of honeydew is especially important in areas where the plants do not produce flowers.

HONEYDEW MELON
see Fruit.

HOPS

The female flowers or cones of a vine which has female and male flowers on different plants. The hops are dried and stored and used in making beer. They are valued for their resins which give beer its bitterness and also for their oil which gives beer its typical aroma. The major resins are humulone and lupulone.

HORMONES

A variety of secretions which include insulin, thyroid hormone, steroids and glucagon as well as hormones such as catecholamines and those involved in the digestion of foods (cholecystokinen and gastrin). All hormones are made of protein.

See also Anabolic steroids.

HORSERADISH

The thick root of the horseradish plant, native to southeastern parts of Europe. When grated, the mustard oils are released. Served with roast beef in England, mixed with vinegar as a dressing for fish in Germany and concentrated into a paste to eat with raw fish in Japan.

Since only very small quantities are normally consumed, its nutritional value has little significance.

HOUMUS
see Hummus.

HUCKLEBERRY
see Fruit.

HUMAN CHORIONIC GONADOTROPHIN (HCG)

A form of growth hormone which can be extracted from the urine of pregnant women. Originally used to treat adolescent boys with a rare hormone deficiency which caused them to accumulate excess fat on their hips, thighs and bottom. In the hope that it may reduce excess weight in any obese people, some doctors began giving daily injections of HCG. Even though studies have shown it to be completely ineffective for weight loss, some doctors continue to use it — together with a 2100 kJ (500 Cals) diet plan!

HUMECTANTS

Food additives used to keep moisture in foods such as icings, spreads, biscuits, cakes and sweetened desiccated coconut. Commonly used humectants include sorbitol, glycerine and propylene glycol.

HUMMUS

A puree of cooked chickpeas and sesame paste, usually with added garlic, lemon juice and olive oil. Hummus (or houmus), is an important part of Middle Eastern meals and a good source of protein, vitamins, minerals and dietary fibre. One tablespoon has 250 kJ (60 Cals).

HUNGER

A sensation of emptiness and a slight pain in the stomach, often combined with a craving for food. Hunger pangs usually occur when the food from the previous meal has been digested and absorbed. The blood sugar level drops slightly, signalling the brain to cause a contraction of the stomach — the common hunger rumble.

If you do not eat when you experience hunger sensations, you will find the pang will disappear for about 40−50 mins and then return. This occurs because the body realises that no food is forthcoming and mobilises some glycogen from the liver to be turned into glucose. This restores the blood glucose level and turns off the hunger signal. Once that glucose has been used, the blood sugar level again drops and another hunger pang arrives. If hunger pangs are repeatedly ignored, the liver glycogen supplies are exhausted and the body begins to break down its lean muscle tissue to supply glucose. At this point, hunger signals usually disappear as the body is literally feeding off itself.

Hunger signals are also absent in those who eat so frequently that the stomach does not have the chance to become empty. Ideally, we should feel hungry 3−4 times a day and eat just enough to last until the next meal before which we should again feel hungry.

HUNZA DIET

Hunza is in the northern part of the Indian subcontinent, high up in the mountains. The Hunza people are reputed to be the world's longest living people and their longevity is often attributed to their diet which consists largely of barley, corn, rice, vegetables, yoghurt and fruit, especially apricots. They also drink a potent home-brewed alcoholic beverage. There is no proof of the age of the people, and it is difficult to divorce the effect of their peaceful surroundings and the hard physical work to produce their food, from the effects of their diet.

HUNZA PIE

A wholemeal pastry with a filling made of spinach, brown rice, onion and egg.

HYDROGENATION

The process whereby the fatty acids in vegetable oils are saturated with hydrogen to turn them from liquids to a solid substance. In making polyunsaturated margarine, only sufficient hydrogen is added to solidify some of the fats. Hydrogenation also produces substances known as trans fatty acids. The effect these fats have on health is not fully understood but they do not appear to play a positive role.

HYDROGEN SULPHIDE

Commonly called rotten egg gas for obvious reasons. Produced in the human intestine during the fermentation of some types of dietary fibre. Also produced when eggs are hard boiled as the sulphur-containing proteins react with hydrogen.

HYDROXYPROLINE

An amino acid which helps make up protein. Not essential in the diet as it can be made from the amino acid proline.

HYPERACTIVITY

Excessive activity, restlessness, short attention span and disruptive behaviour observed in some very unruly, disturbed children. Some people dispute the fact that such as condition exists; others have experienced it. The diagnosis is clouded by many parents who find their offspring 'difficult' and ascribe their exuberance to hyperactivity. (Sometimes called hyperkinesis).

In controlled trials of children who have been clinically diagnosed as hyperactive, various food sensitivities have been noted. The most common reaction occurs with salicylates present quite naturally in many fruits and vegetables. Red colouring and some other food chemicals (both natural and added) may also be responsible for hyperactivity in some children.

Diagnosis of hyperactivity linked with diet is best carried out in allergy clinics where the suspected substances are given in capsule form.

See also Allergies.

HYPERGLYCAEMIA

High blood sugar levels. This condition occurs in diabetics who are not being given sufficient insulin. If untreated, this condition can lead to disturbances in sodium, potassium and water and, eventually, coma. Hyperglycaemia is treated by giving insulin.

HYPERPHAGIA

Abnormally large appetite. May occur because of some rare hormonal imbalance.

HYPERTENSION

A condition in which the heart must continually pump against increased pressure in the arteries. Hypertension may be secondary to severe kidney disease but, in most cases, its cause is unknown. Typically, there are no symptoms associated with it until damage in a major organ occurs.

High blood pressure does not occur overnight but develops gradually as the arteries become stiffened or partially clogged with fatty deposits. Excess weight and nicotine also raise blood pressure. A high-salt diet is considered a major risk factor for many people. Other factors include a high intake of alcohol and, possibly, a lack of calcium in the diet.

Hypertension greatly increases the chances of heart disease and stroke — major causes of death in many countries, and almost unknown in others. Most of the epidemiological evidence points to differences in sodium and potassium intake as being the relevant factors in these distinct regional differences. Others dispute this and maintain that there is still no known cause.

Medical research has clearly established that hypertension can be reduced either by drugs or with a low-salt diet. Weight reduction and eating less fat are also important. The degree to which the salt intake must be lowered is still not entirely clear. However, it does entail eating unsalted processed foods in place of the regular salted varieties. Whether a low-salt diet begun early in life would prevent hypertension is not yet known (see also Salt).

See also Blood pressure.

HYPERURICAEMIA

High levels of uric acid in the blood which occurs in gout. Also associated with high blood pressure or high levels of blood fats. A slow reduction in weight coupled with a low-fat diet and avoidance of alcohol is needed.

HYPOGLYCAEMIA

Low blood sugar level. Normal fasting blood glucose level is 3.6−6.1 mmol/L. After sugar is digested and absorbed into the blood, the blood sugar level rises and the body produces insulin to clear the sugar out of the blood. If an excess of insulin is produced, the blood sugar level may fall below normal levels. This can also occur in diabetics if their insulin dose is too high or if they miss a meal. Exercising without taking extra carbohydrate can also cause hypoglycaemia in diabetics.

Symptoms of low blood sugar level include shakiness, weakness, headache, inability to think clearly, crankiness and sweating. Most of these symptoms also occur from other causes, and it can be difficult for those without diabetes to know the true cause.

Some people have such symptoms before meals, even though tests of their blood sugar levels show them to be within normal limits. It may be that the symptoms develop because of a temporary slight drop in blood sugar level. The only treatment needed is to have something to eat.

Hypoglycaemia has become a rather trendy diagnosis, yet the true condition is fairly rare.

Those who really do have low blood sugar levels need to avoid refined sugar and eat slowly absorbed carbohydrates such as oats, high-fibre cereals, vegetables (including legumes), wholegrain products and fruits. Small frequent meals and snacks are more appropriate than 2 or 3 larger meals per day.

HYPOTHALAMUS

A small region at the centre of the brain which is thought to control hunger, thirst and the production of saliva.

HYPOTHYROIDISM

A condition caused by a deficiency of iodine. Known as myxoedema in adults and cretinism in children. Characterised by an enlarged thyroid gland and a sluggish metabolism.

ICECREAM

A mixture of milk, cream, sugar, eggs and flavourings first produced centuries ago by the Chinese and Arabs. Icecream was introduced into Europe in 1533 by Catherine de Medici. This was followed by two other Italians bringing icecream to the court of Charles I in the seventeenth century. The first commercial icecream appeared in Paris in 1670 and was followed by 'cream ices' about a hundred years later.

Today, icecream is popular in the United States, Australia and parts of Europe, especially Italy. The United States is the world's greatest consumer of icecream.

Regular icecream has about 10 per cent fat and 16 per cent sugar. Richer icecreams and 'natural' icecreams generally have more fat

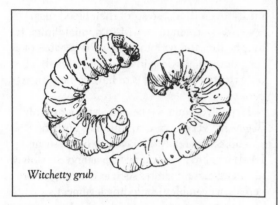

Witchetty grub

from a higher percentage of cream. Most commercial icecreams contain emulsifiers to keep the fat evenly distributed. Many also contain stabilisers which hold air in the icecream foam. The cheaper icecreams tend to contain the most additives and the most air — and the least kilojoules. Most have an overrun of 100−135 per cent, meaning that the original mixture has been increased by this amount by incorporating a lot of air. Richer, more expensive icecreams have an overrun of about 25 per cent. This makes them taste better but increases the kilojoules considerably.

Every now and then a report circulates that icecream contains paint stripper, lice killer and anti-freeze. This has become an urban myth and these substances are not used in any Australian icecream. The major nutritional problem with icecream is its high content of fat and kilojoules.

There are also icecreams made from tofu. Their main claim to fame is that they do not contain any dairy products. This is a definite advantage for those who are intolerant to lactose. However, these products have little advantage for others. Most tofu icecreams contain vegetable fat, usually hydrogenated, with almost as much saturated fat as milk and cream. They have as much sugar as regular icecream, much less protein and calcium and almost as many kilojoules as the regular product. Frozen yoghurts or soft serves made

from frozen fruit juice and gums have less fat and kilojoules than tofu or regular icecreams.

2 rounded scoops (150 mL) of regular icecream have 585 kJ (140 Cals). The same volume of rich icecream has 1070 kJ (255 Cals). Tofu icecream varies in different regions but has an average of 670 kJ (160 Cals) per serve.

ICTHYOSARCOTOXIN
see Food poisoning.

ILEUM
The lower part of the small intestine. Bile salts, vitamin B_{12} and some minerals are absorbed from this area.

IMMUNE SYSTEM
The body's defence against infection is referred to as the immune system. It is influenced by nutrition in that infections and illness are much more common in those who are poorly nourished.

Deficiencies of vitamins A, C, riboflavin, B_6, folic acid, iron or zinc, are known to affect the immune system. However, this does not mean that taking massive doses of these nutrients will provide super-immunity. Excesses of iron and some polyunsaturated fatty acids may also have adverse effects on the immune system. In the absence of valid scientific evidence suggesting super-immunity from any nutrient supplement, it is better to make sure foods are well chosen to supply a wide range of nutrients than to take supplements with unproven effects.

The body's immune system is also involved in food allergies. Immune responses are caused by special proteins called antibodies reacting to foreign substances (called antigens). The immune response is very valuable in protecting us against further attacks by an antibody. For example, once you have had measles, your body develops antibodies which will fight any future invasion by measles and prevent a second dose of the disease.

Sometimes, however, the immune response can cause a release of histamine which will damage the tissues, producing skin rashes and other symptoms.

See also Allergies.

INDIAN FIG
see Fruit, Prickly pear.

INDIAN NUT
see Nuts, Pine nut.

INDIGO CARMINE
see Colourings.

INDOLES

Substances present in cabbage and similar vegetables, contributing to their typical odour. There is some evidence that the presence of indoles may be responsible for the anti-cancer effects of these vegetables. Indoles are also present in faeces.

INGREDIENTS
see Labels, food; Breakfast cereals.

INJERA

The name given to the national flat bread of Ethiopia. The dough is made from millet, yeast, salt and water. It is poured onto a griddle in a large spiral starting at the outside and working inwards to produce a large flexible pancake about 25 cm in diameter.

INOSITOL

Once thought to be part of the vitamin B complex, but then found not to be essential in the diet, since ample supplies can be made in the body from glucose. Inositol is a phospholipid (a combination of phosphorus and a fat) and is part of the structure of cell membranes. High concentrations are found in the heart, brain and liver. Inositol helps prevent fat accumulating in the liver. Good

food sources include liver, meats, milk, wholegrain cereals, nuts, fruits and vegetables.

See also Myoinositol.

INSECTS, EDIBLE

There are a number of insects which are not only edible, but are regarded as delicacies by some people. Many of these insects had a valuable role in the diet of the Australian Aboriginal people before white people disturbed their traditional lifestyle. In some areas, people are again examining insects as possible food sources.

Some of the edible insects include ants and moths. Green tree ants are regarded by some as a gourmet treat. They are gathered by cutting the ants' nests from the trees they inhabit and collecting the white pupae which are considered to be delicious. Honey ants are also highly prized with their marble-sized abdomens full of sticky honey-like food.

Cicada nymphs and wasp larvae are also popular foods and the Bogong moths which fly from northern parts of Australia to the southern states can be roasted and pounded into a 'cake'. One of the most famous insect delicacies in Australia is the witchetty grub. These are the larvae of a moth and are considered by many people to be delicious when roasted. They are rich and rather fatty with a slightly nutty flavour.

See also Aboriginal diet; Bush food.

There are many other people throughout the world who also eat insects. Caterpillars are among the most popular. One group of people in the Philippines also eat locusts and dragon flies. They boil and dry them and grind them into a powder. Red ants, water bugs and various beetles also find themselves being regarded as culinary delights. In parts of Thailand, moths are eaten and the giant water bug is said to taste as good as gorgonzola cheese.

Nutritionally, all these insects are good sources of protein and contain a wide variety of vitamins and minerals.

INSOMNIA

An inability to sleep. One of the most common causes of insomnia is caffeine from coffee or tea. This drug affects different people to varying extents and tolerance to it can develop. Nevertheless, those who have trouble sleeping should avoid caffeine-containing beverages in the late afternoon and evening. Children who have difficulty sleeping should avoid cola drinks.

INSULIN

Insulin is a hormone secreted by cells in the pancreas known as the islets of Langerhans. It is produced whenever the level of glucose in the blood rises. Insulin then removes glucose from the blood and allows it to pass into cells and muscles. It therefore lowers the level of sugar in the blood (see page 39).

In untreated diabetes, the production of insulin either stops, is produced in insufficient quantities or there is some resistance to it from the cells. Whatever the exact mechanism operating in a particular diabetic, the result is that the level of glucose in the blood rises. Eventually it 'spills over' into the urine. When insulin is injected, it is slowly released into the blood and the diabetic must ensure a steady supply of food so that the insulin has something to work on.

Insulin is also involved in the movement of amino acids into the tissues and fatty acids and triglycerides into fat cells. Recent research indicates that insulin is involved in the functioning of the body's immune system.

See also Hyperglycaemia.

INTERNATIONAL UNITS

Some vitamins were once technically difficult to measure so they were measured in terms of their biological activity and this was expressed in International Units (IU). These were discontinued in 1974 when it was possible to measure exact quantities of different vitamins required.

See also Vitamins.

INTESTINE, LARGE
see Large intestine.

INTESTINE, SMALL
see Small intestine.

INTOXICATION

A state when more alcohol is present than can be metabolised (see Alcohol).

IODINE

An essential nutrient for humans, iodine was first identified in seaweeds in 1811. By 1820, iodine-deficiency goitre was being successfully treated with iodine, although there are references that seaweed was known as a treatment for goitre in China some 4000 years ago.

Iodine is concentrated in the thyroid gland and forms part of the thyroid hormone, thyroxine, which controls the body's metabolic rate.

A lack of iodine leads to goitre where the thyroid enlarges to the well known protrusion in the neck. Goitre still occurs in some mountainous areas where the soil lacks iodine, but it is usually recognised and treated with thyroid hormones.

See also Goitre.

There is a common misconception that taking extra iodine (usually from kelp or seaweed) will make the thyroid work harder and speed up the body's metabolic rate, leading to loss of weight. In fact, giving extra iodine can have the opposite effect. The thyroid, detecting so much extra iodine, believes it must stop producing so much thyroxine. The effect can be quite the opposite from that intended by the kelp eater.

Iodine is toxic in large doses. High levels of iodine can cause thyroid diseases. These occur in some areas in Japan where seaweeds are a prominent feature of the diet. There have also been babies born with iodine excesses due to their mothers taking extra iodine during pregnancy. It is best to obtain the small quantities of iodine needed from the diet.

Daily requirement for iodine

mcg IODINE/DAY

Infants 0–6 months	50
7–12 months	60
Children 1–3	70
4–7	90
Boys 8–11	120
12–15	150
16–18	150
Girls 8–11	120
12–15	120
16–18	120
Men	150
Women	120
Pregnancy	150
Lactation	170

Food source of iodine

Seafoods are rich in iodine, including fish, molluscs and shellfish. Vegetables and dairy products are also sources, the amount depending on the soil in which they are produced. Milk products often contain iodine because the sterilising solutions used in dairies contain iodine and traces get into the milk. Iodised salt is another way to take in iodine. It can be useful in areas where goitre is common but is not required in other areas.

IRISH COFFEE
see Drinks, Alcoholic.

IRISH MOSS
see Seaweed.

IRISH STEW

A traditional Irish stew contains potatoes, onions and meat, usually lamb, in the ratio of 1 part of onions to 2 parts of meat to 4 parts of potato. It is flavoured with pepper and herbs and has a thick creamy texture. Sliced potatoes are placed under the meat as well as on top. An average serve (2 cups) has 2370 kJ (565 Cals).

IRON

The amount of iron stored in the body is the equivalent of a large nail. It is vital for good health and peak performance, and is needed in red blood cells to form haemoglobin, which carries oxygen to all body tissues and takes back carbon dioxide to the lungs. In muscles, iron is an essential part of a compound which provides oxygen for strenuous physical activity. Iron is also involved in chemical reactions which produce energy.

About 75 per cent of the body's iron is found in haemoglobin. A small amount is in the cells and the rest is stored in the liver, spleen and bone marrow in the form of ferritin. The red blood cells have a life cycle of 120 days and around 2000 million red blood cells die each day. Their iron becomes available for the 2000 million new cells which are formed in the bone marrow. Some iron is lost from the skin and the intestine each day. Losses for men are quite small; women lose much more because of menstruation. Pregnancy and lactation impose even greater losses, so does taking aspirin. A lack of iron is the most common nutritional deficiency in the world.

The first signs of iron deficiency are a washed-out feeling, weakness, fatigue and a decreased ability for physical activity. Iron deficiency leads to anaemia with symptoms of weakness, shortness of breath, coldness, palpitations and pins and needles in the feet. In extreme cases, anaemia can cause difficulty in swallowing and even death.

A doctor can tell if you lack iron with a simple blood test. Measuring the ferritin stores is also important as these closely reflect the amount of available iron in a person's diet. Women generally have lower ferritin levels than men. Those who have had a number of pregnancies tend to have the lowest iron stores.

A recent report has linked iron deficiency in children with restlessness, inability to concentrate and irritability. Treatment with iron rapidly reversed these problems.

In spite of their much greater need for iron, women have traditionally taken the smallest share of the best food source of iron — lean meat. We have campaigns to 'Feed the Man Meat' and even small boys are encouraged to eat more meat than their sisters. Women need the iron; men eat the meat.

Many women are so obsessed with achieving extreme slenderness that they eat very little and take in insufficient iron. It is almost impossible for any very strict diet to supply enough iron. Even those who are simply health conscious can go to extremes.

Daily requirement for iron

The recommended daily intakes of iron are as follows:

		mg
Women, 18–54 years		12–16
54 +		7
during pregnancy		22–36
during lactation		12–16
Men		5–7
Boys, 1–11 years		6–8
12–18 years		10–13
Girls, 1–11 years		6–8
12–18 years		10–13

Types of iron

Iron is present in foods in two main forms. Haem iron is in meat, seafoods, and poultry. Non-haem iron is in cereals, fruits, vegetables and eggs. Haem iron is absorbed much better than the non-haem variety. Most women will find it easier to meet their iron requirements if they include some meat, seafoods or poultry.

The non-haem iron is absorbed to a much greater extent if some haem iron is present at the same meal or a food containing vitamin C is eaten at the same meal. For this reason alone, it makes good sense to include a fruit or vegetable at each meal so that the vitamin C present will assist the body to absorb iron from other foods.

The amount of iron absorbed depends on how much is needed. If you lack iron, you absorb more. During pregnancy, when needs are especially high, iron absorption can almost double. Children who are finicky eaters and appear to eat very little also absorb much more iron from foods.

Large quantities of unprocessed bran may interfere with iron absorption because of the phytic acid in the bran (see page 63). 1–2 level tablespoons of unprocessed bran a day is fine; more is not.

Oxalic acid in spinach stops iron being well-absorbed. Popeye should probably have tried broccoli! The tannin in well-brewed tea can interfere with iron absorption. Unless you like your tea fairly weak and poured quickly from the pot after it is made, it is best to confine tea drinking to between meals.

Food sources of iron

FOOD	IRON CONTENT (mg)
Kidney, 100 g	9.2
Liver, 100 g	8.8
Oysters, 1 dozen	7.2
Steak, lean, 150 g	4.5
Veal steak, 150 g	2.7
Liverwurst, 40 g	2.1
Lamb loin chops, 2 av.	2.0
Fish, average fillet, 150 g	2.1
Chicken or turkey, 150 g	1.4
Salmon, canned, 100 g	1.4

Pork steak, av. size	1.2
Egg, 1	1.1
Breakfast cereal, av. serve	2.5
Rolled oats, av. serve	1.8
Wholemeal bread, per slice	1.0
White bread, per slice	0.4
Wheatgerm, 1 tablespoon	0.8
Lentils, dried beans, cooked $\frac{1}{2}$ cup	1.8
Broccoli, 100 g, steamed	1.0
Salad vegetables, average plate	1.2
Peas, fresh, frozen or canned, $\frac{1}{2}$ cup	1.1
Vegetables, av. per serve	0.8
Potato, 1 medium	0.8
Carrot, 1 small	0.6
Dried apricots, 50 g	2.0
Fruit, av. piece	0.5
Orange juice, 200 ml glass	0.6

Iron supplements

Women who have heavy periods may need an iron supplement. Those containing vitamin C will help to absorb the iron best. Many people find that iron tablets upset their digestive system and cause either diarrhoea or constipation. Some of the newer iron supplements do not cause this problem.

IRRADIATION

The technique of using gamma rays from cobalt-60 or caesium-137 can destroy micro-organisms which make foods go bad, prevent insect attack, stop foods such as potatoes and onions sprouting and extend the shelf life of many foods. Irradiation can also take away the need to use pesticides.

On the down side, irradiation can give some food an off-flavour, destroy small quantities of some vitamins and, in very large doses, it would be harmful. The doses proposed for foods appear to be safe; some difficulties may be encountered with disposal of radioactive material.

Opponents of irradiation are concerned that it may induce changes which could cause cancer. Food scientists disagree and maintain that irradiation is safer than using pesticides.

IRRITABLE BOWEL SYNDROME

A syndrome characterised by bouts of diarrhoea or constipation. Some cases of irritable bowel have been found to be due to food sensitivity; some are due to tension; a few have no known cause. Treatment is with a high-fibre diet and bulking agents, if necessary. Relaxation techniques may also be useful.

See also Anaemia.

ISOLEUCINE

An amino acid found in most foods.
See also Amino acids.

ISOMERS

Molecules which have the same atoms arranged in different ways. For example, sugars occur naturally in the D isomer form. 'Left-handed' sugars (the L isomer) are not digested in the human intestine since the enzymes which break down sugars do not recognise them.

ISPAGHULA

A gummy type of fibre from the husk of the seed of *Plantago ovata*. Has a possible use as a thickener in some foods but is currently used in bulking agents to treat constipation and other bowel disorders (see Mucilages). Some people are allergic to ispaghula.

ISRAELI ARMY DIET

A popular diet in which the would-be slimmer has 2 days of eating apples, 2 days of chicken, 2 days of salad and 2 days of chicken. No other foods are consumed.

Like most fad diets, this pattern of eating produces an unbalanced diet. Most of the lost weight will consist of water. The diet has been disowned by the Israeli army.

J

JACK CHEESE
see Cheese.

JACKFRUIT
see Fruit.

JALAPENO PEPPER

A variety of hot chilli pepper used in South American and Mexican cooking.

JAM

Product made from chopped or crushed fruits, cooked with sugar until the pectin in the fruit and the sugar form a thickened gel. Fruits which have a low pectin content (strawberries, peaches, figs, pears, grapes or pineapple) may need added pectin. Overripe fruits have lost some of their pectin and are not suitable for making jam. Pectin is also well supplied by lemons. Jams can be made at home by cooking fruits in water (with lemon, if appropriate), adding an equal quantity of sugar and boiling until the mixture gels. Using a microwave eliminates burnt jam saucepans!

It is also possible to make jams by using more fruit with added pectin or other thickeners and an artificial sweetener. In some countries, such as Australia, such jams without sugar do not fit the food regulations and are, technically, illegal. This is somewhat ironic when there is also a call for people to 'avoid eating too much sugar'. A tablespoon of regular jam has 220 kJ (52 Cals). A tablespoon of low-kilojoule jam has 15−30 kJ (4−7 Cals).

See also Pectin.

JAMBO
see Fruit.

JARLSBERG
see Cheese.

JASMINE TEA
see Tea.

JAUNDICE

The condition in which the whites of the eyes, the skin and urine all turn yellow. It is due to high levels of the bile pigment, bilirubin (see page 37), in the blood. Causes include hepatitis, an excessive breakdown of red blood cells, an obstruction in the duodenum or liver damage. If the cause is liver damage or hepatitis, the faeces are a pale colour.

JEJUNUM

The middle section of the small intestine between the ileum and the duodenum (see Digestion, page 94). The jejunum is approximately 2.5 m long and is responsible for the production of digestive juices. Many nutrients are absorbed from this section of the intestine.

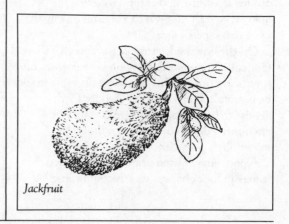

Jackfruit

JELLY

Jellies are like jams but are made from the strained juice of the fruit. They are therefore clear. Their sugar content is the same as that of jam. Fruits with a high content of pectin such as apples, guavas, quinces, red currants, gooseberries and cranberries make good jellies. A tablespoon of any of these jellies has approximately 230 kJ (55 Cals).

Jelly is also a term applied to a mixture of gelatin, sugar and colouring, flavouring or fruit which is set and used as a dessert. In the United States, such a product is known as strawberry (or other flavour) gelatin. An average serving of jelly has 375 kJ (90 Cals). It has little nutritional value. Low-kilojoule jelly has 40 kJ (10 Cals) in an average serve.

JELLYFISH SEAWEED
see Seaweed.

JERKY

Jerky is a dried meat product, usually made from beef strips which are left to dry high over a smoky fire or in the sun. Once the water content is lost, jerky is too dry for bacteria to survive and so it does not go bad. A similar product to pemmican (see page 263).

JERUSALEM ARTICHOKE
see Vegetables, Artichoke.

JEWFISH
see Fish.

JEW'S EAR MUSHROOMS
see Vegetables, Mushrooms.

JICAMA
see Vegetables.

JOHN DORY
see Fish.

JUICES
see Drinks, Non-alcoholic; Fruit juices.

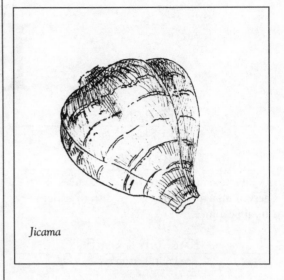

Jicama

JUJUBE
see Fruit.

JUNIPER
see Spices.

JUNKET

An English dessert made by setting sweetened warmed milk with rennet or junket tablets. The rennin in the tablet turns the milk into curds and whey which remains set until the mixture is disturbed.

See also Rennin.

JUNK FOODS

A term applied by nutritionists to foods which contribute kilojoules but few nutrients. Examples are sugar, soft drinks and cordials, most lollies (candies) and other foods made largely from sugar, many fats and snack foods.

Consumers have widened the term junk foods to include many fast foods which are less 'healthy' than home-cooked meals.

Food manufacturers dislike the term junk foods and refer to 'junk diets'. Presumably this is a diet made up largely of what others call 'junk foods'.

K

KABANA

see Sausages.

KAISEKI

A Japanese meal of several light courses, each served on a specially selected dish to enhance its appearance.

KAKI OR KAKEE

see Fruit, Persimmon.

KALE

see Vegetables.

KANOY

see Tea.

KARAYA GUM

see Sterculia.

KASHA

A gruel or porridge made from coarse or cracked wholegrain and commonly served in Eastern European countries. Buckwheat is the usual grain for kasha, but barley, millet, rye, wheat or even rice are sometimes used. To make kasha, cook the grain and seasonings in stock or water until the liquid has been absorbed and the grain is fluffy. The nutritional value depends on the grain used, but most forms are high in complex carbohydrates and dietary fibre.

KASSERI

see Cheese.

KEBAB

Also known as shish kebab, this is the term for bite-sized pieces of meat threaded onto a skewer. The meat is usually marinaded before cooking to provide flavour. Popular in Middle Eastern countries and Greece.

KEDGEREE

A dish made from smoked fish (usually cod) and rice. Often has hard-boiled eggs added.

KEEMUM

see Tea.

KEFIR

An alcoholic beverage made from fermented milk and containing up to 1.5 per cent alcohol. The term also applies to a non-alcoholic liquid yoghurt sold in the United States. It can be used as a refreshing drink or made into desserts or a frozen icecream-like product.

KELLOGG, DR JOHN HARVEY

The founder of the Kellogg company, the American Dr John Harvey Kellogg was a medical graduate who believed that nutrition was important to fight and prevent disease. He took over a Seventh Day Adventist sanatorium to put his principles into practice and determined to liven up the vegetarian menus being used. In 1895, Kellogg developed his first flake cereal by partly cooking wheat grains, rolling them flat and baking them. His product was not highly popular and in 1902 he had much more success with his corn flakes. He was not concerned with the product's lack of dietary fibre as he believed a food which was totally digested and left no residue was highly desirable.

KELP

see Seaweed.

KERATIN

The major protein in hair and nails. Also in animals' hoofs, horns, feathers and scales. Keratin is high in amino acids (see page 21) which contain sulphur. However, eating lots of foods with sulphur-containing amino acids will not build thicker hair or nails. The strength of hair and nails is largely determined by heredity.

KERNEL

Either the inside (edible) part of a nut or the whole of a grain.

KETCHUP

The term used in the United States for processed tomato sauce. The name comes from a Chinese word for 'pickled fish sauce'. Tomato ketchup has 85 kJ (20 Cals) per tablespoon. It is high in salt (except for salt-reduced varieties).

See also Sauces, Tomato.

KETONES

Substances formed when the body uses fats for energy in the absence of carbohydrates. Ketones such as acetoacetic acid and its derivative acetone are toxic substances which cause headaches, nausea, giddiness, fainting or lightheadedness and bad breath (rather like nail-polish remover). The 'spiritual' feelings which some people experience during fasting may well be due to the effects of ketones.

Ketones can cause kidney damage, and in untreated diabetics, can lead to coma. They are also dangerous in a pregnant woman, as their presence indicates that the blood glucose level is low.

The idea that ketones can cause great weight loss from body fat is false. With the maximum production of ketones (before serious toxicity resulted), a maximum of 400 kJ (95 Cals) a day could be lost. Since a kilogram of body fat represents some 32,000 kJ (7700 Cals), it would take a long time to lose substantial amounts of body fat by these methods. Most of the weight lost with such diets comes from loss of muscle glycogen and its attendant water. Diets which produce ketones are not recommended.

KETOSIS

The term given to the condition in which ketones are being produced. In spite of the enthusiasm of some 'diet doctors' for ketosis, it is an unhealthy condition. The Atkins Diet statement that ketosis is a 'state devoutly to be desired' is absurd. It is dangerous to health and useless for permanent weight reduction.

KIDNEY

The kidneys act as an automatic cleaning and filtering system for the body, removing waste products from digestion and metabolism, surplus nutrients and vitamins (water-soluble varieties), water and many toxic or unwanted substances. The kidneys also regulate the balance of water and electrolytes (sodium, potassium, chloride and magnesium) in the body and produce some hormones. We do not need to worry about the balance of acids in the body, the kidneys do it for us. All we need do to keep normal kidneys functioning well is to drink plenty of water.

KIDNEY, AS FOOD

The kidneys of lambs, calves, oxen and pigs are part of the meats which are collectively called offal. Ox kidneys are normally used in steak and kidney while pig's kidneys are eaten less often.

Kidneys should be cooked quickly so that they do not become tough. They are rich sources of nutrients, especially iron and all the B vitamins (especially pantothenic acid and B_{12}). They also supply protein, vitamin E and many minerals. 100 g of kidney have approximately 400 kJ (95 Cals). Their fat content is low but kidneys do contain about 300 mg/100 g of dietary cholesterol. As explained (see Cholesterol, page 72), this is only a problem in those who are eating a high-fat diet or are very sensitive to dietary cholesterol.

KIDNEY BEANS
see Legumes.

KIDNEY STONES
see Renal calculi.

KILOJOULES
see Energy.

KINGFISH
see Fish.

KIPPERS
see Fish.

KIRSCH
see Drinks, Alcoholic.

KISHK
see Cheese.

KIWI FRUIT
see Fruit.

KNOBLAUCHWURST
see Sausages.

KOHLRABI
see Vegetables.

KOJI
An enzyme produced from a mould, *Aspergillus oryzae*, which grows on rice. Used to prepare rice for sake (see page 104) or to make miso (see page 231).

KOLA NUT
see Nuts.

KOLBASS
see Sausages, Csabai.

KOMBU
see Seaweed.

KOSHER FOODS

Foods which meet the requirements of the dietary laws of the Jewish faith. Applied to foods, kosher indicates that the item is permitted. When applied to anything other than food, kosher means 'unfit'.

Kosher foods must not be from animals, birds or fish which are prohibited in the Old Testament. The animals must have been slaughtered by ritual method which involves a qualified person slitting the animal or bird's neck with a special knife with an ultra-sharp blade without nicks. The aim is to sever the main carotid artery and jugular vein in one quick movement. The animal is then bled. After the animal has been examined for blemishes, the meat is salted to remove all blood. Kosher food also means that meat and milk must not come into contact with each other. Separate utensils for cooking meat and milk are kept.

Kosher meats tend to have a high salt intake.

KRANSKY
see Sausages.

KRUPUK

Crisp prawn-flavoured wafers served with Malaysian and some Thai dishes. Made from rice flour with added prawn meal. Deep fried in oil.

KUDZU
see Vegetables.

KULICH

A yeasted bread with eggs, butter and cardamom added for flavouring. Often baked in a wreath shape at Christmas.

KUMMEL
see Drinks, Alcoholic.

KUMQUAT
see Fruit, Cumquat.

KVAS
A mixture of beetroot, milk and rye bread, left to ferment, strained and used as a food colouring.

L

LABAN
A drink made from yoghurt in Middle Eastern countries.

LABELS, FOOD
Labelling laws vary in different countries and even between states in the same country. The net weight of contents, the name and address of the manufacturer, the country of origin of the product and, in some places, a 'use by' date are legal requirements on processed foods.

In general, ingredients must be listed on a label in their order of prominence in the product. In the United States, all ingredients must be listed by name. In Europe and Australia, major ingredients must be listed, while additives are given a number. A guide to the additive numbers is available for consumers and is useful for those who need or want to restrict certain substances. However, even with this system there can be problems. For example, margarine must list its ingredients, but when margarine becomes an ingredient in another product, it may appear as margarine and its additives will not necessarily be included.

Another example occurred with the labelling of some snack foods. The ingredient list mentioned corn, rice, flavouring and a specific colouring number. Even though the product had a high salt content, there was no mention of salt in the ingredient list because the salt was part of the flavouring.

Listing specific nutrients, either in 100 g or in a specified serving of a food product, is called nutritional labelling. It is required in some countries and plans are under way to make it compulsory for certain foods in others. In countries such as Australia, nutritional labelling on human foods has lagged behind nutritional information on dog and cat food. We might well ask why we care more about the nutrition of our pets than what we feed humans?

Ingredient listing does not tell you how much of a particular ingredient is present. Even priority listing can be abused. For example, if a manufacturer is making a fruit bar with 60 per cent sugar and 40 per cent fruit, the ingredients will be listed as 'sugar, fruit'. Since it does not look good for the product to have sugar as its main ingredient, many manufacturers will use, perhaps, 20 per cent each of 3 different sugars so that the fruit can be listed first. For example, the ingredient list for the fruit bar could now read 'fruit, glucose, raw sugar, honey'.

See also Additives, food.

LACTASE
The enzyme which splits the lactose (page 201) in milk to its component sugars of glucose and galactose. Some humans are unique among

mammals in continuing to produce lactase after the usual weaning period. If other mammals are given lactose-containing products after weaning, they no longer have the lactase to break down the lactose. The latter accumulates and is fermented in the small intestine causing bloating, flatulence and stomach cramps. This is why veterinarians advise people not to give dogs or cats milk.

Most humans of Anglo-Saxon origin continue to produce lactose throughout life. On a world scale, however, about 60—70 per cent of the human population do not produce significant amounts of lactose after weaning. For those who do produce lactase, milk continues to be a useful food to supply calcium. For those whose lactase production decreases, milk is not a suitable food and causes abdominal cramps, diarrhoea and flatulence. Most cheeses contain only small amounts of lactose and are well tolerated by those who are lactase deficient. Ricotta and the Norwegian gjetost are among the few cheeses which contain lactose since they are made from the whey portion of milk.

Those who are deficient in lactase should avoid milk and foods containing milk, as well as the cheeses mentioned above. Many pharmaceutical preparations use lactose as a filler and will also need to be avoided.

A very small number of people are totally lactase deficient from birth. They need a synthetic diet and will need to avoid all lactose throughout life.

See also Enzymes.

LACTATION

During lactation, the mother's diet must provide the extra protein, minerals and vitamins which will pass to the infant. Extra energy is also required although fat stores built up during pregnancy will provide some of this. In general, the daily diet should contain plenty of fruits and vegetables, approximately 4—6 slices of wholegrain bread (or other cereal

products), a litre of milk (low fat, if desired) and at least one serving of a high-protein food (fish, chicken, lean meat, eggs, legumes, cheese). Plenty of fluid is also important since the infant will be taking up to a litre of fluid from the mother.

Many women find they are very hungry during lactation. This is quite normal and occurs because the production of milk may take up to 2500 extra kilojoules (600 Cals) a day. Providing fatty and/or sugary foods are not consumed in excess, most women find the lactation helps them return to their pre-pregnant size.

Alcohol and drugs (or products from their metabolism) find their way into breast milk. Women who are breast feeding should consume only small amounts of alcohol and should avoid taking any drug unless strictly necessary. Large doses of vitamins should also be avoided as the high levels passing to the infant may make the child dependent on receiving continued high doses.

See also Breast feeding.

LACTIC ACID

An acid which forms in muscles during short sharp bursts of anaerobic physical activity (without the use of oxygen). Once the lactic acid concentration in blood and muscles reaches a certain level, fatigue occurs and further exercise is impossible until some of the lactic acid is converted by the liver back to glucose. Trained athletes have a greater tolerance to a build up of lactic acid than those who are not used to physical exertion.

Lactic acid is also a by-product of bacterial fermentation. This is used in making sauerkraut, yoghurt and cheese, and results in the characteristic flavours of these products. The production of lactic acid also lowers the pH of the food and makes it less hospitable for other microbes. For this reason, sauerkraut, yoghurt and cheese keep better than the fresh products from which they are made.

LACTOBACILLUS

A species of bacteria which convert lactose to lactic acid. Used in making yoghurt and cheeses. There are various type of lactobacillus. Lactobacillus acidophilus and lactobacillus bulgaricus are used to make sour milk and yoghurts. Lactobacillus bifidus is secreted in human milk and produces lactic acid in the baby's digestive tract, making life difficult for other harmful bacteria.

There is no strong evidence that lactobacillus acidophilus products promote superior health. However, the lactobacilli can preserve milk and hence reduce milk-borne diseases. Those who cannot digest lactose (because of a lactase deficiency) can also eat some yoghurt since the bacteria will have converted the lactose into lactic acid.

LACTOSE

The sugar present naturally in milk. When digested by the enzyme lactase, lactose separates into its component sugars, glucose and galactose.

See also Carbohydrates; Dissacharides; Lactase.

LADY'S FINGERS

A long, slender-shaped pastry with a filling made from minced lamb, onion, tomatoes, spices and pine nuts. Popular in Middle Eastern cuisine. Two lady's fingers contain 1000 kJ (240 Cals).

The name lady's fingers is also given to okra pods (see Vegetables) and to a type of banana (see Fruits).

LAETRILE

Sometimes called vitamin B_{17}, laetrile is extracted from apricot kernels. Although it is reputed to cure cancer and boost muscle development in athletes, it has not been shown to have these effects. In fact, laetrile contains dangerous quantities of cyanide and is therefore not permitted for sale. There have been a number of deaths from its use.

LAGER
see Drinks, Alcoholic, Beer.

LAMB
see Meat.

LAMB LIGHTS

The lungs of a lamb. In most Western countries, these are used only for pet foods, but they are eaten by humans in parts of Asia. Nutritional value is low.

LAMB'S FRY
see Liver, as food.

LAMB'S LETTUCE
see Vegetables.

LAMB'S WOOL
see Fruits, Crabapple.

LAMINGTON

A cake which is popular in Australia. Made from squares of sponge or butter cake, dipped in chocolate icing and then rolled in desiccated coconut. An average lamington has 1260 kJ (300 Cals).

LANGOUSTE
see Seafood, Lobster.

LAOS
see Spices, Lengkuas.

LAPSANG SOUCHANG TEA
see Tea.

LARD

The fat from pigs. Lard makes the best quality pastry because it forms large crystals which separate the starch granules and protein strands in the dough from each other, providing a light flaky result.

Lard has virtually no minerals or vitamins. It is almost 100 per cent fat, of which 46 per cent is saturated, 44 per cent is monounsaturated and 10 per cent is polyunsaturated. This is not significantly different from the fats found in solid vegetable fats. 100 g of lard have 3725 kJ (890 Cals).

LARGE INTESTINE

The portion of the gastrointestinal tract which includes the colon and rectum. It extends from the end of the small intestine to the anus and is about 1.8 m in length. About 1.5 l of fluid plus dietary fibre and any indigested carbohydrates enter the large intestine. Bacteria break down the fibre (see page 92) and also ferment any remaining carbohydrate. All except 100–200 ml of the water is reabsorbed through the colon.

If there is insufficient dietary fibre present over many years, the muscular walls of the large intestine become weak. Small pouches called diverticula may develop and can be painful if material becomes trapped in them.

LASAGNE

An Italian dish made from layers of wide flat noodles, meat sauce and a cheese sauce. Once the layers are assembled, the dish is topped with cheese and baked. A typical serve (400 g) has 2850 kJ (680 Cals).

LASSI

see Drinks, Non-alcoholic.

LAVER

see Seaweed.

LAXATIVES

Instead of eating sufficient quantities of dietary fibre, some peope take laxatives to stimulate bowel motions. Laxatives may be either bulking agents which absorb water and provide softer and more bulky stools, or they may contain chemical substances which irritate the wall of the bowel. Frequent use of laxatives can reduce the muscle tone of the bowel walls so that constipation becomes chronic. Some laxatives, particularly those which contain anthroquinone, should be avoided as they may produce serious damage to the nerves in the walls of the bowel. Laxatives which contain anthraquinones include some of the widely available laxative pills, some senna preparations, cascara and a variety of herbal preparations.

A study in Strathalbyn, South Australia, found that laxative use decreased dramatically after a 6-month intensive education campaign on the benefits of dietary fibre. 2 years later, laxative use was still low.

At best, laxatives provide temporary relief of constipation. At worst, they may inflict permanent damage to the bowel.

The use of laxatives for weight reduction is foolish and of little use for losing body fat. Taken in large doses, laxatives promote a loss of water from the body. They may also cause a loss of minerals and vitamins and general feelings of weakness.

See also Constipation; Faecal softeners.

LDL CHOLESTEROL

see Lipoproteins.

LEAD

A toxic mineral for humans, lead from traffic exhaust and industrial contamination enters and accumulates in the body. Lead is more easily absorbed from liquids than solids. However, there have been cases of lead poisoning from people taking supplements of bone meal. The World Health Organisation recommends that a weekly intake of 50 mcg of lead per kilogram of body weight is tolerable for adults. Smaller intakes are obviously much better.

LEATHERJACKET

see Fish.

LEAVES

Green leafy edible plants are excellent sources

of vitamins, especially vitamin C, carotene (which is converted to vitamin A in the body) and folacin (another of the B vitamins). They also supply dietary fibre.

Edible leaves contain some protein and this can be separated from the fibrous section of the plants. The process involves mashing the leaves and squeezing out the juice to separate it from the fibrous residue. By heating the extracted juice, the protein coagulates and can form a food source. While leaf protein has not yet been widely used, it represents a possible future food source.

LECITHIN

A combination of a fat, phosphorus and choline, lecithin is known as a phospholipid (see page 265). The fatty acids in lecithin may be saturated, monounsaturated or polyunsaturated depending on their source.

Lecithin is widely distributed in natural foods such as eggs, fish, legumes, vegetable seeds and oils, chicken and meats. It is also used extensively as an emulsifier to keep fats evenly distributed through processed foods such as icecream, mayonnaises, margarines, chocolate, cakes and desserts. Eggs are a natural source of lecithin and this contributes to the physical properties of egg yolk in making mayonnaise.

The body also produces its own lecithin. It is used in the structure of cell membranes and lipoproteins (protein-fat combinations). Lecithin is also used to make bile and helps keep the cholesterol in bile in solution rather than allowing the cholesterol to settle out as gallstones. This fact has been extrapolated by some to assume that taking extra lecithin will stop cholesterol being deposited out of the blood into fatty deposits in the arteries. Unfortunately, this does not occur and those who take extra lecithin are merely supplying themselves with extra fat.

The choline in lecithin has been shown to have value in people with neurological disorders. However, this does not mean that taking extra lecithin will be of benefit to others.

See also Choline.

LECTINS

Toxic substances in legumes which cause vomiting, diarrhoea and blood cells to clump together. Destroyed when legumes are cooked.

LEEKS
see Vegetables.

LEGUMES
See following pages.

LEICESTER
see Cheese.

LEMON
see Fruits.

LEMONGRASS
see Herbs.

LEMON VERBENA
see Herbs.

LENGKUAS
see Spices.

LENT

The period of 40 days before Easter; a time of abstinence. For some people, this means omitting meat from the diet. Fish is eaten instead.

LENTILS
see Legumes.

LETTUCE
see Vegetables.

LEUCINE

One of the amino acids in protein foods. Well supplied by many foods.

See also Amino acids.

· LEGUMES

Dried beans and peas, also known as pulses, are among the most valuable foods available for human consumption. They are rich in protein and complex carbohydrate, provide very useful types of dietary fibre and are very good sources of many minerals and vitamins. Legumes can be stored easily and retain most of their nutritional value through storage and cooking. If they are eaten raw, some, such as kidney beans, contain factors which can destroy vitamins. When cooked, however, these factors are themselves destroyed.

Dried beans are cooked by first soaking in water and then simmering until tender. An alternative method is to cover the beans with water, bring them to the boil, cover tightly and allow to stand for about an hour. They can then be boiled. Beans do not soften once they are in an acid solution, so in dishes containing beans and acid vegetables such as tomatoes, the beans must be pre-cooked before being added to the tomato-based mixture. Beans in tomato sauce are thus cooked first and then added to the tomato sauce.

Aduki beans

Also known as the azuki, adzuki or feijao bean, these small, round, reddish-brown beans are popular in Japan and China. They have a light, nutty, slightly sweet flavour and are often made into candied bean cakes which are served as a dessert with green leaf tea. Cooked with rice, they impart a pink colour to the grain. Legend has it that the aduki bean was a gift from a benevolent god to an evil world.

Nutritionally, the beans are a source of protein, iron and the B group vitamins. They have almost no fat.

Baked beans

see Haricot beans.

Black beans

A small kidney-shaped bean with a shiny black skin and creamy-coloured flesh. Used in South American and Caribbean cooking, especially in a spicy black bean soup. Also called 'Mexican blacks' or 'frijoles negros'.

In China, the black bean is small and round, and has a greenish-coloured flesh. It is most commonly salted and fermented and used in strongly-flavoured sauces.

Black-eyed beans

Small, white kidney-shaped beans with a black spot at the sprouting point. Sometimes called black-eyed peas, cow peas or black-eyed Suzies, they have a thinner skin than many beans and therefore cook quite quickly without needing to be soaked. Although they originated in Africa, they are widely used in Middle Eastern, Indian and Greek cookery.

Borlotti beans

Also known as Roman, cranberry, saluggia or rosecoco beans, these plump beans may be beige or brown or, most commonly, speckled pink. The smooth texture and slightly ham-like flavour of the cooked beans makes them popular in soups and Italian dishes. Borlotti beans are very similar to pinto beans and can be substituted in the same recipes.

Boston baked beans

A dish made from haricot beans cooked in a rich, dark sauce. Includes mustard and molasses.

Broad beans

Commonly believed to have been the first cultivated legume, broad beans can be eaten fresh or dried. When very young, the green pod can be eaten along with the pale green beans. Dried broad beans have a very tough skin and need a long soak and long slow cooking to soften. Also known as fava beans and, if eaten uncooked, may cause a form of anaemia known as favism in some Mediterranean people with a specific sensitivity to a toxin found in the beans. In spite of this, broad beans are popular in Europe, the Middle East, Egypt and India.

Fresh broad beans are a good source of dietary fibre, riboflavin and a useful source of iron and niacin. 100 g have 170 kJ (40 Cals).

Butter beans

There are two varieties of butter bean: a large plump white bean which originated in Peru (also known as Lima bean); and a smaller bean from Mexico which cooks much more quickly.

The butter bean is popular in soups, stews and casseroles and goes well with pork. With sweetcorn, butter beans also make up the traditional South American dish Succotash.

Bean sprouts

see Vegetables.

Cannellini beans

These white, oval, slightly nutty-flavoured beans are a member of the haricot bean family and were first cultivated in Argentina. In many countries, a bean properly known as the Great Northern bean is sold as a cannellini. The beans need to be cooked for $1\frac{1}{2}$ hours, after soaking.

Chickpeas

see Garbanzos.

Cranberry beans

see Borlotti beans.

Fava beans

see Broad beans.

Flageolet beans

A type of haricot bean, harvested while young, small, green and tender. More expensive than most beans, sometimes available only in cans and used in French and Italian cookery, often as a salad. Can be cooked without soaking and take about 1 hour to reach tenderness.

French beans

see Vegetables, Beans.

Ful medames

A small round brown bean popular in the Middle East. Baked with eggs, cumin and garlic, they are an Egyptian national dish.

Garbanzos

A round, light-brown coloured pea with a chicken-beak point at one end, garbanzos are widely used in Middle Eastern countries, India, Spain, Italy, Greece, Asia and North Africa. They were known in Rome as *Cicer arietinum*, meaning 'a ram's head legume', because they were thought to resemble the head of a ram with curling horns. Garbanzos are also called chickpeas or Bengal gram.

Commonly used in Middle Eastern countries as hummus — a ground paste made of chickpeas, garlic, olive oil, sesame seeds and lemon juice. In both Israel and Egypt, chickpeas are made into small flat savoury cakes known as felafel. Throughout Europe, they are made into stews and soups. In India, the chickpea is boiled, roasted, fried, sprouted, stewed into the familiar dhal and ground into a flour (called besan).

Garbanzos have a more nut-like texture and taste than most beans and this may be responsible for their popularity. After soaking, they take about $1\frac{1}{2}$ hours to cook. (Felafel are made from raw soaked beans.)

Nutritionally, garbanzos are an excellent source of dietary fibre, a good source of protein and iron, and provide smaller quantities of other minerals and vitamins. They are low in fat. 100 g of raw garbanzos have 1340 kJ (320 Cals) while 100 g of the cooked beans have 610 kJ (145 Cals).

Great northern bean

Similar to cannellini beans but slightly smaller. Cooking time, after soaking, is $1-1\frac{1}{2}$ hrs.

Haricot beans

The most commonly used beans for the familiar canned baked beans. Small, white oval-shaped beans, also known as navy beans. Widely used in the Middle East and Mediterranean countries. Cooking time, after soaking, is $1-1\frac{1}{2}$ hrs.

Nutritionally, haricot beans are an excellent source of dietary fibre, iron, protein and potassium and a good source of zinc and several vitamins of the B complex. 100 g of raw beans have 1130 kJ (270 Cals) while 100 g of the cooked beans have 395 kJ (95 Cals). Canned baked beans in tomato sauce provide smaller quantities of the same nutrients; 100 g have 270 kJ (65 Cals).

Kidney beans

Red kidney beans are the most commonly used variety but these beans also come in brown, black and white. The beans originated in the West Indies but are now used throughout the world, especially in South America in the well-known dish of chilli con carne. Canned kidney beans are a convenient product and the raw beans take $1-1\frac{1}{2}$ hours gentle boiling after an initial soaking.

Nutritionally, kidney beans are an excellent source of dietary fibre, iron, protein and potassium and a good source of other minerals and vitamins of the B complex. 100 g of raw kidney beans have 1135 kJ (270 Cals).

Lentils

One of the first legumes to be cultivated, lentils are mentioned in the Old Testament. They are thought to have originated in Syria and are now a major part of the diet in India, the Middle East and parts of Eastern Europe.

There are many varieties, the most common being red, green or brown; both red and brown becoming a brownish yellow colour when cooked.

Lentils are popular because they need no soaking, cook in 20−30 mins and can be used in a variety of ways. A lentil puree called dhal is the major source of protein in India. Lentils are also used in soups and stews and make excellent vegetarian burgers.

Nutritionally, lentils are an excellent source of protein, iron and zinc and a good source of dietary fibre, pantothenic acid and potassium. They also supply vitamins of the B complex and various minerals. 100 g of raw lentils have 1275 kJ (305 Cals) while 100 g of cooked lentils have 420 kJ (100 Cals).

Lima beans

A bean which originated in Peru, and is a larger variety of the butter bean. When young, the beans are small and green or white; older beans are larger, flat and slightly kidney-shaped. The flavour is slightly sweet and rather floury. After soaking, they take $1-1\frac{1}{2}$ hours to cook.

The nutritional value of the Lima bean varies according to the extent it has been dried. Raw beans are a good source of vitamin C but much of this is lost in the dried bean. The beans are also a good source of iron and contribute protein, B complex vitamins and minerals. 100 g raw or cooked Lima beans have 480 kJ (115 Cals).

Lupins

The use of these legumes is limited because they contain bitter alkaloids which can cause liver damage. In some areas, lupins are placed in a running stream for 2 weeks to remove the alkaloids. Soaking, boiling and then soaking in salt water for several days can also remove the alkaloids. These legumes are really only worth eating if foods are scarce.

Mung beans

Native to India, the tiny green mung beans are also used throughout Asia. The beans do not need to be soaked and can be eaten whole (after cooking), ground into flour, or used as the familiar mung bean sprouts.

Nutritionally, mung beans (also called green gram) are a good source of dietary fibre, iron and protein and also contribute other minerals and vitamins of the B complex. When sprouted, they provide vitamin C. 100 g of raw mung beans have 960 kJ (230 Cals) while cooked beans have 440 kJ (105 Cals) per 100 g.

Navy beans

see Haricot beans.

Peas, dried

Dried peas are available as blue peas or as split green or yellow peas. They have a long history, originating in the Middle East, and were used by the Romans. They soon spread to India, China and Europe since they could be stored and used throughout the winter months when fresh peas were unavailable. The old English pease pudding was made from dried peas. Dried blue peas take about 1 hr to cook, after soaking. Split peas need no soaking and cook relatively quickly. They are widely used in soups and stews.

Dried whole peas have more dietary fibre than the varieties of peas used for split peas. In other nutritional respects, all peas are similar, providing a source of protein, zinc, iron, vitamins of the B complex and various minerals. 100 g of dried or split peas have 1195 kJ (285 Cals). When cooked, 100 g have 440 kJ (105 Cals).

Pink beans

Medium sized kidney-shaped beans with a deep pink skin, sometimes called red Mexican beans. Popular in southern parts of the United States.

Pinto beans

These creamy-coloured beans are speckled with beige and pink and look most attractive. They turn a dusky pink when cooked. Pintos originated in Mexico and are commonly used in Mexican recipes for both hot and cold dishes. After soaking, they take about 2 hrs to cook.

Like most legumes, pinto beans are a good source of protein, dietary fibre, iron and other minerals and vitamins.

Rosecoco beans

see Borlotti beans.

Roman beans

see Borlotti beans.

Saluggia

see Borlotti beans.

Soya beans

Probably one of the most important food crops throughout the world, soya beans originated in China and have been a staple food throughout Asia for over 5000 years. The beans themselves are eaten, and they are used to produce soya bean milk, soya bean curd (tofu), soya bean flour, soy sauce, soy paste (tempeh) and soya bean oil (which is then made into margarine). Soya beans have also been spun into fibres to use as a meat substitute. Soya bean meal has been extensively used for animal feed, although there is an enormous wastage in converting a perfectly good source of food into animal flesh. Soya beans represent the largest cash crop in the United States.

Soya beans are particularly valuable because of their oil and protein. They contain much more oil than most beans, with about 17 per cent of the dried bean being fat — mostly polyunsaturated fat. The protein in soya beans has a selection of amino acids which are much closer to human requirements than any other single vegetable food. They are also a very good source of dietary fibre, iron, zinc and other minerals, and provide a wide selection of vitamins of the B complex. Even vitamin B_{12}, found mainly in animal foods, is produced in fermented soya bean products such as tempeh while vitamin C is available from sprouted soya beans. 100 g of raw soya beans provide 1680 kJ (400 Cals); 100 g of cooked soya beans have 545 kJ (130 Cals).

Soya beans are small, oval, light brown in colour and need to be soaked and then boiled for about 2 hrs to become tender.

See also Miso; Soya bean milk; Sauce, Soy; Tempeh; Tofu.

LEVULOSE
see Fructose.

LEYDON
see Cheese.

LICORICE
see Liquorice.

LIGNIN

This substance is one of the major constituents of wood. It is also part of the structure of plant cell walls and is a valuable form of dietary fibre. It is found in older, more woody vegetables and seems to be resistant to any type of fermentation or digestion in the human intestine. Its value lies in its ability to hold water and give bulk to faeces, thus preventing constipation. Lignin also has some ability to bind and remove bile salts from the body — a feature which may be of benefit in preventing bowel cancer. Unprocessed bran contains more lignin than most commonly consumed foods. Moderate quantities of unprocessed bran (1–2 tablespoons a day) supply a useful quantity of lignin. Larger amounts of bran are not advisable.

See also Bran; Dietary fibre.

LILLIPILLI
see Fruit, Jambo.

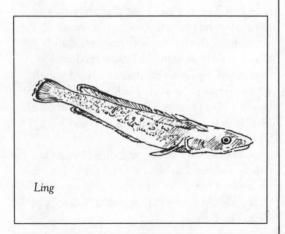

Ling

LIMA BEANS
see Legumes.

LIMBURGER
see Cheese.

LIME
see Fruit.

LIMPETS
see Seafood.

LING
see Fish.

LINOLEIC ACID

A polyunsaturated fatty acid which is essential to humans. Sometimes abbreviated as C18:2, meaning it has 18 carbon atoms and 2 double bonds. Belongs to the omega 6 series of fatty acids, indicating that it has one of its double carbon bonds situated on the sixth carbon from the end of its carbon chain.

Linoleic acid is sometimes called vitamin F, but it does not function in the way that vitamins do. It plays an important role in the formation of prostaglandins (see page 281), helps remove some undesirable very low density (VLDL) fats from the circulation and is an important part of cell membranes.

The quantity of linoleic acid needed by the body has not yet been specified. It is generally accepted that a total of 4–10 g of essential fatty acids are required each day. Medical researchers in this field also suggest that the ratio of the omega 6 to omega 3 fatty acids be around 5:1. It can thus be argued that the appropriate linoleic acid content of the daily diet should be around 3–8 g per day.

The idea that one must eat some obviously fatty food to obtain essential fatty acids such as linoleic acid is incorrect, as the table below shows.

Major food sources of linoleic acid are:

FOOD	LINOLEIC ACID CONTENT (g)
Safflower oil, 1 tablespoon	15.0
Sunflower oil, 1 tablespoon	10.4
Soya bean oil, 1 tablespoon	10.4
Corn oil, 1 tablespoon	10.0
Cottonseed oil, 1 tablespoon	9.8
Peanut oil, 1 tablespoon	5.8
Linseed oil, 1 tablespoon	2.8
Olive oil, 1 tablespoon	2.2
Palm oil, 1 tablespoon	1.7
Coconut oil, 1 tablespoon	0.4
Polyunsaturated margarine, 1 tablespoon	10.2
Hard margarine, 1 tablespoon	0.7
Butter, 1 tablespoon	0.2
Walnuts, 50 g	15.5
Brazil nuts, 50 g	12.0
Peanuts, 50 g	7.1
Almonds, 50 g	5.1
Peanut butter, 30 g (amount on sandwich)	4.2
Hazelnuts, 50 g	1.9
Chestnuts, 50 g	0.5
Avocado, $\frac{1}{2}$	1.8
Tuna in oil, 100 g	8.1
Liver, calves' or chicken, 150 g	1.5
Chicken or turkey, lean, 150 g	1.0
Pork, lean, 150 g, cooked	0.8
Beef, lean, 150 g, grilled	0.2
Lamb, lean, 150 g, cooked	0.1
Egg, 1	0.7
Milk, 250 mL glass	0.1
Oats, 60 g raw weight	2.1
Wholemeal bread, 2 slices	0.8
Brown rice, 60 g raw weight	0.7
Barley, 60 g raw weight	0.6
Rye crispbread, 4	0.6
Wheat bran, 2 tablespoons	0.5

LINOLENIC ACID

A polyunsaturated fatty acid (abbreviated as C18:3) which may be essential in the human diet. Linolenic acid has 18 carbon atoms and 3 double bonds and exists as both alpha and gamma forms. Alpha linolenic acid belongs to the omega 3 family of fatty acids while the gamma type belongs to the omega 6 series. The two fatty acids have different roles in the body. Linolenic acid is sometimes incorrectly referred to as vitamin F. It is not a vitamin.

Alpha linolenic acid can be converted into eicosapentaenoic acid (EPA) and docosahexaenoic acid (DHA), both of which are omega 3 fatty acids. This conversion occurs slowly, especially when levels of linoleic acid are high. This is because linoleic acid (which is converted to arachidonic acid) competes for the same enzymes. It is now thought that the ideal ratio of omega 6: omega 3 fatty acids (the latter include not only linolenic acid but also the fats found in fish) is 5:1 (see page 254). Omega 3 fatty acids are also used to make hormone-like substances called prostaglandins. Linolenic acid itself is also needed by the retina of the eye.

The daily requirement of linolenic plus omega 3 fatty acids in fish is estimated to be 1−2 g per day (see also Omega 3 fatty acids, page 254). Linolenic acid is found in the leaves of plants. Linseeds and walnuts are also good sources.

Major food sources of linolenic acid are:

FOOD	LINOLENIC ACID CONTENT (g)
Oats, 60 g raw	0.12
Barley, 60 g raw	0.06
Rye crispbread, 4	0.06
Wholemeal bread, 2 slices	0.05
Unprocessed bran, 2 tablespoons	0.03
Linseed oil, 1 tablespoon	10.00
Rapeseed oil, 1 tablespoon	2.10
Soya bean oil, 1 tablespoon	1.48
Corn oil, 1 tablespoon	0.32
Cottonseed oil, 1 tablespoon	0.20
Peanut oil, 1 tablespoon	0.16
Olive oil, 1 tablespoon	0.14
Safflower oil, 1 tablespoon	0.10
Sunflower oil, 1 tablespoon	0.06
Palm oil, 1 tablespoon	0.06
Polyunsaturated margarine, 1 tablespoon	0.14
Walnuts, 50 g	2.94
Peanuts, 50 g	0.20

Hazelnuts, 50 g	0.04
Chestnuts, 50 g	0.06
Mushrooms, 100 g	0.33
Baked beans, 150 g	0.29
Spinach, 75 g	0.23
Banana, 150 g	0.10
Avocado, $\frac{1}{2}$	0.09
Liver, lamb, 150 g	0.59
Rabbit, 150 g	0.59
Crab, 100 g flesh	0.24
Herring, 100 g	0.22
Beef, lean, 150 g, grilled	0.17
Chicken or turkey, lean, 150 g	0.10
Lamb, lean, 150 g, cooked	0.10
Milk, 250 mL glass	0.14

LINSEED

Also known as flaxseed, the small brown shiny seeds of the linseed plant are used to produce linseed oil, or are added to foods such as breads. The meal remaining after the extraction of the oil is an important animal feed. Linseed oil is the richest food source of alpha linolenic acid (see page 209).

LINSEED OIL
see Oils.

LINZER TORTE

A rich dessert named after the Austrian town of Linz. It is made from a ground nut pastry base, spread with jam with a criss-cross pattern on the nut pastry topping. An average serve has 1340 kJ (320 Cals).

LIPASES

Enzymes which split fats into fatty acids and glycerol. They occur in pancreatic juices, intestinal juices and the blood. Most of the action of the lipases occurs in the small intestine where bile salts reduce the surface tension of the fat droplets so that the lipases can split the fat molecules. There is also some action by lipases within the cells of the membranes lining the walls of the intestine.
See also Enzymes.

LIPIDS

The correct name for fats (see Fats).

LIPOIC ACID

A fatty acid containing sulphur, discovered in the late 1940s, and now known to be involved in the metabolism of proteins, fats and carbohydrates in the body. Lipoic acid is essential for the growth of some micro-organisms but has not been shown to be a dietary necessity for growth in humans. It is found in liver and yeast.

LIPOPROTEINS

Substances which contain both fat and protein. Since fats are insoluble in water, they attach themselves to protein molecules in order to be transported in the plasma portion of the blood and in cell membranes.

Lipoproteins come in different sizes and densities. The largest are called chylomicrons and have very little protein and lots of fat. Most of the fat in the chylomicrons is triglyceride but they also carry some cholesterol and phospholipids (such as lecithin). Fat is taken from the intestine through the lymph to the great veins of the neck and then into the blood as chylomicrons which can be used for energy or stored as body fat.

In the blood, the density of the lipoproteins can decrease as fatty acids are dropped off to the tissues or deposited in the arteries. Very low density lipoproteins (VLDLs) go to the muscles and fat depots to deposit their triglycerides. They then become low density lipoproteins (LDLs) with their core of triglyceride being replaced by cholesterol. The LDLs set off to all the body cells to deliver their cholesterol package. In theory, the cells having received their cholesterol can then cease making it themselves. In practice, this system may go astray. LDLs also deposit cholesterol into the walls of the arteries.

High density lipoproteins (HDLs) are made in the liver and small intestine and are almost entirely composed of phospholipid. Known as the 'good guys', HDLs travel through the blood picking up cholesterol and taking it to the liver for excretion.

LIPTAUER

see Cheese.

LIQUEURS

see Drinks, Alcoholic.

LIQUORICE

The extract of a leguminous plant native to the Middle East, liquorice was used for medicinal purposes in Egypt from about 2000 BC. Liquorice extract is made by boiling the yellow roots of the plant in water and then evaporating the water until a sticky black residue remains. The extract contains an oil, anethole, which provides an aniseed flavour and also glycyrrhizic acid, which tastes sweet. The latter is used to flavour and sweeten chewing, pipe and cigarette tobaccos, and also confectionery. Root beer, some chocolates, vanilla and liqueur flavourings also use liquorice. The ammonium salt of glycyrrhizic acid is considered a safe sugar substitute or food additive in some countries; it is 50 times as sweet as sugar.

Liquorice, eaten in excess, can cause hypertension and potassium deficiency. This is unlikely to be a problem unless very large quantities are consumed.

LITCHEE

see Fruits, Lychee.

LITHIUM

Lithium carbonate, a salt of the element lithium, is used as an anti-depressant and as a treatment for some cluster headaches. Among its side effects are diarrhoea, nausea, drowsiness, fluid retention and weight gain. Those using lithium compounds should also be aware that caffeine speeds up the clearance of lithium from the body. Changing one's usual coffee or tea intake could therefore affect the quantity of the drug required.

LIVER, AS FOOD

The livers of calves, chickens, pigs and cattle are eaten by humans. With its role as the storehouse and processing centre of an animal's body, liver is a rich source of nutrients. It is high in vitamin A, riboflavin, niacin, B_6, pantothenic acid, biotin, folacin, B_{12} and vitamin C. It supplies protein, linoleic acid (see page 208) and zinc, and is the richest food source of iron. Lamb's liver (also known as lamb's fry) is a good source of linolenic acid (see page 209).

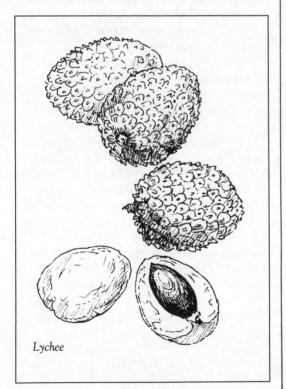

Lychee

Liver also contains dietary cholesterol and a 100 g serving of liver has almost as much cholesterol as 2 egg yolks. Since liver is not rich in saturated fats — the major source of high levels of cholesterol in the blood (see page 72) — its cholesterol content is only likely to be a problem if it is fried or eaten as part of a high-fat diet. A low-fat diet, with the occasional serving of liver, will provide a rich source of nutrients and should not increase blood cholesterol levels in most people.

Before cooking, the thin membrane on the outside of liver should be removed, except in the case of chicken livers where this is unnecessary. Liver should be cooked (by pan frying, char grilling or braising) for only a short time. Long cooking makes it tough and dry since, unlike meat muscle, it has little connective tissue.

100 g of liver have 670 kJ (160 Cals). This amount also contains more than 10 days' supply of vitamin A and almost a whole day's supply of several vitamins and minerals.

LIVER, HUMAN

The largest glandular organ in the body, the liver is the major site for metabolism of nutrients and alcohol. It also detoxifies unwanted substances.

The liver is involved in:

- Protein metabolism — Amino acids are broken down to form glucose for energy or are used to make body proteins; the ammonia produced from the breakdown of amino acids is converted by the liver to urea, which is then excreted in urine. The liver also produces enzymes, blood serum proteins and some clotting factors from amino acids.
- Fat metabolism — Fats are oxidised to produce energy, especially if no carbohydrate is available, as occurs during fasting or in untreated diabetes. Cholesterol and phospholipids such as lecithin are also made in the liver. The liver makes 800–1000 mL

of bile each day and despatches it through the bile duct to the small intestine (at meal times) or to the gallbladder (in between meals). If the liver is not functioning properly (as occurs in hepatitis), bile will not flow to the intestine, fats will not be digested and the person will feel sick. Bile is also used for the excretion of some waste products.

- Carbohydrate metabolism — Sugars such as fructose are converted to glucose; excess glucose is converted to glycogen. If blood sugar level drops, this glycogen is converted back to glucose. Approximately 85 g of glycogen are stored in the liver — sufficient to provide about 1428 kJ (340 Cals) of energy (see also Hunger).
- Vitamins — A, E and K, B_{12} and folacin are all stored in the liver.
- Alcohol — Initial oxidation of alcohol occurs in the liver.
- Detoxification — Drugs, harmful or unwanted chemicals, some food additives, are altered to a safer form or to a compound which can be excreted.
- Blood chemistry — The liver synthesises substances involved in blood clotting, removes waste products from the blood and breaks down old red blood cells, allowing their iron to be re-used.

The liver has great powers of regeneration after slight damage. However, once it is damaged, it has enormous implications for health. Both alcohol and toxic chemicals can destroy the liver cells. Initially, there is an infiltration of fat into the liver, followed by hardening of the soft tissues. As the liver is progressively damaged, it can no longer process the nutrients. One of its major functions — the conversion of ammonia (from amino acids) to urea — ceases, and the build up of ammonia causes mental confusion and eventually, death.

LIVERWURST

see Sausages.

LOAF SUGAR

Another name for cubes of sugar.

LOBSTER

see Seafood.

LOCUST BEAN GUM

see Carob.

LOGANBERRY

see Fruit.

LOLLIES

see Confectionery.

LONGAN

see Fruit.

LONGEVITY

Many factors, including genetics and environmental influences, obviously influence how long one lives. Nutrition is also important but attempts to unravel the secrets of the diet most likely to produce longevity have not yet come to a definite conclusion.

Experimental work with rats has shown that those on minimal diets which provide enough nutrients but no excess energy, have the longest life expectancy. Whether this applies to humans — or even whether we want it to — is not yet known.

At this stage, it appears that greater longevity is achieved by reducing risks of the common killers, heart disease and cancer. The simplest way to reduce the risk of such conditions is to adopt a low-fat diet with increased quantities of wholegrain products, fruits, vegetables and legumes.

The increased use of antioxidants, or foods containing these substances, may also play a part in longevity (see Ageing).

LONG-LIFE MILK

see Milk.

LOQUAT

see Fruit.

LOTUS ROOT

see Vegetables.

LOVAGE

see Herbs.

LOVE APPLES

The name given to tomatoes in England in the sixteenth century when they were thought to be suitable only as an ornamental fruit.

LOW-DENSITY LIPOPROTEINS

see Lipoproteins.

LOW-KILOJOULE FOODS

Low-kilojoule (or low-calorie) foods have a reduction in their energy levels, usually by having artificial sweeteners replacing sugar. In some foods, fats are also reduced. Some countries have set standards for what constitutes a low-kilojoule food; others accept a certain reduction (usually one-third) compared with the regular food.

Debate continues as to whether low-kilojoule foods are a good idea for overweight people. On one hand, there is the argument that it is better to lose one's taste for sweet and/or fatty foods than to trick the body by using artificially sweetened products. The opposing point of view is that some people have no right to dictate what others should be eating and that the low-kilojoule foods offer an alternative for those who want the sweet taste but not the kilojoules of sugar.

LUCERNE

see Vegetables, Alfalfa.

LUFFA

see Vegetables.

LUPINS
see Legumes.

LYCHEE
see Fruit; Nuts.

LYSINE

An essential amino acid, well supplied by animal protein foods but missing from cereals such as wheat, rice, and especially from corn. Wild rice has a higher content of lysine than other varieties. Most nuts are also relatively deficient in lysine. Legumes are high in lysine and so make a good protein combination when combined with cereals. For example, soya beans and rice or tortillas and kidney beans together provide a better set of amino acids than either food alone.

When foods are browned, lysine contributes to the production of the more intense flavour. Unfortunately, in doing so, the lysine content of the food decreases. In a mixed diet which contains animal proteins, this is unimportant as the total amount of lysine supplied is well in excess of requirements. In a limited vegetarian diet, lysine is likely to be the scarcest of the amino acids and its loss through baking or browning may cause problems.

See also Amino acids.

M

MACADAMIA NUTS
see Nuts.

MACARONI
see Pasta.

MACAROON

A meringue with ground almonds, coconut or other nut.

MACE
see Spices.

MACKEREL
see Fish.

MACROBIOTIC (ZEN) DIET

The word macrobiotic comes from a Greek word meaning 'long life'. The original macrobiotic diet was devised by Georges Ohsawa from Japan and was based on the division of foods into two basic groups, Yin and Yang, which represented negative and positive forces.

Yin foods include sugar, all liquids, alcohol, dairy products, fruits and any food chemicals. Yang foods include meat and other animal products and salt. Grains and vegetables are neither yin nor yang and therefore represent balance. In cold climates, more yang foods are to be eaten while the yin foods are for hotter areas. Creative people are supposed to choose more yin foods while physical work requires the yang foods.

The macrobiotic diet offers a series of programs, each a little closer to the ultimate diet consisting only of brown rice. The early stages of the macrobiotic diet are quite well-

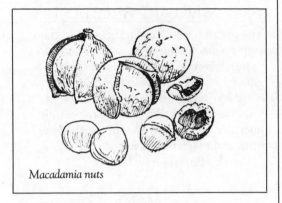

Macadamia nuts

balanced; the later stages may or may not bring spiritual enlightenment and harmony but will almost certainly bring malnutrition and death.

The yin and yang philosophy is just that — a philosophy. There is no nutritional basis for most of the ideas in the upper levels of the macrobiotic diet.

See also Yin and Yang.

MACROCYTIC ANAEMIA

An anaemia in which young red blood cells do not develop properly. Most commonly due to a deficiency of the B complex vitamin folacin.

MACRONUTRIENTS

Protein, fats and carbohydrates are known as macronutrients, as they are required in relatively large quantities. Vitamins and most minerals are known as micronutrients since they are needed in small quantities.

MADEIRA

see Drinks, Alcoholic.

MADEIRA CAKE

A British cake made with butter, sugar, flour, eggs and lemon or orange peel. Traditionally served with a glass of madeira.

MADELINES

Small, light cakes traditionally baked in scallop-shaped madeline tins. Can also be made in shallow muffin pans.

MAGNESIUM

About 60 per cent of the 25 g of this mineral present in the body is in bones; most of the remaining magnesium is within cells where it plays an important role in the biochemistry of the body. A small amount of magnesium is in nerves, muscles and body fluids.

Magnesium is essential for all reactions involving the release of energy from ATP (see page 11). It is thus important in the way the body uses proteins, fats and carbohydrates and plays an important role in muscle contraction.

Between 25−75 per cent of the magnesium we eat is absorbed, depending on how much we need. Any excess is excreted by the kidneys.

Magnesium deficiency rarely arises because of a dietary lack of the mineral. Magnesium is part of chlorophyll in plants and is also found in many other foods (see table below). A deficiency is more likely to be due to excessive losses in the urine or faeces, for example, with diarrhoea. Alcoholism also causes great losses. Symptoms of a lack of magnesium include muscular weakness, apathy, and in extreme cases, convulsions. This has led some people to believe that supplements of magnesium might help those with conditions such as epilepsy. There is no evidence to support this notion.

Magnesium deficiency has been shown to be involved in some cardiac conditions and some researchers have pointed to the difference in heart disease rates between areas of hard water, which has a high magnesium content, compared with soft water areas, where the magnesium is low. However, there are many areas where the hardness of the water (and hence the magnesium level) does not correlate with the incidence of heart disease. Magnesium is probably involved in the action of the heart muscle, but is not the only factor of importance.

Daily requirement for magnesium

mg MAGNESIUM/DAY

Infants 0—6 months	40
7—12 months	60
Children 1—3	80
4—7	110
Boys 8—11	180
12—15	260
16—18	320
Girls 8—11	160
12—15	240
16—18	270
Men	320
Women	270
Pregnancy	300
Lactation	340

Food sources of magnesium

FOOD	MAGNESIUM (mg)
All Bran, 40 g	148
Wheat bran, 2 tablespoons	104
Oats, 50 g	55
Bread, wholemeal, 2 slices	47
Bread, white, 2 slices	13
Milk, 250 mL glass (regular or skim)	30
Chicken, 150 g	40
Meat, average serve	32
Prawns, 100 g flesh	110
Sardines, canned, 100 g	52
Oysters, 1 dozen	50
Crab, 100 g flesh	48
Fish, av. fillet	45
Chickpeas, 1 cup cooked	108
Haricot beans, 1 cup cooked	72
Spinach, 100 g	68
Banana, 1 medium	28
Vegetables, av. serve	25
Avocado, $\frac{1}{2}$	20
Fruit, dried, 50 g	40
Fruit, av. piece	15
Brazil nuts, 50 g	205
Almonds, 50 g	130
Peanuts, 50 g	90
Walnuts, 50 g	65
Chocolate, 100 g	55

MAILLARD REACTION

The reaction which occurs between certain amino acids and sugars in foods, causing foods to turn brown. The maillard reaction can be either desirable or undesirable. The browning of toast is desirable, whereas the maillard reaction which produces browning of fruit juices, or the loss of colour from dehydrated fruits and vegetables, is not.

See also Browning (of Foods).

MAIZE
see Corn.

MAIZE OIL
see Oils, Corn oil.

MALABSORPTION

An inability to absorb one or more nutrients. Usually occurs because of some defect in the lining of the intestine, the lack of an enzyme, or because of competition from bacteria for the particular nutrients. Malabsorption is characterised by loss of weight, failure to grow (in children), diarrhoea, abdominal pain and signs of vitamin deficiencies in skin, mouth or muscles. The cause must be found and fixed for recovery to occur.

MALBEC
see Wine, Varieties.

MALIC ACID

An acid present in some fruits and vegetables. The products with the highest content of malic acid include rhubarb, plums, cherries, quinces, apricots, nectarines, sugar bananas, apples, grapes, passionfruit, peaches, Jerusalem artichokes, limes, loquats and lychees. Malic acid has some degree of sourness and wines with a high content of malic acid tend to taste sour. Some winemakers add particular strains of bacteria to convert malic acid to the less sour-tasting lactic acid.

MALNUTRITION

A condition resulting from an inadequate supply of total food or nutrients. Protein, vitamins and minerals are usually limited in the diet of those suffering from malnutrition. The condition occurs in countries where the food supply is inadequate and is only found in developed countries in those who follow bizarre diets, or have anorexia nervosa (see page 24).

Malnutrition is reversed by providing food. If severe malnutrition occurs in a young child, there can be permanent brain damage.

MALT

A product made by taking a grain (usually barley), soaking it in water and allowing it to germinate or sprout so that the complex carbohydrate in the grain is converted to maltose. This is dried to produce malt which is then used as the basis of brewing (see Beer).

Malt extract is made by soaking powdered malt in water and heating the mixture until some of the water evaporates and the malt becomes a dark sticky mass. Since malt extract attracts water, its addition to bread or cakes gives a moist product. Malt extract can also be used as a topping for bread.

Malt is a good source of iron and niacin and also provides other vitamins of the B complex. 20 g of dried malt extract have 315 kJ (74 Cals). One tablespoon (25 g) of the dark-coloured syrupy malt extract has 315 kJ (75 Cals).

MALTASE

The enzyme produced in the intestine to digest maltose.

See also Maltose.

MALTED MILK

A combination of maltose, glucose and dried milk powder. Supposed to promote sleep, malted milk may achieve its reputation from its content of tryptophan (see page 349). The addition of maltose increases the carbohydrate in malted milk and when compared with regular milk, it has lower levels of all nutrients. Two level teaspoons of malted milk powder (10 g) have 170 kJ (40 Cals).

MALTODEXTRINS

Used as thickening agents in foods, maltodextrins consist of partially digested starch. They can be used to modify texture of foods or to slow down the rate at which sugars will be absorbed.

MALTOSE

A double sugar (or disaccharide) consisting of two molecules of glucose linked together. Maltose is found in malt and in malted milk and is also produced during the digestion of complex carbohydrates (see page 55) and glycogen (see page 165). It is about half as sweet as sugar. In the intestine, maltose is split by the enzyme maltase into its component glucose molecules.

MAMMEE
see Fruit.

MANCHEGO
see Cheese.

MANDARIN
see Fruit.

MANDARIN ORANGE
see Fruit.

MANGANESE

In 1931 it was recognised that manganese was an essential mineral. The human body contains 10—20 mg of manganese, mainly in bones and in the liver. It has been difficult to study the effects of a deficiency of manganese since it is so rare. However, it is known that the mineral is essential for several enzymes to bring about chemical reactions in the body. Manganese seems to be particularly important in bones and cartilage and also plays a role in brain function.

A recommended intake for manganese has not been established, but 2.5−5 mg is generally considered a desirable level. The mineral is widely distributed in foods with the highest levels in nuts, wholegrain products, vegetables and fruits. Tea is a particularly rich source.

MANGE TOUT
see Vegetables, Peas.

MANGO
see Fruit.

MANGOSTEEN
see Fruit.

MANIOC
see Vegetables, Cassava.

MANNITOL

A sugar alcohol which provides a sweet taste to foods such as jellies, drinks and desserts. Mannitol has been used in place of sugar in some foods and has the advantage of being absorbed into the bloodstream more slowly than sugar. However, mannitol has only 70 per cent of the sweetness of sugar, still contributes kilojoules and has the disadvantage of causing diarrhoea and stomach cramps if used in high doses. It is shown on food labels as additive number 421.

MANNOSE

A constituent of the gummy type of dietary fibre in plants. The highest food sources are red currants, gooseberries, blackcurrants and soya beans. Other sources of mannose include canned and fresh tomatoes, green beans, eggplant, cabbage, swedes, turnips and capsicums.

MAPLE SYRUP

A syrup extracted from the North American maple tree. Before European settlement in America, the Indians used to tap the maple trees and collect the clear-coloured sugar solution. The sugar solution is evaporated to about one-thirtieth of its volume to produce the familiar, thicker, brown-coloured maple syrup. The syrup can be collected from the trees for about 6 weeks a year. It is traditionally used on pancakes, hotcakes, cakes, baked beans, bacon and ham, sweet potatoes and apples.

Maple syrup has some calcium and iron as well as small quantities of potassium. Two tablespoons of syrup have 585 kJ (140 Cals).

The imitation maple syrups have similar kilojoule content but little nutritional value.

MARASCHINO
see Drinks, Alcoholic.

MARENGO

Chicken marengo was a dish created for Napoleon after his victory in the Battle of Marengo in 1800. The surrounding countryside offered chicken, garlic, tomatoes, mushrooms and herbs. These were cooked with some oil and wine and the term marengo is now applied to dishes which use these flavourings.

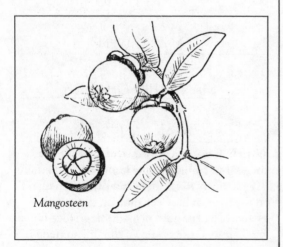
Mangosteen

MARGARINE

Napoleon is credited with being the father of the margarine industry. A French chemist produced the first margarine for him in 1869 in France from animal fats with some added milk to provide better flavour. The product was patented in 1873 and further improved by churning it with milk and salt. In many parts of the world, legislation forbade the addition of yellow colouring to margarine and it was not until such restrictions were lifted that margarine became more popular.

Various vegetable oils are now used to make many margarines. These liquid oils are hardened by the process of hydrogenation (see page 185) so that they become solid. This processing also alters the chemical nature of the products so that their original polyunsaturated fats become saturated. In margarines labelled as polyunsaturated, only sufficient oils are hydrogenated to produce a spreadable product. Fish oils can also be deodorised to produce margarines. This practice is used in the United Kingdom to some extent.

Margarine undergoes a lot of processing. The vegetable oils are first degummed to remove any off flavours. They are then neutralised by mixing with an alkali such as caustic soda, separating out the soap and leaving an oily residue. This is then bleached to remove any colour pigments and hydrogenated to harden the product to a spreadable form. More bleaching, filtering and deodorising, plus the addition of salt, colouring, flavouring, preservatives, emulsifiers and some vitamins, gives us the familiar spread.

Many people believe margarine is a healthier and less fatty product than the butter it replaces. In fact, margarine and butter have an equal quantity of fat and the same high kilojoule count. Polyunsaturated margarines do, however, have a higher percentage of polyunsaturated fats than other margarines or butter. They also have the advantage of being more easily spread so that, in theory, a smaller quantity can be used. In practice, those who replace butter with margarine, continue to use similar or even slightly greater amounts.

All margarines have 615 kJ (147 Cals) per tablespoon. Most have vitamins A and D added to the same level as present naturally in butter.

The choice between butter and margarine can be difficult. Most people with discriminating palates can taste the difference between the two products, and are likely to prefer butter. Those with high levels of cholesterol in their blood are usually advised to switch to polyunsaturated margarine. However, although the fats in this product may benefit the arteries, there is little evidence that margarine is of value to the rest of the body. Margarines have the same potential to increase body fat as butter, and since extra body fat can increase cholesterol levels, the end effect of switching to margarine may be less positive than once believed. It is probably best to eat as little as possible of either butter or margarine.

MARGARITA
see Drinks, Alcoholic.

MARINADE

A solution in which meats, fish, chicken or fruits are soaked to provide flavour and increase tenderness before cooking or eating. Popular marinades include wine, oil, lemon juice, vinegar, herbs and spices for savoury foods. Wine or acid (such as lemon juice or vinegar) breaks down some of the surface proteins giving a softer consistency. However, this process can also produce a drier product when the meat is cooked. For practical nutritional purposes, when meat or other marinaded food is grilled, the nutritional contribution and kilojoules from the marinade is very small.

MARJORAM
see Herbs.

MARMALADE

A conserve made from citrus fruits, water and sugar and popular in England and most English-speaking countries of the world. The French marmelade, the Italian marmalata and the Portuguese marmalada do not contain any citrus fruit.

Marmalade contains small quantities of minerals but most of its vitamins are lost during its preparation. However, marmalades do contain pectin, a valuable form of dietary fibre. Those varieties containing the most peel have the most pectin. One tablespoon of marmalade has 210 kJ (50 Cals).

MARMITE

A yeast and vegetable extract originally made in the early 1920s. Rich in vitamins of the B group, Marmite also contains salt. It is low in kilojoules and a typical spread (3.5 g) has only 25 kJ (6 Cals).

See also Vegemite.

MARRON

The French word for chestnut (see page 244). See also Seafood.

MARROW

see Vegetables.

MARROW BONE

The soft fatty interior of the thigh bones of beef cattle which can be extracted from the bones after steaming or scooped out of cracked bones. Used as a spread or as an addition to soups, hors d'oeuvres or specialty dishes. Bone marrow is very high in fat and contains some of the B complex vitamins. 20 g of bone marrow have 735 kJ (175 Cals).

MARSALA

see Drinks, Alcoholic.

MARS BAR

A popular chocolate caramel bar. A 70 g Mars bar has 1340 kJ (320 Cals).

MARSHMALLOW

Marshmallow was originally the root of the marshmallow plant which contained gelatinous substances as well as some fat and carbohydrate. The root was used as a confection. These days, marshmallow is made from a mixture of sugar, egg white and gelatine which is allowed to partially set and is then beaten to a light frothiness. Individual pieces of marshmallow are rolled in finely powdered sugar or rice flour. 100 g of marshmallow have 1360 kJ (325 Cals). Most of the kilojoules come from sugar; there is almost no fat.

MARTINI

see Drinks, Alcoholic.

MARZIPAN

Probably one of the earliest confections known, marzipan originated in the Middle East. It is made from a mixture of ground almonds (or almond paste), sugar and egg white. A soft marzipan mixture is used as a filling for pastries and cakes, while a firmer mixture is often modelled into various shapes which are used as decorative forms of confection. German marzipan is made from ground almonds and sugar heated until dry and then moistened to a thick paste with icing sugar and glucose. French marzipan is made from more finely ground almonds and egg white mixed with a sugar syrup to give a finer, whiter product. 50 g of marzipan have 905 kJ (215 Cals). These kilojoules come from sugar and also from the fat from the almonds.

MARZOUM

A yoghurt drink which is popular in Armenia.

MASA

A mixture of corn meal and an alkaline solution. By soaking corn in alkali, some of the amino acids are made less available to the body. This improves the balance of the remaining amino acids (see also Corn).

MASAI

A nomadic East African tribe whose diet consists mainly of milk and blood taken from the jugular vein of their cattle. In spite of this diet with its high content of fat and pre-formed cholesterol, the Masai tribe are strong, healthy and have low levels of serum cholesterol. The reason for this is unknown but it is thought that milk may contain some factor which prevents a rise in serum cholesterol.

MASCARPONE

see Cheese.

MATARO

see Wine, Varieties.

MATJES HERRINGS

see Fish.

MATZO

Also called matza, matzoth or matzot, matzo is an unleavened bread eaten by Jewish people during Passover in commemoration of their rapid exit from Egypt when there was no time to allow bread to be fermented. Matzo meal is made by grinding unleavened crispbread made from wheat flour and water. It can be used in place of breadcrumbs. Matzo has approximately 1470 kJ (350 Cals) per 100 g. It is a source of complex carbohydrate and has some vitamins of the B complex, protein and dietary fibre.

MAYONNAISE

A densely-packed emulsion of oil and egg yolk, usually flavoured with lemon juice. An important accompaniment to salads and other cold savoury dishes, it was first made by Cardinal Richelieu in the seventeenth century. To make true mayonnaise, egg yolks and a little lemon juice (both at room temperature) are whisked together. A good quality vegetable oil (preferably olive) is added very slowly, while the mixture is beaten continuously, so that the oil droplets will be incorporated into the liquid

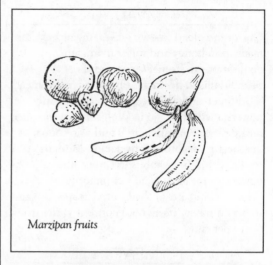

Marzipan fruits

ingredients rather than rising to the top. Once the volume of oil added approximates the volume of the liquid ingredients, the oil can be added a little faster. A mayonnaise can separate during beating if the oil particles are too large and rise to the top of the mixture. This problem can be corrected by taking another egg yolk, plus some mustard (which contains natural emulsifiers) in a clean bowl and slowly adding the curdled mayonnaise mixture. With constant beating, the mayonnaise will once again thicken.

Commercially prepared mayonnaises have a much lower percentage of oil and use various emulsifiers to keep the oil and water phases of the mixture together. In some countries, there is a legal limit on the minimum quantity of oil in a mayonnaise; in others, such as Australia, the oil content can vary from 15−80 per cent. In general, cheaper products have less oil.

The kilojoule content of mayonnaise varies considerably. For a true mayonnaise, each tablespoon will have about 630 kJ (150 Cals). For cheaper products with less oil, a tablespoon has 170 kJ (40 Cals).

MCT (MEDIUM CHAIN TRIGLYCERIDES)

see Triglycerides.

MEAD

One of the oldest known wines, mead was made from honey and water in ancient civilisations in Rome, Greece and Scandinavia. The ancient Romans called mead 'Hydromel' and believed it had therapeutic powers. Centuries ago in Wales, mead was also regarded as being medicinal and was known as 'metheglin', meaning 'physician'. Modern medicine has not established any curative powers for mead. It is now commonly consumed in parts of the United States and also in Scandinavia. Its alcohol content varies from 6–12 per cent.

MEAT

See following pages.

MEDIUM CHAIN TRIGLYCERIDES (MCT)

see Triglycerides.

MEDLAR

see Fruit, Azarole.

MEGAVITAMINS

Doses of vitamins at least 10 times the recommended daily intake. At these levels, many vitamins act quite differently and function as drugs rather than playing their normal role. Unlike vitamins, however, megadoses of vitamins can be sold without health warnings or any testing (see also Vitamin supplements).

MEKABU

see Seaweed.

MELANIN

see Copper.

MELBA TOAST

Dame Nellie Melba, the great opera singer, gave her name to Melba toast which is made by slicing bread very thinly and allowing the slices to dry to a golden crispness in a moderate oven. Often served with pâté, mousse or soups. The kilojoule value will vary with the product, but a typical slice of Melba toast will have about 105 kJ (25 Cals).

MELONS

see Fruit.

MELT

The spleen of an animal. Not commonly eaten in Western societies although it may find its way into sausages. More likely to be used for pet food.

MENSTRUATION AND NUTRITION

The blood loss during menstruation means that iron will be lost from the body. This can be replaced throughout the month if the diet contains sufficient iron. Because of menstrual iron loss, the recommended daily intake of iron for women is more than twice that for men (see page 191). Those who have heavy periods usually need to aim for the top of the range of iron, that is, 16 mg/day.

Just before menstruation, changes in hormone levels may cause a temporary increase in sodium levels. This sodium (which comes from salt) keeps extra fluid in the body and produces the well-known bloated feeling many women experience just before their period.

Some take vitamin B_6 or other B complex vitamins in an attempt to correct the fluid retention and related symptoms (headache, irritability, swelling of the tummy). Properly controlled studies have shown that taking extra B_6 is no better than a placebo. The best cure for the fluid retention is to drink extra water to flush out the retained sodium. Eating less salt may also help.

Many women also find they have a craving for carbohydrate just before or during their period. Although the phenomenon is common, the reasons for it remain obscure. It does not seem to be related to any abnormality in blood sugar level.

MEAT

The flesh of animals, usually taken to mean the muscle of the animal. Red meat is taken to mean the flesh of beef cattle, buffalo and sheep while white meat includes pork and veal, and, in many cases, fish and poultry. No one seems too sure just where game meats such as venison fit into this classification. Venison is often taken to be red meat while hare and rabbit are seen as white.

Most humans consider it quite moral to kill animals for food although some religious groups find the practice offensive. Although there are many vegetarian populations throughout the world, most are vegetarian because they do not have the facilities to keep, kill and store meat (see also vegetarian diet, page 374). Meat probably became more important in the diet when animals were first domesticated some 10,000 years ago. During the Middle Ages, larger quantities of meat were consumed in Europe; consumption decreased rapidly as the population increased.

In countries such as Australia and the United States, a high meat consumption has always been a dominant feature of the diet.

From the nutritional point of view, meat contains an excellent selection of the amino acids which make up protein. It is also a good source of minerals such as iron and zinc and provides vitamins of the B complex, especially niacin, thiamin and B_{12}. It takes a relatively long time to be digested by humans and so provides satiety.

The major nutritional problem with meat concerns the large amount of fat in many of the cuts of meat from domesticated animals. Most of this fat is saturated. As people have realised the high fat content of large serves of meat, consumption has dropped in countries such as Australia, although it is still very high by world standards. Large fatty steaks still hang over the dinner plates of many Australians and servings of 250—300 g are not uncommon. It would be better for health if we could persuade people to eat only small portions of the leaner meats available and to trim off all visible fat. Many people claim to remove the fat from their meat; fewer actually do so.

Production of leaner animals and less fatty meats would also be a forward nutritional step. Recently, there have been some attempts to produce leaner animals and less fatty cuts of meat. Unfortunately, the leaner cuts of meat tend to be more expensive than the fattier portions and the processed meat products such as sausages.

Meat is made up of water, protein and fat. Lean raw meat has 65—70 per cent water, about 20 per cent protein and 10—15 per cent fat. Lean cuts of meat may have as little as 4 per cent fat. The kilojoule level has a wide range depending on the quantity eaten, the cut, the cooking method and the fat content.

In general, cooked lean beef has about 775 kJ (185 Cals) per 100 g. If both lean and fat are eaten, the value for 100 g increases to 940 kJ (225 Cals). For lamb, if only the lean portion is eaten, 100 g will have 820 kJ (195 Cals). If both the fat and the lean portion of lamb are eaten, 100 g will contribute 1280 kJ (305 Cals). As can be seen from this, average cuts of lamb are much fattier than beef.

These figures cannot be taken to indicate the contribution meat makes to the kilojoules in the diet since many people in countries such as Australia and the United States will eat 200−300 g of meat at a meal. Steaks this size are the norm in some areas and contribute a large number of kilojoules.

On the other hand, those who keep the size of their meat servings moderate (less than 100 g) will not find that their meat is fattening.

If meat is omitted from the diet, the major nutrients which may be lacking will be iron and zinc. (See pages 191 and 407 for details of other sources of these nutrients.)

The more active the animal, the lower the fat content both on the edge of the cut of meat and within the muscle fibre. Game meats such as venison, hare or rabbit therefore have little fat. Domesticated animals which are kept in a confined space have much higher levels of fat. Range-fed animals which can walk and graze at will are leaner than lot-fed animals.

In general, the more a muscle is used, the tougher the muscle fibre and the longer it takes to cook. This is why fillet steak (which comes from the back of the animal) is much more tender after cooking for a few minutes than the shank meat from the leg (which requires long slow cooking to soften the connective tissue).

Lean meat was once regarded as less tender than fattier meats. However, with modern methods of butchering and the use of electrical impulses to soften muscle fibres, this is no longer necessarily true.

Meat can be kept refrigerated for several days, or frozen for much longer periods. Once cooked, it should either be consumed or refrigerated to prevent spoilage by micro-organisms.

Suitable cooking methods for different cuts of meats include grilling, braising, barbecuing, roasting, casseroling, stewing and frying. Meats can also be micro-waved but a browning dish will be required to produce the normal flavoursome browning of the outside parts of the meat.

Beef

Beef refers to the muscle from cattle and various cuts have different nutritional value, with the major variation occurring in the fat level. In general, older beef has more fat than younger beef (sometimes called yearling). However, lot-feeding, where animals are provided with food rather than having to walk around and graze, can markedly increase the fat content. Beef from grain-fed cattle may have a higher fat content than that from range cattle.

Ground beef is the term used in the United States for minced steak.

Nutritionally, beef is an excellent source of protein and a good source of iron, zinc and several of the B complex vitamins. Its fat content ranges from 6−24 per cent. Energy content also extends over a wide range with very lean cooked beef having 800 kJ (190 Cals) per 100 g while a good sized steak may have more than 2940 kJ (700 Cals).

Lamb

Meat from young sheep, especially popular in New Zealand, Australia, the Middle East and France. Most cuts of lamb have more fat than beef. Of the fat present, 57 per cent is saturated, 41 per cent is monounsaturated and only 2 per cent is polyunsaturated. If all visible fat is removed from lamb, the lean cooked meat can have as little as 8 per cent fat. If both lean and fat are eaten, the fat in cooked lamb cutlets is 28 per cent, in lamb loin chops 31 per cent, and in leg of lamb 12 per cent.

Lamb is a good source of protein, zinc, iron and the B group vitamin, niacin. Two grilled lamb loin chops have 1550 kJ (370 Cals) while a 100 g portion of roast lamb has 520 kJ (125 Cals).

Mutton

Meat from sheep which are more than 2 years old. Mutton has a darker colour and a stronger flavour than lamb. It also needs longer, slower cooking to break down the tougher muscle fibres. For practical purposes, its nutritional value can be considered approximately the same as for lamb.

Pork

Pigs were first used for food in China and they were probably the only domestic animals of Neolithic times. In some areas pork has never been used for food since it is forbidden by the laws of both Judaism and Islam. The major pork-eating countries include Germany, Denmark, Poland and Austria.

Pigs, like humans, are omnivorous animals. They are also known for their willingness to overeat and so are often high in fat. Some pigs, however, are kept under controlled conditions and have less fat than the traditional 'porky pig'. The pork from these animals is very low in fat.

In some areas of the world, pig flesh can carry a parasite known as trichinosis. Thorough cooking is necessary to kill this organism. In other countries, including Australia, trichinosis does not exist and so the emphasis on longer cooking times is unnecessary.

More than half the pork produced in countries such as the United States or Australia is cured (using saltpetre) or smoked for ham and bacon. These products have a higher salt level and a variable fat content.

Different cuts of pork can be roasted, boiled or stewed, stuffed and baked, stir-fried, made into sausages or roasted on a spit. The meat is usually tender. The most popular cuts are the leg (as a joint or in leg steaks), the loin (usually as loin chops), the ribs (as spare ribs) and the shoulder (cut into chops or left whole for roasting). A fairly fatty cut from the fore end of the animal is known as the 'hand'. It is braised or roasted.

Do not be tempted by 'long pork' — it is the name given by cannibals to human flesh!

Salt pork was once the staple diet of the poor, the sailor and the settler. The pork was soaked in a strongly salted solution to kill any micro-organisms and could be kept without refrigeration. Once a certain income level was reached, salt pork was generally rejected in favour of fresh meats.

The nutritional value of pork is different in some respects from other meats. Pork is particularly rich in thiamin having up to 7 times the level found in lean beef. It is also a good source of protein and niacin and has much less saturated fat than lamb or beef. Of the fat in pork, 38 per cent is saturated, 50 per cent is monounsaturated and 12 per cent is polyunsaturated. The higher content of unsaturated fats in pork is the reason why pork fat stays fairly soft, even in the refrigerator.

Tradional cuts of pork can be very high in fat and kilojoules. A cooked forequarter pork chop, for example, has a massive 41 g of fat and 2075 kJ (495 Cals). The newer leaner cuts of pork, however, are much more nutritionally desirable. The lean portion of a typical serve of cooked pork leg steak has just 3 g of fat and 545 kJ (130 Cals).

Silverside

Lean boneless cut of beef, available either fresh or corned. The silverside is corned in a brine solution with sodium nitrate added to make it pink and preserve it. Corned silverside is much leaner than corned brisket.

Steak

A cut of meat. Usually beef although pork and lamb and even fish 'steaks' are also marketed.

Veal

The meat from young dairy cattle, usually killed before the animals are about 3 months of age so that their flesh is tender. Milk-fed veal is sold in Europe and is a very light colour. Veal in countries such as Australia is pinker but does not have the red colour of the meat from older animals.

Veal has very little fat and needs to be cooked using moist heat so that it does not dry out. Grilling is not always suitable and roasting, pan frying or braising may give juicier results.

Veal scallopine is one of the best known ways of preparing veal. The basic cut is a piece of leg steak and it earned both its fame and its name in Milan in the sixteenth century. Milan at this time was part of the Spanish empire and the scallop shell was the emblem of Spain's patron saint, St James. It was also featured on homes in Milan at the time. Later, when Milan was occupied by Austrian soldiers, the scallopine became the famous *wiener schnitzel*. Other famous veal dishes include *blanquette de veau*, the French white veal stew and *vitello tonnato*, the Italian dish of cold veal with tuna sauce.

Most cuts of veal have 2−4 per cent fat — much less than beef or lamb. Veal is an excellent source of protein, a good source of niacin and also supplies some other B complex vitamins, zinc and iron. The iron content is lower than in beef but is still significant. 100 g veal leg steak have 590 kJ (140 Cals).

MENTHOL

Also known as peppermint camphor, menthol comes from a variety of mint which grows in Japan. Added to medicines, sweets and cosmetics.

MERCAPTANS

Products from the breakdown of sulphur-containing amino acids. In the intestine, mercaptans are broken down by bacteria to form methane and hydrogen sulphide. These substances are responsible for the odour of intestinal gas. Asparagus has a high content of sulphur-containing amino acids. Sulphur compounds released from cabbage may also form mercaptans in the intestine.

MERCURY

A mineral which has no known function in humans and is toxic. Mercury poisoning has occurred from eating fish from contaminated waters. Few foods other than seafoods contain any mercury. It causes damage to the brain and kidneys. Regular checks on mercury levels in foods are carried out by regulatory authorities.

MERINGUE

A mixture of egg white and sugar which is baked. Meringue may be lightly baked so that it is soft or it may be left in a slow oven until it is dry and crisp. The basic mixture for meringue uses 2 tablespoons of sugar for each egg white. For a lighter softer meringue, as in a topping on a pie, less sugar can be used.

MERLOT

see Wine, Varieties.

MESOMORPH

Within a system of categorisation of the shape of the human body originally devised by the American psychologist W. H. Sheldon, a mesomorph has greater than average muscle development. The extreme mesomorph has a large head, broad muscular chest and shoulders and heavy muscular arm and leg development.

METABISULPHITE

Usually present in foods as sodium or potassium metabisulphite (Additive nos. 223 and 224). Acts as a source of sulphur dioxide which acts as a preservative and antioxidant and is commonly used in wines, beer, fruit juices, sausages, soft drinks, some dried fruit and frozen potato products. Some people are sensitive to these additives, especially asthmatics.

METABOLIC RATE

see Basal Metabolic Rate.

METABOLISM

The sum of all the chemical reactions which occur to keep the body alive. Metabolism involves the use of energy for growth and maintenance of all body tissues. Both the building up of new tissue and the removal of the old are included in metabolism. The rate at which the body's metabolism proceeds can be measured from the amount of energy taken in and given out. It is expressed as basal metabolic rate (see page 33).

The greater the quantity of muscle tissue, the higher the rate of metabolism. Those who are active enough to build up greater muscle fibre therefore use more energy than those whose body has a higher degree of fat.

METCHNIKOFF, ILYA

A distinguished Russian pathologist who won the Nobel Prize in 1908 for his discovery that white blood cells fight infection. Metchnikoff believed that the colon was 'useless in the case of man'. He maintained that the colon harboured great numbers of bacteria which he believed produced toxins which slowly poisoned the body. To counteract the bacteria, Metchnikoff thought yoghurt held the key, assuming that the lactic bacteria in yoghurt would overcome the colonic bacteria. Unfortunately, the yoghurt bacteria will not live in the human intestine. Metchnikoff's theory has sold a lot of yoghurt but has done little else.

METHANOL

Also known as methyl alcohol, this product is the simplest alcohol. It has many industrial applications but is quite toxic to humans. Methanol is present in methylated spirits. In the body it is metabolised in the liver to form formaldehyde which can damage the retina in the eye, leading to blindness. Once obtained commercially from the distillation of wood, methanol is now made chemically. Very small quantities of methanol are found in foods, but it would not be possible to consume adequate amounts for foods to be a harmful source.

METHIONINE

An essential sulphur-containing amino acid in protein foods. Some vegetarian diets lack methionine as it is present in inadequate quantities in vegetables and legumes. Eggs are a rich source and sufficient methionine is also found in cereals. Thus beans and rice or corn, or beans on toast, can supply a full complement of amino acids.

METHYL CELLULOSE

A vegetable gum produced by chemical alteration of cellulose. Acts as a form of dietary fibre and is used as a thickener in cakes, biscuits, salad dressings and toppings. Additive no. 461.

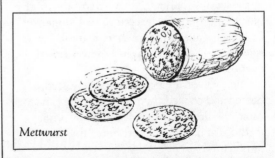
Mettwurst

METTWURST

see Sausages.

MICROWAVE COOKERY

The high energy electromagnetic radiation in a microwave oven comes from a magnetron tube. This converts electricity into microwave energy which is reflected, absorbed and transmitted within the food. Since microwaves are reflected away from metals, food in a metal container will not heat in a microwave oven. The oven walls are also metal so that energy is reflected away from them and comes into contact with the food.

All foods contain some water (even meat is about 70 per cent water). Microwave radiation causes the water particles to vibrate at the astounding rate of over 2400 million times per second. The friction caused by this vibration produces heat energy which is then conducted throughout the food.

Microwaves were first used for cooking in 1945 when a scientist, Dr Percy Spencer, used them to pop corn. They became popular as a domestic appliance in the 1970s and are now found in 50 per cent of homes in countries such as Australia.

Microwave ovens are made to produce a certain amount of energy. A 700 watt oven, for example, sends 700 watts of energy into the oven. If the oven is operating on full power, the 700 watts enter continuously over the period chosen. If the oven is programmed to operate at 50 per cent power, 700 watts will enter for 50 per cent of the cooking time chosen. This allows rest periods when the heat in the food is conducted throughout the food. Not all foods should be cooked on high power in a microwave any more than all foods are suitably cooked at 250°C in a conventional oven.

Microwaves allow foods to be defrosted, heated and cooked. In most cases, the time for these operations is much less than by other methods and the results are generally very satisfactory.

Usually, there is less loss of vitamins in microwaved food than in foods cooked by conventional methods. Reheating usually means some loss of nutrients from foods. Using the microwave for reheating reduces these losses to a minimum.

There is also a greater retention of the natural flavours so that microwaved foods require less salt than foods cooked by other methods. Since foods do not burn in the microwave, less fats can also be used. Perhaps, most importantly, microwave cookery often takes less time than is needed to visit a fast food outlet. This gives microwave cookery an indirect health advantage.

Microwaves do not brown foods. Since the browning reaction is responsible for some of the most desirable flavours in foods such as meats or chicken, a special browning dish is needed when cooking these foods. Browning dishes have impregnated into their base a special layer of material which becomes very hot in the microwave. Chicken, fish or meats placed onto this material brown and develop the same flavours as with conventional cookery.

MIGRAINE

A headache usually characterised by severe pain in one part of the head, visual disturbances, nausea and vomiting. Stress and changes to the body's environment can sometimes trigger an attack in susceptible people. Changes in female hormones are another cause. Some people also find that they are sensitive to certain foods. Common culprits include monosodium glutamate (occurring naturally in foods such as mushrooms and tomatoes, as well as being present as food additive no. 621), and naturally occurring amines (in red wines, chocolate, bananas, avocado, cheeses, yeast extract).

Food sensitivities are usually dose-related and it may be that at certain times a lower dose will produce a reaction than at others. For example, some women find that at times of hormonal change (such as ovulation, just before a period or at menopause), foods to which they are not normally sensitive will produce a reaction.

If food sensitivity is suspected as being related to migraine, or any other condition, it is important to contact a dietitian who specialises in this area. Most allergy tests will not pinpoint all the problem foods and they may give false results.

See also Allergies.

MILK

The secretion from the mammary glands of animals is the young animal's sole source of nutrients (see Breast feeding).

Humans continue to drink the milk of other species of animal after they are weaned — a practice not natural to any other animal. However, humans are the only mammals who continue to produce lactase, the enzyme needed to digest the lactose sugar present in milk. In some parts of the world, lactase production decreases after weaning and is almost absent after puberty. For these people, milk is not a suitable food since its undigested sugar ferments and causes abdominal pain and diarrhoea (see page 199).

The milk of cows, goats, sheep, yaks, buffaloes or horses is used as a food by people in different parts of the world. The nutrient content of these products is fairly similar, although there are some differences. Goat's milk, for example, has less vitamin B_6 and folic acid than cow's milk, and these nutrients must be supplied in some other form for a human infant being given goat's milk (see also page 166).

Milk is an ideal medium for bacteria, and in times past, many health problems were spread through milk. The process of pasteurisation, developed by the great scientist Louis Pasteur, has virtually wiped out many of these problems, at little nutritional cost. During pasteurisation, milk is heated rapidly for a very short time to kill microbes. It is then rapidly chilled. The process destroys some of the vitamin C and

thiamine (vitamin B_1) in milk but as raw milk is a poor source of these nutrients, the small losses have little practical significance. Other nutrients for which milk is a prime source (calcium, protein, riboflavin) are unaffected. Pasteurised milk must still be refrigerated — a problem for people in many parts of the world.

In countries such as Spain, Italy, the Middle East and many other areas, most of the milk now available is long-life milk. This is produced by heating milk rapidly to a high temperature to sterilise it, then cooling it quickly. As its name suggests, long-life milk keeps at room temperature — with no additives of any kind — for many months. Once opened, bacteria can enter and long-life milk must then be refrigerated. In countries where people do not have access to a refrigerator, these ultra heat-treated milks have dramatically reduced the incidence of milk-borne diseases. The nutritional value of long-life milk is the same as regular milks.

Since milk contains fat (in the form of cream) and fat has a lower density than milk, cream rises to the top of milk. To prevent this occurring, some milk is homogenised by forcing it at high pressure through a very small nozzle to break up the fat particles to a smaller size (see page 183). This produces a uniform product with the cream evenly distributed throughout.

Fat content of milk

The usual fat content of cow's milk varies from 3.2−4.5 per cent, depending on the breed of cow being used. Australian milk has a fat content of 3.6−3.8 per cent. Most goat's milk has a fat content of 4.5 per cent.

In many areas, low-fat, reduced fat or skim milks are also available. Skim and low-fat milks have all the fat taken out; reduced fat milks generally have 50−60 per cent of the fat removed.

Fortified milks are also becoming popular. These consist of either skim milk or a mixture of skim milk and whole milk, with some

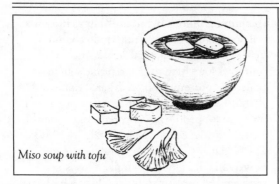

Miso soup with tofu

concentrated skim milk added. The fat content ranges from 0—1.8 per cent, and the greater skim milk concentration increases the protein, calcium and other nutrients. The natural lactose content also increases, giving the products a slightly sweeter flavour. These milks are ideal for those who need extra calcium without fat.

Low-fat milk compared with regular milk has:

- less fat
- fewer kilojoules
- lower levels of vitamins A and D
- the same amounts of calcium, protein and riboflavin

The first two differences are usually considered desirable for adults in Western countries. The loss of vitamins A and D is fairly unimportant for those on a mixed diet. Vitamin A is obtainable from foods such as fish, cheese or liver or from the carotene present in brightly coloured fruits and vegetables. Vitamin D comes from the action of sunlight on skin. For most of the population in developed countries, reduced fat milks make good sense.

For children, low-fat milks may not always be suitable. A warning to this effect is placed on the label of low-fat milk products sold in countries such as Australia. The reasons why these products are not considered a good idea for small children are as follows:

- Since low-fat milk has fewer kilojoules, young children who are dependent on milk for most of their energy will take in less energy.
- If children drink a greater quantity of low-fat milk to make up for the lower energy content, they will also be taking in a larger protein load. Immature kidneys may have difficulty coping with the greater quantity of protein break down products.
- The loss of vitamin A may be a problem for those children who do not yet eat sufficient fruits and vegetables.
- The fat in milk may be an important source of energy for a young child. Breast milk is high in fat and also contains more cholesterol than cow's milk. This may be important in setting up a feedback mechanism within the child so that the body knows when to turn off its cholesterol production mechanism.

Milk can be made into yoghurt (see page 406) or cheese (see page 62). Like milk, these are highly nutritious products and, together with milk, they provide most of the calcium in the Western diet.

See also Calcium; Drinks, Non-alcoholic; Soya bean milk.

MILLE FEUILLES

Literally 'a thousand leaves', mille feuilles consist of layers of light, crisp puff pastry. To achieve the many layers, the pastry has a high content of fat.

MILLET

see Grains.

MILT

The secretions of the sex organs of the male fish, equivalent to the roe in the female fish.

MINCE

Finely chopped or ground meat. Different grades of mince exist; the cheaper varieties have a higher fat content.

MINCEMEAT

Not meat at all, but a mixture of dried fruits, spices and brandy or rum mixed with suet or butter and used to fill small pies served at

Christmas. Mincemeat is usually made ahead of time and left for the flavours to mature for a month or two. A quarter of a cup has 740 kJ (175 Cals).

MINERALS

Many minerals are required for good health, some only in minute amounts. They are important in bones, teeth, in the blood and connective tissues. Minerals are important components of the enzymes which allow many of the body's chemical reactions to proceed. Some are also involved with hormones and vitamins.

Trace minerals are those which are required only in minute quantities. They are more difficult to study since the amounts needed within the body are so small. Deficiencies are also rare and difficult to detect. By the same token, excessive doses of these minerals are easily possible from uncontrolled use of supplements.

Minerals occur in foods, as food additives or as part of food additives, and some come from contamination during production or processing of foodstuffs.

Some minerals are likely to be in short supply in some people's diets. A lack of iron, calcium and zinc represent the most common deficiencies in the Western diet. For some unknown reason, vitamins have always been given more attention than minerals and many people whose diets contain perfectly adequate amounts of vitamins take supplements while neglecting their mineral requirements.

A diet chosen from a wide range of foods can meet the body's mineral requirements. However, if any commonly eaten class of food is omitted (such as milk or meat or seafoods), it is possible that inadequate quantities of some minerals may result.

The minerals known to be essential include calcium, chlorine, iron, magnesium, phosphorus, potassium, sodium, sulphur and sinc. Trace minerals which are also necessary include cadmium, chromium, cobalt, copper, fluorine, iodine, manganese, molybdenum, nickel, selenium, silicon, tin and vanadium. (See individual entries for details.)

MINERAL WATER
see Water.

MINESTRONE

A thick Italian soup usually containing a variety of vegetables, pasta and beans and served with Parmesan cheese. In Italy, minestrone is usually eaten as a meal in itself. One large bowl has 600 kJ (145 Cals).

MINT
see Herbs.

MINT JULEP
see Drinks, Alcoholic.

MINT SAUCE
see Sauces, Other.

MIRABELLE
see Fruit.

MIRIN
see Drinks, Alcoholic.

MIRROR DORY
see Fish.

MISO

A fermented soya bean product with a full flavour which is usually used in miso soup but can also be incorporated into sweet dishes. Widely used in Japanese cooking. Most varieties of miso have added salt and this may vary from 5-18 per cent. A tablespoon of miso has 150 kJ (35 Cals). Powdered miso has 18 per cent salt and 20 g provide 250 kJ (60 Cals). Miso also supplies some iron.

MIXED SPICE
see Spices.

MOCHA

One of the world's most highly esteemed coffees, mocha has a strong flavour and comes from the old port of Yemen. Since the beans

231

are so strongly flavoured and have a limited production, they are usually blended with other beans.

Mocha flavouring usually refers to coffee-flavoured products and is sometimes used to denote a mixture of coffee and chocolate.

MOCK CREAM

A cream substitute made from butter and sugar or from a beaten custard mixture. It is usually somewhat heavier than whipped cream and has about $1\frac{1}{2}$ times as many kilojoules as regular cream.

MOLASSES

A dark-coloured syrup produced in the early stages of the refining of sugar cane. Molasses may be dark or light, according to its degree of refinement. The first extraction of sugar crystals produces a light molasses. Very dark concentrated molasses is known as blackstrap. It has a strong bitter flavour and has high levels of iron and potassium as well as some B vitamins from the original sugar cane. Blackstrap molasses is sometimes used as a 'health food'. However, its nutrients can easily be obtained from more palatable sources.

Molasses is used in some recipes for dark moist cakes, Boston baked beans and some desserts. Light molasses is sometimes used as a syrup for pancakes.

A tablespoon of molasses has approximately 190 kJ (45 Cals); this quantity of the blackstrap variety has 3.2 mg of iron — as much as a typical serving of meat.

MOLE

A mole (abbreviated to mol) represents the molecular weight of a compound in grams. A millimole (mmol) is the molecular weight of the compound in milligrams (mg).

There is sometimes confusion when levels of different substances are expressed in millimoles or milligrams. To convert millimoles into milligrams, multiply the molecular weight of the compound by the number of moles. For example, the recommended daily intake for sodium is 40–100 mmols. To convert this to milligrams, you need to know that the molecular weight of sodium is 23. Forty mmols of sodium is thus 23×40 mg, or 920 mg. 100 mmols sodium is 23×100 mg, or 2300 mg. Thus the RDI for sodium is 40–100 mmol, or 920–2300 mg.

MOLLUSCS

Creatures which inhabit shells, mostly acquatic. The shells may be hinged (clams, mussels, oysters or pipis) or may be a single shell (abalone, winkles, limpets and whelks). There are also other classifications of molluscs, including squid, cuttlefish and octopus. For details, see individual entries.

Nutritionally, molluscs are good sources of protein, minerals (especially iron) and vitamins. They have little fat and are generally low in kilojoules. The common belief that they should not be included in a cholesterol-lowering diet is incorrect (see Cholesterol).

MOLYBDENUM

An essential mineral which takes part in many of the body's chemical reactions. As with many minerals, it has been difficult to study the effects of a deficiency as it is so rare. There is no established daily intake but the generally recommended level is 150–500 mcg a day. High doses are not recommended as too much molybdenum interferes with the body's ability to use copper.

The level of molybdenum in foods depends on the levels found in the soils in which foods grow. Neutral or alkaline soils with a high content of organic material have the highest molybdenum levels. Acid sandy soils have much less. In general, root vegetables, other vegetables, legumes, fruits and cereal grains are good sources of molybdenum.

MONOAMINE OXIDASE

An enzyme which takes part in chemical reactions with substances known as amines, the

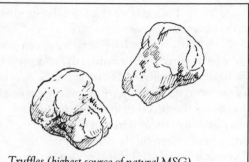

Truffles (highest source of natural MSG)

best known being the amino acid called tyramine. This enzyme is important since amines can constrict blood vessels and raise blood pressure. Some drugs used to treat depression prevent monoamine oxidase performing its normal function. This means levels of amines build up and cause symptoms ranging from headaches to dangerously high blood pressure. Anyone taking drugs which fall into the class known as monoamine oxidase inhibitors must therefore avoid foods containing high levels of amines (see page 21).

MONOGLYCERIDES

Fats which contain glycerol, alcohol and 1 fatty acid. They occur during the break down of fats and are also used in foods such as margarines, dessert mixes, instant mashed potato and soups where they reduce stickiness and keep fats evenly dispersed throughout the product (additive nos. 471, 472).

MONOSACCHARIDES

The simplest sugars containing only one carbohydrate unit. Examples are glucose and fructose. These sugars can be used by the body without further digestion. The five-carbon sugar ribose which is part of riboflavin and RNA is also a monosaccharide.

See also Carbohydrates; Disaccharides.

MONOSODIUM GLUTAMATE

Commonly called MSG, this substance is the sodium salt of the amino acid, glutamic acid.

It has a strong salt flavour and is supposed to enhance other food flavours. For this reason, it is widely used in processed and take-away foods, especially Chinese foods. For most people, it simply adds an extra source of sodium. Some people, however, are sensitive to MSG, and develop a series of symptoms including headache, dizziness, nausea or migraine after consuming it.

MSG is not only added to foods, but occurs quite naturally in some foods. Truffles are said to be the highest source. Mushrooms, tomatoes, tomato paste, puree or juice, strong cheeses, yeast, vegetable or meat extracts and some wines are high in natural MSG.

There is a set of symptoms called Chinese restaurant syndrome characterised by a burning sensation in the back of the neck, a headache and, possibly, a tight feeling in the chest. It occurs in susceptible people after eating some Chinese foods. MSG (monosodium glutamate) is usually blamed for the symptoms although there are those who dispute this.

MONOUNSATURATED FATS
see Fats.

MONSTERA
see Fruit.

MONTEREY JACK
see Cheese.

MOOD, AND FOOD

There is an increasing body of evidence that what we eat may alter levels of chemical substances in the brain which affect our moods. There is no question that food does affect mood; but the mechanisms are not fully known.

For some effects there are simple explanations. A cup of tea or coffee, for example, contains caffeine which is a stimulant for the central nervous system, including the brain.

With other foods the situation is more complex and is complicated by interactions between physiology and psychology. For example, if you were fed lollies, biscuits or cakes as rewards or bribes during your childhood, you may well feel comforted, happy and in a better mood every time you eat sweet foods. This may be due to the psychological memories that sweet foods have for you, or the sugar may trigger brain chemicals which affect your mood and behaviour.

It would appear that just as some drugs can alter behaviour, so the chemicals (both natural and added) in some foods affect the functioning of the brain. Some people find sweet foods relax them; others claim that sugar excites the brain and produces hyperactivity in children. Some people develop migraines or become irritable and depressed after eating certain foods; others become fired with enthusiasm and energy.

Researchers have now found links between certain amino acids in the blood and reactions which affect mood. Amino acids not required to repair tissues throughout the body, or for production of the body's hormones and enzymes, can be converted into glucose or body fat. Some amino acids can also be carried into the brain where they stimulate the production of chemical messenger substances called neurotransmitters. So far, about 50 of these neurotransmitters have been found. They are so tiny that more than 20,000 could fit onto the head of a pin.

Eating large amounts of sugar triggers the release of insulin which allows some of the sugar to pass into the body cells (the excess is converted into body fat). The insulin also causes most amino acids in the bloodstream (from protein foods) to be absorbed into body tissues. However, one amino acid, called tryptophan, doesn't get absorbed and may enter the brain. Tryptophan then stimulates the production of a neuro-transmitter called serotonin which has a calming effect on the body. From this, scientists conclude that it is more likely that sugar will have a calming effect rather than causing hyperactivity.

Parents who report hyperactivity after a party may be incorrect in attributing the effect solely to sugar. It is impossible to separate the effects of one food from another. Few people eat single foods and the effects of foods eaten together may be quite different from individual ingredients eaten on their own. The hyperactivity which parents notice in their offspring after a party may be related to the mixtures of foods eaten or to the colourings in sweet foods, or even to the preservatives in the cocktail frankfurts. Or it may be purely a way of a child letting off steam and have nothing to do with the foods eaten.

About 45 per cent of people suffering from depression have been found to have a low level of serotonin in the brain. Eating more sugar may make these people very calm and even drowsy. By contrast, eating more protein may increase their alertness.

Food sensitivities may also play a part in altering mood. Preservatives or other substances added to foods or natural components of foods such as the salicylates present in fruit and vegetables, the amines in bananas or the monosodium glutamate which occurs naturally in tomatoes, may produce mood changes in some people.

It is known that food sensitivities can relate to the brain and thus influence behaviour. Depression and irritability are both symptoms of brain changes which may also be caused by extreme sensitivity to particular amino acids or chemical substances found in foods. Further research is needed to clarify these issues.

See also Allergies; Amino acids; Hyperactivity.

MOON FISH
see Fish.

MORELLO
see Fruit

MORELS
see Vegetables, Mushrooms.

MORETON BAY BUG
see Seafood, Lobster.

MORNAY SAUCE
see Sauces, White sauce.

MORNING SICKNESS
see Pregnancy.

MORTADELLA
see Sausages.

MORWONG
see Fish.

MOULDS
A variety of moulds can develop on foods. Some moulds are quite harmless and many are even useful. For example, blue vein cheese uses a mould to impart the characteristic flavour and moulds can be used in producing some alcoholic beverages.

Many moulds, however, produce toxins which cause illness and even death (see Mycotoxins and Aflatoxins).

Mould tends to develop on the surfaces of plants, especially in the presence of acids. The spores of moulds are present in the atmosphere but they usually only grow to any extent on old or damaged produce, or in the case of peanuts, legumes and grains, in the absence of oxygen.

When a fruit or vegetable is damaged, the cell walls break and fluids which are nutritious to moulds are released. One patch of mould encourages other patches to develop.

In the domestic situation, moulds can be avoided by using fresh products, throwing out any damaged foods and keeping foods at the correct storage temperature.

In food production, moulds can be eliminated by good handling practices, and by the use of preservatives and mould inhibitors. These substances are much less harmful than the moulds they prevent. In Australia, mould inhibitors are added to bread (usually additives 280–283) during the summer months when mould infestation is more likely.

MOUSSAKA
A Mediterranean dish containing layers of egg plant (aubergine) and minced lamb, topped with a savoury custard or yoghurt mixture. An average serve (250 g) has 1600 kJ (382 Cals).

MOUSSE
A light airy mixture, either sweet or savoury and served hot or cold. The lightness is usually achieved from beaten egg whites and/or cream. The nutritional value will depend on the ingredients. A seafood mousse may be quite low in kilojoules whereas a chocolate mousse may provide many hundreds of kilojoules per serve.

MOUSSELINE
A very light dish, named after the very light fabric, muslin. Mousselines are usually made with seafood, poultry or a vegetable pureed, with added whipped cream and beaten egg whites, placed in individual moulds and baked in a water bath until set.

MOZZARELLA
see Cheese.

MSG
see Monosodium Glutamate.

MUCILAGES
Forms of dietary fibre which are soluble in water. Derived from seeds and seaweeds, mucilages are used in some laxatives (see Ispaghula and Psyllium) and faecal softeners. Mucilages can form complexes with bile acids and increase their excretion. Since bile acids are one of the body's chief ways of disposing of cholesterol (see page 72), mucilages can be beneficial in the diet. They are also used as thickening agents in foods such as cream,

desserts, low-kilojoule foods and salad dressings. They have additive numbers from 400−416.

MUCIN

A complex mixture of protein and carbohydrate which protects various body membranes. The stomach walls secrete a mucin which protects them against attack by the hydrochloric acid also produced by the stomach.

MUCUS

Secretions from body cells which protect the body against infection. Mucus is essential in the eye, the nose, the digestive tract, the respiratory tract and the urinary system. An excessive amount of mucus may occur in the respiratory tract in response to infection or some sensitivity.

After drinking milk, some fruit juices or tea, some people believe the thick viscous feeling in the back of the throat is harmful mucus which will cause respiratory problems. While there is no doubt that a few asthmatics are sensitive to milk protein, there is no evidence that the temporary thick feeling after drinking milk has any undesirable or harmful effect. One study found a greater incidence of the problem in those who had not consumed sufficient water.

Most of the various diets promoted as anti-mucus diets have no scientific backing.

MUESLI

A breakfast food which takes different forms according to the country in which it is served. The original Swiss Bircher muesli was made by Dr Bircher-Benner at his sanitarium in Switzerland. It consists of rolled oats soaked overnight in water and then mixed with grated apple, honey, cream or yoghurt. Nuts are sometimes added. It is served either for breakfast or as an evening snack.

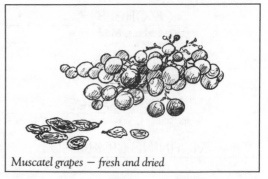
Muscatel grapes — fresh and dried

In Australia, muesli is a cereal made from oats, other grains or wheatgerm, plus dried fruits, seeds and nuts. Most commercial varieties have about 25 per cent added sugar. In toasted mueslis, the oats are mixed with oil (usually the highly saturated coconut oil) and sugar and are baked until crisp. Dried fruits, seeds and nuts may then be added.

The nutritional value of muesli varies with the ingredients. Most toasted mueslis have a sugar and fat content which is approximately the same as that found in sweet biscuits. The so-called 'natural' mueslis usually have better value although this varies with the brand. For an average natural muesli, a 60 g serve has 940 kJ (225 Cals). Toasted muesli is even higher with 1120 kJ (265 Cals) per 60 g serve. An average serve of commercial toasted muesli has 12 g of fat — as much as in 2 eggs.

Toasted muesli

500 g rolled oats
$\frac{1}{4}$ cup sesame seeds
$\frac{1}{2}$ cup coconut flakes
250 g rolled rye or barley flakes* (or use a mixture)
1 cup oat bran (processed product is suitable)
1 cup wheatgerm
1 cup dried fruit medley (apricots, apples, pears, sultanas)
1 cup sultanas
$\frac{1}{2}$ cup pepitas*
1 cup sunflower seeds
$\frac{1}{2}$ cup roasted buckwheat*

* available from health food stores

Toast oats by placing them on a flat, ungreased oven tray in a moderate oven for about 10 mins, stirring occasionally until oats brown (some oats take longer than others). Toast sesame seeds and coconut by the same method. While toasted ingredients are cooling, mix remaining ingredients together. Add cooled oats, seeds and coconut.

MUFFINS

English muffins are round yeasted cakes which are pulled apart, toasted and eaten while hot, usually with butter and honey, jam or a savoury topping. They were originally sold by a muffin man who would walk around the streets, ringing his bell to attract potential customers. They now come in a variety of flavours, including wholegrain and spicy fruit and are sold in supermarkets. One English muffin has much the same nutritional value as 2 slices of bread. They contain almost no fat or sugar. Each muffin half has approximately 295 kJ (70 Cals).

American muffins are like large cup cakes and contain both sugar and butter. They are eaten for breakfast and are much more filling than an English muffin. Corn, blueberry and bran muffins are especially popular. They are either made at home or are sold in specialty muffin shops. An average American muffin has 1240 kJ (295 Cals).

MULATO

A pungent red chilli pepper.

MULBERRY
see Fruit.

MULLET
see Fish.

MULLIGATAWNY

A thick spicy soup served in India. It may contain meat or chicken, curry spices, onions and other vegetables, and coconut milk. It is usually served with rice.

MULLOWAY
see Fish, Jewish.

MULTIPLE SCLEROSIS

A disease of the brain and spinal cord caused by some unknown substance attacking the nerve cells. Hard areas (sclerosis) eventually lead to loss of function of various parts of the body.

Those with multiple sclerosis often have a remission of their symptoms. If these periods coincide with including or omitting certain foods in the diet, there is a tendency to assume that particular foods are related to multiple sclerosis. At this stage there is no good evidence that the condition can be cured by any combination of foods. Studies using fish oils are examining any possible implications of the omega 3 oils found in seafoods. Large doses of vitamins have not been found to have any effect on the disease.

MULTIVITAMINS
see Vitamin supplements.

MUNG BEANS
see Legumes.

MUNSTER
see Cheese.

MUSCAT
see Drinks, Alcoholic.

MUSCATEL

A dried grape with a full flavour.

MUSCOVADO SUGAR

A soft moist brown sugar which is slightly coarser and darker than regular brown sugar. Used in cakes to maintain moisture and also used in many Indian dishes. Its nutritional value is similar to that of brown sugar and its nutrient content is insignificant in the diet as a whole.

MUSHROOMS

see Vegetables.

MUSKMELON

see Fruit.

MUSSEL

see Seafood.

MUST

In making wine, the initial step is to crush the grapes. This produces a mixture of 85 per cent liquid and 15 per cent skins and seeds. The liquid portion is called the 'must'.

MUSTARD

The seeds of the black or white mustard plant can be ground to produce a powder which can be hot and spicy or mild, depending on the variety of mustard seed used. Most mustards are quite mild; English, Chinese and Japanese mustards being the hottest.

The pungency of mustard is due to mustard oil which forms when the ground seeds are mixed with water. Mustard powder should be mixed about 10—15 mins before serving to achieve its strongest pungent flavour. For this

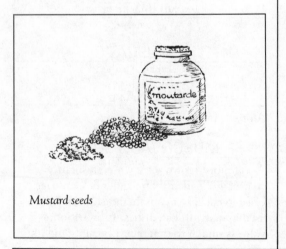

Mustard seeds

reason, much of the mustard used in England is prepared from a dry powder. The milder prepared mustards of France and Germany often have herbs, vinegars, lemon or spices added to provide different flavours.

Mustard was used by the ancient Greeks and Romans who introduced it to Britain. The popular mustard of medieval times was a coarsely ground product mixed with grape juice. The fine yellow powdered mustard was only introduced in the eighteenth century by a lady called Mrs Clements from Durham.

Today, many of the world's finest mustards are produced in Dijon in the Bordeaux region of France. These products vary in their strength and are used with meats but also in sauces and mayonnaises. The mustard oil actually acts as an emulsifier to prevent mayonnaise from separating.

- *Dijon* mustard is a pale colour because it is made from mustard seed without its husk. It can be fairly hot and is available with white wine or green peppercorns added. Dijon mustards containing whole mustard seeds are also available.
- *Bordeaux* mustard is darker than the Dijon style (it contains the seed husk) and has a slightly sweet-sour flavour from the vinegar and sugar added. It is usually flavoured with tarragon. German mustard resembles the Bordeaux variety.
- *American* mustards are made from white mustard seeds and usually contain sugar, vinegar and salt. They do not have the subtlety of the French mustards.
- *English* mustards are made from a mixture of black and white mustard seeds. They are hot and may have added turmeric to produce a bright yellow colour.
- *Chinese* mustard is made from dry mustard mixed with water or beer. It is very hot.
- *Whole seed* mustards, known as *moutarde de meaux*, have a mild flavour but release an intensity when one bites on the seeds.

Nutritionally, mustard seeds are rich in

protein, dietary fibre and various vitamins and minerals. In practice, few people eat sufficient mustard for this to have any dietary significance. One teaspoon of mustard powder has 85 kJ (20 Cals).

MUSTARD GREENS
see Vegetables.

MUSTARD OIL
see Oils.

MUTTON
see Meat.

MYCOTOXINS

Toxins produced by fungi which may grow on foods. Ergot, the rust which attacks wheat and rye is a mycotoxin. Aflatoxin (see page 14) on peanuts is also a mycotoxin. Mycotoxins affect the liver and the nervous system and some are known to cause cancer. They are found in some moulds on foods and for this reason, mouldy foods (especially grains and nuts) should not be eaten (see Moulds).

Control of moulds on foods and animal feeds is a major public health problem. Although many people dislike the use of preservatives and mould inhibitors in foods, these added chemicals are much safer than the natural toxins which can be produced by plants.

MYOCARDIUM

The thick muscular wall of the heart. A myocardial infarction (abbreviated as MI) is the correct term for a heart attack and occurs when the heart muscle is starved of oxygen. This usually occurs because of a blockage in one of the coronary arteries which supply blood to the myocardium. The area of the heart deprived of its oxygen dies. The victim may die or the infarction may heal leaving a scar.

MYOGLOBIN

A protein which stores oxygen in muscle tissue and, hence appears bright red. Iron in the diet is needed in the myoglobin molecule so that it can attract and hold oxygen. Athletes, with their higher body content of myoglobin, thus need plenty of iron.

Animal tissues with a higher myoglobin content have a greater blood flow and look darker than those with less. This is why the leg meat on chickens (where the muscle is more active) is darker than the breast meat (where the muscle is used to a lesser extent).

When a piece of meat is freshly cut, the myoglobin picks up oxygen from the air and appears bright red. After some time, this red colour loses its oxygen and reverts to a grey colour. Fresh meat thus has a reddish colour from its myoglobin plus oxygen.

MYOINOSITOL

A form of inositol (see page 189), regarded by some people as a vitamin. Myoinositol is found in many foods, usually with substances such as phospholipids and is important in the structure of the membranes which surround cells. However, there is currently no evidence that it functions as a vitamin. It is widely distributed in foods and a normal mixed diet contains 300—1000 mg.

Phytic acid (see page 266) consists of myoinositol joined with 6 phosphate molecules.

MYRISTIC ACID

A saturated fatty acid with 14 carbon atoms. Widely distributed in foods.

MYRISTICIN

A hallucinogenic compound found in nutmeg (see page 327).

MYXOEDEMA
see Hypothyroidism.

NAAN

A yeasted Indian bread which contains yoghurt. Usually cooked in small individual loaves in a hot oven so that it puffs up to form a light product which is eaten with curries. A 50 g naan has 710 kJ (170 Cals) and supplies some dietary fibre, vitamins and minerals.

See also Tandoori.

NACHOS

A Mexican dish made from corn chips served with melted cheese. Avocado, chopped tomato and sour cream are also often served with nachos.

NACNE REPORT

A British report from the National Advisory Committee on Nutrition Education which attempted to identify problems in the British diet and suggested ways to remedy these. Their proposals called for a reduction of fat intake from its present level of 38 per cent to 34 per cent in the short term and 30 per cent of the energy in the longer term; increase in dietary carbohydrate from its present level of 45 per cent to 50 and then 55 per cent of the energy; and a reduction of alcohol from 6 per cent to 5 and then to 4 per cent of the kilojoules in the average diet.

NAM PLA

A shrimp paste used in Asia, especially in Thailand. The paste is made by cleaning small whole shrimp, mixing them with salt and pressing the resulting mixture. Nam pla has very few kilojoules and is high in both calcium (50 mg/teaspoon) and salt.

NASEBERRY

see Fruit, Sapodilla.

NASHI FRUIT

see Fruit.

NASI GORENG

An Indonesian dish consisting of fried rice with small pieces of fried meats, onion, eggs, garlic and, usually, shrimp paste, chilli and seafoods.

NATTO

A fermented soya bean product which looks like a dark sticky paste. Used in Asian cooking in place of salt.

NATURAL FOODS

A somewhat vague term, generally taken to mean foods which have had minimal

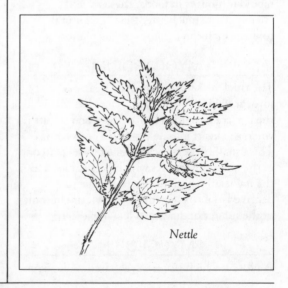

Nettle

HERBS

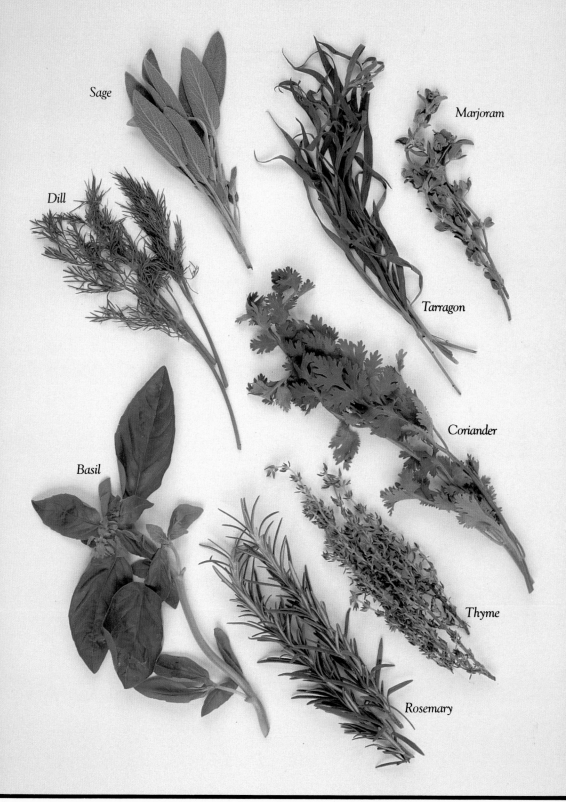

Sage

Marjoram

Dill

Tarragon

Coriander

Basil

Thyme

Rosemary

LEGUMES

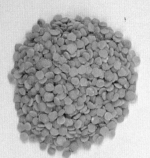

Toor dhal (lentil)

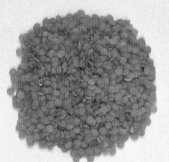

Red lentils

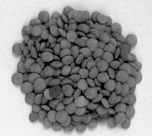

Brown lentils

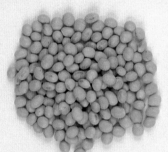

Soya beans

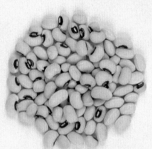

Black-eyed beans

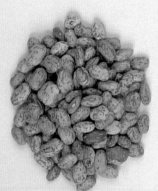

Pinto beans

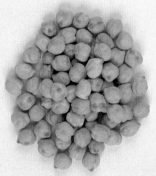

Chickpeas

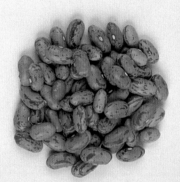

Borlotti beans

processing. Fruits, vegetables, grains, legumes, eggs, meat, poultry and fish are usually described as natural foods. Others would add milk, cheese, yoghurt, wholemeal bread and wholegrain cereal products, although none of these is strictly natural. In general, the word 'natural' is now so overused that it has little meaning.

NATUROPATHY

A system of medicine which aims to use heat, light, water, diet, massage and other healing methods in place of drugs or surgery.

NAVARIN

A French stew made with lamb, potatoes, turnips, carrots and onions.

NAVY BEANS
see Legumes, Haricot beans.

NECTAR

Flowers produce nectar — a solution consisting mostly of sugars and gathered by bees. A few nectars contain substances which are toxic to humans and honeys from such areas are poisonous. In the beehive, nectar is concentrated to a point where it is inhospitable for bacteria and can be stored without going bad. Initially, a bee will pump nectar in and out of its body until it becomes more concentrated. The nectar is then deposited in a thin film on the honeycomb and left to dry to about 20 per cent moisture.

The concentrated juices from fruits such as apricots and peaches is also referred to as nectar. These products have a relatively high solids content and less water than most juices.

NECTARINE
see Fruit.

NEENISH TART
see Tarts.

NEROLI

An Italian concentrate of orange flowers which is used to flavour desserts and cakes.

NESSELRODE DESSERT

A rich frozen concoction containing icecream, glace fruits, nuts and liqueur. A nesselrode pie may have an unfrozen creamy filling containing fruits, chocolate and liqueur.

NET PROTEIN UTILISATION (NPU)

This refers to the amount of protein consumed which is retained by the body cells. Foods with a high NPU have a balance of amino acids which can be well used by the body. Eggs, for example, have a high NPU since virtually all their amino acids can be used by the body. Wheat protein, by contrast, has a much lower NPU since its amino acids are present in such proportions that less than half are utilised by the body. In general, animal protein foods have a higher NPU than vegetable-based foods. When mixtures of vegetable foods are eaten, their combined NPU is often higher than either food eaten alone, since one will supply an amino acid missing from another.

See also Vegetarian diet.

NETTLE
see Vegetables.

NEUFCHATEL
see Cheese.

NEURITIS

Inflammation of a nerve. Occurs in vitamin B_6 deficiency but a polyneuritis of the nerve endings in the fingers and feet may also occur with large doses of supplementary B_6.

NEURO-TRANSMITTERS

Substances which carry impulses from one nerve to another. Some of the more familiar neuro-transmitters include serotonin, acetylcholine and histamine.

NEW ZEALAND GROPER
see Fish, Cod.

NIACIN
see Vitamins, Vitamin B_3.

NICKEL

A mineral which is thought to be essential to humans (in very small doses). May have a role in maintaining the structure of cell membranes and as a coenzyme in various chemical reactions. Found mainly in green leafy vegetables with smaller quantities in fruits and grains.

NICOISE

Coming from Nice, dishes with the nicoise tag usually contain garlic, tomatoes, olive oil and black olives.

NICOTINAMIDE

A form of niacin.
See Vitamins, Vitamin B_3.

NICOTINE
see Smoking.

NICOTINIC ACID

Another name for niacin.
See Vitamins, Vitamin B_3.

NIGHTSHADE FAMILY

The family of plants which includes the potato, eggplant, capsicum and tomato. The tobacco plant also belongs to this family. Deadly nightshade is a plant with poisonous black berries. It contains the alkaloid drug atropine and also belladonna.

NITRATES

Chemical components of many foods and also used in fertilisers and as curing agents in meat where they act as preservatives, colouring and flavouring agents. Sodium nitrate (additive no. 251) or potassium nitrate (additive no. 252 and also known as saltpetre) are used in ham, bacon, sausages, salamis, corned and pickled meats. The nitrate undergoes a series of chemical reactions with myoglobin (the red pigment in the meat muscle) to produce the characteristic pink colour of cured meats. In the process, nitrates are reduced to nitrites. Some people are sensitive to high levels of nitrates in foods and develop symptoms such as asthma, headaches or eczema. Most people, however, have no obvious reaction to nitrates. Small quantities of nitrates are found in vegetables.

NITRITES

Sodium or potassium nitrite (additives nos. 249 and 250) are used as preservatives in meats (in addition to, or in place of, nitrates). They inhibit the growth of the bacteria which cause the fatal disease, botulism.

In the acid environment of the stomach, nitrites react with amino acids (from food proteins) to form nitrosamines. These have been shown to cause cancer in laboratory animals. In humans, stomach cancer occurs most commonly in populations who consume a lot of nitrites or nitrates. With the use of refrigeration for keeping meats, smaller quantities of both these substances are now used in making smallgoods.

NITROSAMINES

Compounds which are found in some pickled foods and also form in the stomach when nitrites react with amino acids from the proteins in foods. If vitamin C is present, the reaction does not proceed. Since large doses of nitrosamines are known to be carcinogenic, it makes sense to have a source of vitamin C such as a tomato or another fresh fruit or vegetable with bacon or ham or any other cured meats.

NON-STICK COOKING

In the 1960s, carbon-fluorine polymers were developed and used to coat frying pans and other cookware. These substances are inert and also have very low friction characteristics so that foods do not stick to them. Non-stick coatings which are sprayed onto cooking surfaces are also used. The propellant in the spray can causes respiratory problems in some people.

NOODLES
see Pasta.

NOREPINEPHRINE

Also known as noradrenaline, this chemical substance may help control appetite. Norepinephrine is released by nerves and increases heat production and basic metabolic rate in the body. Studies have shown that changes in norepinephrine levels alter daily food intake. Reduced levels occur in anorexia nervosa and starvation although whether they are the cause or the effect of the lack of food is not yet understood. Further research into the release of norepinephrine in the body is occurring and this should help us understand how the body controls food intake.

NORI
See Seaweed, laver.

NOUGAT

A rich variety of candy containing sugar, eggs, butter and nuts. 100 g have 1740 kJ (415 Cals).

NUCLEIC ACIDS

DNA (deoxyribonucleic acid) and RNA (ribonucleic acid) contain genetic material to control growth and development.

They do not come directly from foods but are made in the human body, and consist of chains of amino acids. Proteins, vitamins B_6, B_{12} and folacin, certain minerals and carbohydrates are used by the body to make its DNA and RNA.

NUOC NAM

A clear brown liquid made in Vietnam from small whole fish which are salted and left to ferment for about 3 months. After this time, the liquid is drained off and used to flavour dishes. 1 tablespoon of high quality nuoc nam has 230 kJ (55 Cals); poorer quality products have 105 kJ (25 Cals) and lower quantities of nutrients.

NUTMEG
see Spices.

NUTRIENT DENSITY

Refers to the nutritional value of a food relevant to the number of kilojoules it supplies, or, to the percentage of the daily requirements of nutrients it supplies. Tends to be calculated in various ways by different people, making comparisons of nutrient density difficult. In general, a food which has a high nutrient density is a good source of one or more nutrients relative to its contribution of energy. Foods such as soft drinks or fats have a very low nutrient density since they contribute energy but few nutrients. Eggs, liver or milk would have a high nutrient density since they contribute a lot of nutrients relevant to their kilojoule count.

NUTRIENTS

Compounds present in foods which are essential to life and health. Generally include proteins, fats, carbohydrates, vitamins and minerals. Some people also include dietary fibre and water as nutrients.

NUTRITION

The science of food and its relation to health. Also involves the processes whereby a living organism receives and processes the nutrients essential for life, growth and physical activity.

NUTRITION, CHILDREN AND GROWTH
see Children, growth and nutrition.

243

NUTS

Nuts are single seeded, dry fruits with a hard shell. The term is also used for any edible kernel in a hard shell. Almonds, coconut, pecans, walnuts and peanuts are usually classed as nuts although none of them fits the true definition of a nut.

Nuts have been part of the human diet since the earliest times and were cultivated by the ancient Romans from the time of Christ.

They are dense sources of nutrients and contain fats, proteins and carbohydrates as well as a wide selection of minerals and vitamins.

Acorn

The acorn is one of the few true nuts (an edible kernel surrounded by a hard shell). It comes from the oak tree and its woody exterior corresponds to the usual fleshy layer of fruits. Acorns have little fat (only 5 per cent) and are high in complex carbohydrate. They can be ground into a coarse flour to use as a porridge or to make into pancakes.

Almond

A popular nut which is really the seed of a fruit, closely related to the plum and peach. Native to southwest Asia, almonds are used in both sweet and savoury dishes including salads, soups, meat or fish dishes, stir-fried Asian-style foods, and in cakes, desserts, biscuits and confectionery. Ground almonds are also used in cakes and desserts.

Almonds have more calcium than any other nut and are also a source of iron, zinc, vitamin E, potassium, dietary fibre, riboflavin and other vitamins of the B group. Of their fat, 72 per cent is monounsaturated, 20 per cent is polyunsaturated and only 8 per cent is saturated. 100 g of almonds have 2340 kJ (560 Cals).

Brazil nut

The edible seed of a large South American tree (about 50 m tall) which grows around the Amazon. The nuts occur in large pods which can weigh over 2 kg. Brazil nuts are eaten as a snack food or may be ground and used in cakes and biscuits. Chopped Brazil nuts also go well with vegetables, in stuffings for meat dishes or in sweets.

Brazil nuts are a good source of vitamin E and several of the B complex vitamins as well as minerals such as iron, zinc, potassium, magnesium. They also supply dietary fibre and protein. Of their fat, 27 per cent is saturated, 34 per cent is monounsaturated and 39 per cent is polyunsaturated. 100 g of shelled nuts have 2595 kJ (620 Cals).

Cashew

A native nut which originally grew near the Amazon but is now grown mainly in India and East Africa. The cashew nut is actually a seed which is related to poison ivy. Its shell contains an irritating oil which is removed (and used for paint, as an insecticide and even as a rocket lubricant) before the nut is extracted. Cashew nuts are eaten as a snack or are added to savoury dishes with vegetables, chicken or various meats.

Nutritionally, the cashew nut is rich in fat and is a good source of protein, iron, the B complex vitamins and vitamin E. Of the fat in cashews, 21 per cent is saturated, 62 per cent is monounsaturated and 18 per cent is polyunsaturated. 100 g of cashew nuts have 2405 kJ (575 Cals).

Chestnut

A nut which comes from several species of trees

in the beech family. The sweet chestnut (also called the European or Spanish chestnut) has glossy brown nuts protected by a green cupule with long spines. This is easily removed but the skin of the chestnut is best removed by heating the nuts in an oven (or fire) for about 10 mins and then rubbing off the skin. Sometimes chestnuts are steamed and eaten as a vegetable. Horse chestnuts, Moreton Bay chestnuts, palm chestnuts and water chestnuts are not true chestnuts; their nuts are also inedible.

Unlike most nuts, the chestnut has little fat and protein and consists mainly of complex carbohydrate. It also has a higher water content than most nuts and this turns it mouldy much faster than most nuts.

Nutritionally, the chestnut is a good source of complex carbohydrate, dietary fibre and potassium. It also has small quantities of many minerals and vitamins. 100 g chestnuts have 570 kJ (170 Cals), about one-third the level of most nuts.

Cobnut

see Hazelnut.

Coconut

The fruit of the coconut palm is one of the oldest food sources and is the most important commercial nut in the world. The coconut originated in Malaysia but is widely grown throughout the tropics. Major coconut producers are the Philippines, India and Indonesia. The coconut provides oil, fibre in the form of copra, and an important food. Coconut oil is now widely used in processed foods such as biscuits, cakes and pastries.

The flesh of the coconut is either eaten fresh or is dried. It has a wide variety of uses ranging from being an essential ingredient in some curries to its use in biscuits, cakes, desserts, muesli and confectionery. The coconut milk in the centre of the nut is a refreshing drink.

Nutritionally, coconut provides fats, dietary fibre and small quantities of protein, minerals and vitamins. Of the fat, over 90 per cent is saturated; 7 per cent is monounsaturated and the rest is polyunsaturated. Much of the vegetable oil used in biscuits, cakes, pastries and for frying fast foods comes from either coconut oil or palm oil. In spite of the label saying vegetable oil, most of these products contain a high level of saturated fat. Coconut flesh is 36 per cent fat. Desiccated coconut has a very low water content and is 62 per cent fat. Fresh coconut has 1465 kJ/100 g (350 Cals) while the desiccated coconut has 2535 kJ/100 g (605 Cals). Coconut milk has little nutritional value, apart from some potassium. It also has little fat and is low in kilojoules with a 200 mL glass having 180 kJ (43 Cals).

Hazelnut

Also known as filberts or cobnuts, these nuts were used in China in 3000 BC. The term filberts probably came from St Philbert, a French abbott whose feast day falls at the same time that filberts are ripe in France.

The nut has a shiny brown shell with a rounded creamy interior. When correctly roasted and fresh, they are crisp and brittle. The skins can be removed from the kernels by heating the nuts in a moderate oven for about 5 mins, placing on a clean cloth and rubbing gently until the skin is loosened. The nuts with their brown skins are often ground and used in cakes, desserts, muesli and icecreams. They can also be added to salads, stuffings, sauces and sandwiches.

Nutritionally, hazelnuts have less protein and fat than some other nuts, are rich in vitamin E, and provide a wide selection of minerals and vitamins, as well as some dietary fibre. 100 g hazelnuts have 1590 kJ (380 Cals). They are about one-third fat, of which 11 per cent is polyunsaturated, 81 per cent is monounsaturated and 8 per cent is saturated.

Hickory

A member of the walnut family, hickory nuts are native to the eastern part of North America. They can be used in much the same way as pecans or walnuts but are usually served salted as a savoury accompaniment to drinks.

Nutritionally, hickory nuts are high in fat and provide a selection of minerals and vitamins as well as some dietary fibre. 100 g hickory nuts (shelled) contribute 2765 kJ (660 Cals). The nuts are about two-thirds fat, of which 36 per cent is polyunsaturated, 53 per cent is monounsaturated and 11 per cent is saturated.

Indian nut

see Pine nut.

Kola

see Drinks, Non-alcoholic, Cola.

Lychee

Usually thought of as a fruit, lychees are also dried and eaten as a nut. The flesh has a nutty fruity flavour.

Macadamia nut

A native of Australia, the nut was introduced to Hawaii and became commercially important in the 1930s. It was not used commercially in Australia until the 1980s when its flavour and texture became popular. The hard shell is difficult to crack, making the nuts expensive. The nuts are considered a very desirable snack food and are also used in icecreams and desserts, cakes, biscuits and confectionery as well as in stuffings and as a garnish for meat or fish dishes.

Nutritionally, macadamias are high in fat and provide small quantities of many minerals and vitamins as well as some dietary fibre. 100 g of macadamia nuts have 2940 kJ (700 Cals). The nut is 74 per cent fat, of which only 2 per cent is polyunsaturated, a high 82 per cent is monounsaturated and 16 per cent is saturated.

Peanut

Although referred to as a nut, peanuts are actually the seed of a legume bush which is native to South America. They grow under the ground. Peanuts were eaten in Peru at least 2800 years ago, but recently they have been mainly fed to cattle. It is only in the twentieth century that peanuts have become an important human food, either as a snack, an ingredient in cooking (both sweet and savoury dishes) or as peanut butter. India and China are now the world's leading producers of peanuts.

Peanut oil has been the predominant oil in Asian cuisine until recent times when it has been largely replaced by the cheaper palm and coconut oils.

Nutritionally, peanuts are much more like legumes than nuts, having a much higher content of protein than any nuts. They are almost 50 per cent fat, and an excellent source of the B group vitamins niacin, folacin and pantothenic aid, and vitamin E. They contain other vitamins, some minerals and dietary fibre. 100 g peanuts have 2385 kJ (570 Cals). Of their fat, 30 per cent is polyunsaturated, 50 per cent is monounsaturated and 20 per cent is saturated.

Pecan

The pecan nut comes from a species of hickory and is native to the Mississippi River area. Its texture is soft but full-flavoured. Toasting the nut improves the crispness and brings out the flavour. They can be used in the same way as walnuts and are delicious in salads, with chicken or in desserts. Pecan pie (a rich shortcrust pastry filled with pecans in a sweet, rich, slightly sticky filling) is very popular.

Nutritionally, pecans supply dietary fibre, protein and a mixture of minerals and vitamins. They are also high in fat, of which 26 per cent is polyunsaturated, 66 per cent is monounsaturated and 8 per cent is saturated. 100 g pecans have 2765 kJ (660 Cals).

Pine nut

The seed of several different varieties of pine, pine nuts are popular in Spain and Italy. Also called pignolia or Indian nut. The small nuts add a delicious and delicate flavour to many foods such as salads, stuffing, fish and chicken dishes, muesli, soups and the famous pesto sauce (see page 265).

Nutritionally, pine nuts have more protein than most nuts. They are also a good source of iron and supply some dietary fibre and a range of minerals and vitamins. About half the nut is fat, of which 44 per cent is polyunsaturated, 40 per cent is monounsaturated and 16 per cent is saturated. 100 g pine nuts have 2155 kJ (515 Cals).

Pistachio nut

An old nut, native to the Middle East and Asia and cultivated in Asia for thousands of years. The pistachio is a relative of the cashew and produces a seed with a greenish interior. When the seed is ripe, the shell cracks open. The nuts must be eaten soon after this stage or they become soft. Pistachios are now grown in the hot dry climates of North Africa and the Middle East, as well as in India, Europe and North America.

The greenish colour of the nuts makes them popular in desserts, confectionery, icecream and in mixed salted nuts. They are also used in stuffings and with meat dishes.

Nutritionally, pistachios are a good source of potassium and provide some protein, vitamins (A, B and E), minerals and dietary fibre. They are approximately 50 per cent fat, of which 16 per cent is polyunsaturated, 71 per cent is monounsaturated and 13 per cent is saturated. 100 g of the nuts have 2415 kJ (575 Cals).

Walnut

A native of Asia, Europe and North America, walnuts are one of the most widely used and popular nuts in the world. They are eaten on their own or added to a range of sweet and savoury dishes, including many sweets, biscuits, cakes and desserts as well as salads (they are a major ingredient of the famous Waldorf salad), meat and vegetable dishes.

Different varieties of walnuts are grown. European walnuts are easier to shell than the native black American variety. France, Italy and the United States are the major walnut-producing countries.

Nutritionally, walnuts are a source of protein, dietary fibre and vitamins B and E, and supply some iron and other minerals. Like most nuts, they are about 50 per cent fat and have a higher percentage of polyunsaturated fat than other nuts. Of their fat, 72 per cent is polyunsaturated 16 per cent is monounsaturated and 12 per cent is saturated.

OAT BRAN

A variety of products are sold as oat bran. Some are just the outside part of the oat; others include varying amounts of the endosperm. These products have become popular since medical researchers found that oat bran can lower blood cholesterol levels. Since the part of the oat which appears to have the greatest effect in lowering cholesterol lies just between the outside and the endosperm, some oat bran products which use only the outside part do not have the desired effect in lowering blood cholesterol levels. With oat bran, it is worth seeking out products from larger companies who have the quality control facilities to ensure that their oat bran always contains the relevant part of the oat. The alternative is to eat rolled oats which always contain the important soluble fibre.

OATS

see Grains.

OBESITY

The term usually used for a state of considerable excess weight. Often taken as being 20 per cent or more above the standard weight for height or W/H^2 greater than 30.

Obesity increases the risks of many conditions to an even greater extent than being overweight. (See Overweight, for a list of the increased hazards of carrying too much body fat.)

OCTOPUS

see Seafood.

OEDEMA

see Fluid retention.

OESOPHAGUS

Sometimes called the gullet, the oesophagus is the part of the intestine between the mouth and the stomach. Cancer of the oesophagus may occur with high intake of alcohol, especially in those who also smoke. A hiatus hernia occurs when a portion of the stomach pushes back into the oesophagus, allowing the strong stomach acid to come into contact with the oesophagus.

OESTROGEN

One of the female hormones. As well as its sexual functions, oestrogen is important in maintaining higher levels of HDL cholesterol (see page 72) and also in keeping a good retention of calcium in bones to prevent osteoporosis.

After the menopause, oestrogen levels fall. At this stage, HDL cholesterol gradually decreases and it becomes difficult to replace lost calcium into bones.

Oestrogen levels also fall with severe or sudden weight loss. This is apparent when periods stop but also has the effect of decreasing calcium retention, a problem which will not be evident until chalky bones break.

See also Calcium.

OFFAL

Sometimes called variety meats, offal is any edible part of the animal other than the muscle meat. The liver, kidney, heart, pancreas, the thymus gland (sweetbreads), brains, stomach lining (tripe), feet and tongue are offal. In some countries, the intestines (pigs' intestines are called chitterlings), eyeballs and other parts such as the head are also eaten.

Liver and kidneys are generally highly regarded; other forms of offal are less popular in Western societies. See individual listings for details.

OGEN MELON

see Fruit, Melons.

OHSAWA, GEORGES

The originator of the Zen macrobiotic diet (see page 214).

OILS

See following pages.

OKRA

see Vegetables.

OLEIC ACID

A monounsaturated fatty acid, the most common naturally-occurring fat. Oleic acid is widely distributed in foods and makes up about 30 per cent of most fats. Abbreviated as C18:1. Makes up 38 per cent of the fat in oats, 28 per cent of the fat in milk, 43 per cent of the fat in eggs, 72 per cent of that in olive oil, around 40 per cent of the fat in meats and poultry, 71 per cent of the fat in almonds and 75 per cent of the fat in avocados.

OLIGOSACCHARIDES

Carbohydrates consisting of several basic sugar units. Examples are raffinose, stachyose and verbacose. Found in seeds and other parts of plants and also formed during the digestion of complex carbohydrates. The human digestive tract does not contain the enzymes needed to split oligosaccharides so they pass through to the large intestine where they are fermented by bacteria, adding to the faecal bulk (see also Dietary fibre). Some faecal bulking agents made from plant seeds have a high content of oligosaccharides.

OLIVE

The origins of the olive are unclear but it probably came from Greece, some part of Asia Minor or Egypt. It has provided a staple food for many thousands of years and is a vital part of the Mediterranean diet, both as the fruits and the oil which is pressed from them. It was the oil which was considered the valuable part of the olive. Not only was it eaten but it was used for religious ceremonies, as fuel for lamps and for rubbing into the skin.

About 90 per cent of the world's olive oil is now produced by Spain and Italy; Greece produces about three-quarters of the world's olives. In most cases, different varieties of olive tree are cultivated for oil or fruit, although a few varieties are good for both purposes.

The fruits are green at first and become black when ripe. They are bitter and generally considered inedible until processed. This is done by first covering the olives with a solution of caustic soda ($\frac{1}{3}$ cup of soda to 4 l of water). If firm olives are desired, add about $\frac{1}{4}$ cup of salt to prevent excessive softening. Keep green olives submerged in the caustic soda solution and cover the vessel. Expose black olives to the air several times to turn the flesh from purple to black. Soak the olives for 8—24 hours until the solution has penetrated about halfway through the flesh. Then wash the olives to remove the soaking solution. At this stage, the olives need to be put through a series of brine baths with the salt solution gradually being made stronger. This stage takes 3—4 weeks, after which the olives are washed and kept in a brine solution.

The Greek method of pickling black olives is to place them into jars, layer with salt and leave them for 2 months. The salt is then washed off and the olives are placed in olive oil, often with some herbs.

Olives are a good source of dietary fibre (10 olives have as much fibre as 2 small apples) and also provide small quantities of potassium, other minerals, and vitamins. Pickled olives are also high in salt. The reputation that olives are fattening is undeserved; 10 olives have just 125 kJ (30 Cals). 10 olives also have 1.8 g of fat, mainly monounsaturated.

OILS

Oils are fats which are liquid at room temperature. They consist of a variety of fatty acids: saturated, monounsaturated and polyunsaturated (see also Fats). Whatever their type of fat, all oils have the same high kilojoule level — 755 kJ (180 Cals) per tablespoon. Depending on the oil, they also contain different levels of tocopherols (vitamin E (see page 392) and essential fatty acids (see Linoleic and Linolenic acids). Oils have no other nutrients.

The flavour of some types of oil is superb. Avocado or almond oil, for example, adds a delicious touch to a salad dressing. When frying, high temperatures will cause most oils to break down, producing off flavours.

Many oils have been used throughout history. The ancient Egyptians pressed oil out of radishes — a feat indeed, while the Greeks used olive oil, the Europeans favoured sesame oil and almond oil was the favoured product in the Middle East.

The chemical composition of oils varies. Contrary to popular belief, all vegetable oils are not polyunsaturated. Some of the most commonly used oils, such as palm or coconut oil, contain mostly saturated fats. These products have no advantages over animal fats. In general, seed oils have a high content of polyunsaturated fats, while fruit and nut oils tend to have more of the mono-unsaturated fats (see page 120). In making margarine from vegetable oils, some of the fats present must be saturated with hydrogen so that the product will be solid enough to spread.

All oils are very high in kilojoules. 100 g of oil have 3705 kJ (885 Cals). A 20 g tablespoon of oil thus adds 740 kJ (175 Cals). Those who believe that it is all right to fry foods as long as oil is used may thus be unwittingly adding a large number of kilojoules.

Oils are extracted by pressing, with or without heat. Virgin oils are cold-pressed without the application of any heat. Oil seeds are generally crushed and great pressure applied to force the oil out. The oil-seed cake usually still contains about 5 per cent oil and this can be extracted using solvents. The solvent is allowed to permeate the cake or meal and dissolves the oil. The solvent itself is then evaporated. In general, the best-tasting oils are the cold-pressed. There is some evidence that these oils also have a higher content of tocopherols.

Almond

A delicately flavoured oil extracted from almonds, this oil is superb with salads or entrees. Of its fat, only about 10 per cent is saturated, 70 per cent is monounsaturated and about 20 per cent is polyunsaturated.

Almond oil is rich in vitamin E and 20 mL (1 tablespoon) would supply the entire day's supply.

Apricot kernel

A few drops of this oil add a delicious flavour to

salads. Like almond oil, most of its fat is monounsaturated. Approximately 7 per cent is saturated, over 60 per cent is monounsaturated and over 30 per cent is polyunsaturated. Apricot kernel oil is especially rich in vitamin E and a tablespoon (20 mL) would more than supply the daily needs.

Borage seed

An oil extracted from the seeds of the borage plant. Rich in polyunsaturated fats, especially gamma-linolenic acid (also found in evening primrose oil).

Coconut

A highly saturated oil extracted from coconuts. Of the fat present, 91 per cent is saturated, 7 per cent is monounsaturated and only 2 per cent is polyunsaturated.

Cod liver

An oil extracted from the liver of the cod. Extremely rich in vitamins A and D, it also contains about 8 per cent of its fat as the omega 3 fatty acid EPA and 9 per cent DHA (see page 96). Because of its very high level of vitamin A, cod liver oil is no longer recommended for most people, especially children, unless given in very small doses.

Corn

An oil extracted from corn or maize. Useful for cooking but usually considered too heavy for salads. Of the fat present about 50 per cent is polyunsaturated, 35 per cent is monounsaturated and 15 per cent is saturated. These proportions can vary somewhat for corn from different areas. Corn oil is rich in vitamin E, although not all is in the form of the most valuable alpha tocopherol (see page 392).

Cottonseed

An oil extracted from cottonseeds. It is used in cooking but has no special flavour to recommend it for salads. Of the fat present, 53 per cent is polyunsaturated, 22 per cent is monounsaturated and 25 per cent is saturated.

Like many other oils, cottonseed oil is rich in vitamin E. Less than 2 teaspoons would supply the day's requirements.

Grape seed

The humble grape seed contains oil which can be extracted. It has a fine light texture and is good in salad dressings. Like other seed oils, it contains largely polyunsaturated fats which make up over 70 per cent of its fats. Monounsaturated fats comprise 17 per cent and saturated fats about 11 per cent.

Hazelnut

Another oil with a flavour which is superb drizzled onto a salad or with poultry or fish. The fat present in hazelnut oil is similar to that in other nut oils: about 11 per cent is polyunsaturated, over 80 per cent is monounsaturated and only 7 per cent is saturated.

Linseed

Most people do not find the flavour of linseed oil acceptable. This is a pity since it is one of the few vegetable sources of alpha linolenic acid which is made into the omega 3 fatty acids found in fish and seafoods. Alpha linolenic acid makes up about 54 per cent of linseed oil. Other polyunsaturated fats contribute a further 15 per cent, making the total polyunsaturated fat level about 69 per cent. Monounsaturated fats comprise a further 21 per cent and saturated fats account for the remaining 10 per cent.

Mustard

Produced from pressing mustard seeds. Used to some extent in Indian cooking, mainly for its flavour. Not used much in other areas, with the exception of rapeseed oil, a relative of the mustard plant.

Olive

The oil extracted from olives has been the major type of oil in the human diet for thousands of years. In fact, it is only very recently that any other oils have become significant in the diet of any human population. Olive oil was firstly popular as an oil for heating and providing the light from oil lamps before it became an important part of the human diet of people in Mediterranean countries.

During the 1960s and 70s, olive oil was largely ignored by many medical researchers since it was not found to have the same power to lower the total level of cholesterol as the predominantly polyunsaturated oils such as safflower and sunflower. During the 1980s, interest in olive oil was renewed when its more favourable effect on the different fractions of blood cholesterol was recognised. Polyunsaturated fats appear to lower cholesterol levels very effectively but they do this by reducing the good HDL cholesterol as well as the bad LDL. Olive oil, by comparison, does not give as great a reduction in total cholesterol because it lowers bad LDL cholesterol but *increases* the protective HDL cholesterol fraction. Thus its effect on *total* cholesterol does not show up its true benefits. Further evidence for the worth of olive oil is provided by the low levels of heart disease and cancer in Mediterranean populations whose major source of fat is olive oil.

Virgin olive oil comes only from the pulp of the highest grade fruit and is never deodorised or bleached. It tends to have a distinctive flavour and a slightly greenish colour. Pure olive oil is pressed from the pulp and kernels of olives.

Of the fat present in olive oil, an average of 12 per cent is polyunsaturated, 73 per cent is monounsaturated, and 15 per cent is saturated. Olive oil is also a good source of vitamin E. 1 tablespoon would supply about one-third of the day's needs.

Palm kernel

One of the cheapest oils, palm kernel oil has largely replaced peanut oil in many parts of Asia. It is also widely used in processed and fast foods. Unlike the oils it has been replacing, only 4 per cent of the fat in palm kernel oil is polyunsaturated, about 15 per cent is monounsaturated and 81 per cent is saturated. The oil is becoming widely used because it is cheap and because saturated fats do not go rancid as quickly as unsaturated fats. It is thus more suitable for food processing but not necessarily more suitable for human consumption. Palm kernel oil has only small quantities of vitamin E.

Peanut

Also known as groundnut oil, peanut oil was once widely used in Chinese cooking. The oil is excellent for frying or for salads. Its fat content varies considerably but, on average, about 32 per cent is polyunsaturated, 55 per cent is monounsaturated and about 13 per cent is saturated. Peanut oil is a good source of vitamin E, with about half its content as the valuable aloha tocopherol. 1 tablespoon (20mL) would supply about two-thirds of the day's requirements.

Poppyseed

Not used to any extent, poppyseeds can be pressed and their oil extracted. The fats are largely polyunsaturated (65 per cent) with some monounsaturated fats (20 per cent) and some saturated fats (15 per cent).

Rapeseed

A member of the cabbage family, rapeseed oil has not been widely used because it contains an acid called erucic acid. A new genetic variety, Canbra, has no erucic acid and is suitable for human consumption.

This new variety contains some alpha linolenic acid — not quite as much as in linseed oil, but a very worthwhile amount which can contribute to omega 3 fatty acids. (see page 254) for details about omega 3 fats). The alpha linolenic acid makes up 11 per cent of the fat; other polyunsaturated fats bring the polyunsaturated level to 34 per cent.

Monounsaturated fats comprise a total of 56 per cent of the fat and saturated fats make up about 10 per cent.

Rice bran

Used in Pakistan to make a margarine to replace ghee, rice bran oil contains 35–40 per cent polyunsaturated fats, 40 per cent monounsaturated fats and 20–25 per cent saturated. This oil is a good source of vitamin E. 1 tablespoon would supply the whole day's requirements.

Safflower

Also known as Mexican saffron, safflower oil has the highest content of polyunsaturated fats of any of the vegetable oils. It is used to make polyunsaturated margarines, for frying and for salads. It has a bland flavour. Of its fat, 75 per cent is polyunsaturated, 15 per cent is monounsaturated and 10 per cent is saturated. Safflower oil is also a good source of vitamin E. 1 tablespoon (20 mL) would supply almost the entire day's needs.

Sesame

This strongly flavoured oil is used in Asian and some Middle Eastern cooking. A few drops added to other oil used for salads provides a delightful lift. Sesame oil has about 45 per cent of its fat in the polyunsaturated forms, 40 per cent as monounsaturated fat and the remaining 15 per cent is saturated. Sesame oil is high in vitamin E, although most is not present as the valuable alpha tocopherol.

Soya bean

The useful soya bean not only provides a wonderful source of protein and other nutrients, it also has far more oil than most other legumes. It is used in margarines, for frying and as a salad oil. Its flavour is not particularly distinctive. Of its fat, about 7 per cent is the valuable alpha linolenic acid, a further 53 per cent is polyunsaturated fat, about 25 per cent is monounsaturated and 15 per cent is saturated. Soya bean oil is rich in vitamin E but not all is in the most valuable form of alpha tocopherol (see page 392).

Sunflower

Sunflower seeds contain about 40 per cent oil which can be pressed out. Sunflower oil is used in many margarines and for cooking and salads. Its flavour is mild. Of the fat present in sunflower oil, 52 per cent is polyunsaturated, 34 per cent is monounsaturated and 14 per cent is saturated. Sunflower oil is a good source of vitamin E, especially alpha tocopherol. 1 tablespoon would supply the whole day's requirements.

Walnut

A delightfully delicate oil, walnut oil is usually kept for use on salads. Most walnut oil is produced in France and Italy. It is high in polyunsaturates, including the valuable alpha linolenic acid which makes up over 10 per cent of the fat. A further 54 per cent of the fat consists of other polyunsaturated fats, 23 per cent is monounsaturated and the rest is saturated. Like walnuts, the oil is a good source of vitamin E, although most of this is not in the form of the valuable alpha tocopherol (see page 392).

Wheatgerm

Wheatgerm is a highly nutritious product and that goes for its oil. An oil with a definite flavour, wheatgerm oil is extremely rich in vitamin E. Just 3 mL would supply the entire day's supply. Most of its fats are present as polyunsaturated fatty acids (65 per cent), including some alpha linolenic acid which the body uses to make omega 3 fatty acids. About 15 per cent of the fat is monounsaturated and the remaining 20 per cent is saturated.

OLIVE OIL
see Oils.

OMEGA 3 FATTY ACIDS

These polyunsaturated fatty acids are found principally in fish and seafoods. They can also be made in the body from alpha linolenic acid found in linseeds and linseed oil, soya bean oil, olive oil, rapeseed oil, walnuts, walnut oil, wheatgerm oil and various vegetables and seeds (see page 209). The terminology, omega 3, comes from the double bond in their carbon chain situated 3 carbons from the end of the chain. Omega 6 fatty acids, the major polyunsaturated fat found in vegetable oils, have a double bond 6 carbons from the end of the chain.

The major fatty acids in the omega 3 family are EPA (eicosapentaenoic acid) and DHA (docosahexaenoic acid). These fats are highly polyunsaturated and are found in cold water fish.

Some years ago medical researchers noted that Greenland Eskimos ate a fairly high fat diet but had arteries which were surprisingly free of the fatty deposits which afflicted much of the Western world. A closer look at the Eskimos' diet showed that fish from the icy waters of the Arctic circle had a much higher level of omega 3 fatty acids than fish from warmer waters.

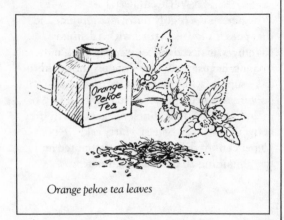

Orange pekoe tea leaves

From the fishes' point of view, these omega 3 fats help prevent their flesh freezing at sub-zero temperatures. For humans their value lies in the effects they have on blood fats and on the formation of blood clots.

After digestion, omega 3 fatty acids follow a different pathway from the omega 6 polyunsaturated fats in vegetable oils. Both omega 3 and omega 6 polyunsaturated fats produce hormone-like substances called prostaglandins. These are then converted into thromboxanes and prostacyclins which are involved in the way platelets in red blood cells stick together and also affect the arteries themselves.

The major difference between the polyunsaturated fats in vegetable oils and fish is in the *types* of thromboxanes and prostacyclins eventually formed.

The products from the omega 3 fatty acids, in general, suppress blood clotting, inflammatory reactions and immune responses. These substances may therefore be useful in controlling or treating some aspects of coronary heart disease, organ transplants and certain types of arthritis, and, possibly, even cancer.

At present, there is no recommended daily intake of omega 3 fatty acids. However, it seems that a greater consumption of fish containing these fatty acids would be beneficial.

Omega 3 fatty acids are found in highest quantity in salmon, ocean trout (especially those from fish farms), mackerel, herring, sardines and tuna. Other fish and seafoods also contain some. Chicken and turkey are also potential sources of omega 3 fatty acids, if their feed contains fish meal.

See also Prostaglandins.

OMELETTE

A mixture of lightly beaten eggs and water, cooked in a greased pan. Usually 2 eggs are used for each omelette and a variety of fillings including herbs, tomato, mushroom or some other vegetables may be added. A plain omelette will have 755 kJ (180 Cals).

ONIONS
see Vegetables.

OOLONG TEA
see Tea.

OPAH
see Fish, Moon fish.

ORANGE
see Fruit.

ORANGE PEKOE TEA
see Tea.

OREGANO
see Herbs.

ORGANICALLY GROWN FOODS

Foods which are grown without fertilisers, pesticides or herbicides. Natural manure and compost may be used. In theory, organic growing makes good sense in conserving resources, re-using materials and avoiding pesticides. In practice, most large farms would be unable to operate without modern methods of soil enrichment and pest control.

Nutritionally, foods grown organically have very little advantage over conventionally-grown products. Plants grow essentially for their own sake and absorb the necessary nutrients to do so. If those nutrients are missing, the plant does not grow properly. Tests on the nutritional value of organically-grown produce show virtually no difference in nutritional value. In some countries where high levels of pesticides are used, organically-grown foods may have lower levels of residues. In places such as Australia where only relatively low levels of pesticides are used, the residues in ordinary or organic produce show no differences.

It would undoubtedly be better to have no pesticide residues in our food supply. If insects are not to eat certain crops, this desirable situation is impossible. As for soil quality and the addition of fertilisers, agricultural experts know much more about the nutrients plants need than nutritionists know about human requirements. Modern soil conservation for efficient farming takes note of plants' nutritional needs.

Organically-grown produce makes good sense for home gardeners. This group tends to abuse pesticides and fertilisers mainly because they are not experts in this field and want to ensure their produce survives. A compost heap and a vigilant eye for pests can be put into practice at home whereas it is impractical in the large-scale farming which our economy currently demands.

ORGANOLEPTIC

Appealing to taste and smell. The taste buds register bitter, sweet, acid and salty tastes. Much of what we attribute to taste is actually provided by smell.

OROTIC ACID

Sometimes referred to as vitamin B_{13}, orotic acid is found in the whey portion of cow's milk. It is not found in significant quantities in human milk.

Orotic acid is important in the chemistry of all body cells but it appears that the body does not need an external source of it. Researchers have tried using supplements of orotic acid to lower blood cholesterol levels and to assist in the repair of heart muscle after a heart attack. At this stage, there is no conclusive evidence that orotic acid should be given as a supplement. If you're tempted to pay large prices for orotic acid as a supplement, you should be aware that it can damage the liver in rats and its full range of actions in humans is not yet understood.

ORRIS ROOT

A substance extracted from the finely ground root of a variety of iris. Sometimes added to confectionery and has a perfumed taste.

ORYZENIN

The major protein in rice.

OSETR

The caviar from the Danube sturgeon. Also found in the Caspian Sea.

OSMOSIS

The process whereby substances of a higher concentration diffuse towards those of a lower concentration in order to bring about an even distribution of ions. This occurs in the body, for example, when too much salt is consumed without extra fluid. Salt contributes sodium and the presence of extra sodium in the blood makes it more concentrated than the fluids in the cells. By the process of osmosis, water will pass from the cells into the blood to even up the concentration. By this means, the body controls undesirably high levels of sodium (or other electrolytes) in different compartments.

OSTEOARTHRITIS

A condition in which there are bony outgrowths at the edges of joints and a degeneration of the cartilage at the ends of the joints. Although there are many theories relating diet to osteoarthritis, there have been few conclusions apart from the general advice to keep active and control weight so that there is not too much stress of the joints.

Many people swear by a particular diet for osteoarthritis. Some maintain that vegetarian food helps; others have found their arthritis goes into remission when they eat a particular food or combination of foods. In general, there is no exact diet which is suitable for everyone who has osteoarthritis apart from general advice to lose excess weight.

OSTEOMALACIA

An adult form of rickets caused by a deficiency of vitamin D. This vitamin is produced in the body when sunlight acts on a substance in the skin and is essential for calcium to be absorbed into bones. Those who have no vitamin D because they do not expose any of their skin to the sunlight cannot absorb calcium into the bones. This causes the bones to become misshapen. Osteomalacia occurs in some countries where it is not considered socially acceptable for a woman's skin to be exposed.

OSTEOPOROSIS

A condition in which the bones become less dense, porous and brittle. It is common in post-menopausal women in Western countries. When oestrogen levels drop at menopause, the amount of calcium retained by bones falls. Gradually the bones becomes less dense.

If bones are strong and dense to start with, the loss of calcium from bones after menopause will not be great enough to cause osteoporosis. If, however, the withdrawal of calcium from bones has been slightly greater than the deposits over the previous 20 or 30 years, the menopausal losses can be sufficient to produce the porous bones of osteoporosis.

See also Bone; Calcium; Sodium.

OUZO
see Drinks, Alcoholic.

OVALBUMIN
see Albumen.

OVERWEIGHT

A condition of excess body fat, usually defined as having a Body Mass Index (see page 40 and the chart on page 7) greater than 25. There is considerable medical evidence that being overweight increases the risks of coronary heart disease, high blood pressure, diabetes (adult onset type), gallstones and certain types of cancer (especially hormone-dependent cancers and bowel cancer). In addition, being overweight makes arthritis and joint problems worse and surgery more hazardous.

OXALIC ACID

An organic acid present in plants, especially rhubarb leaves, celery leaves, spinach, beetroot, parsley and tea leaves. Oxalic acid forms insoluble complexes with calcium, making the calcium unavailable to the body. Calcium oxalate is the major component of kidney stones.

Excessive quantities of vitamin C are also metabolised to oxalic acid. Megadoses of vitamin C (several grams a day) are probably a greater hazard than foods containing oxalic acid, with the exception of rhubarb leaves which have a high enough concentration to be toxic.

See also Food poisoning.

OXIDATION

The loss of hydrogen or the gaining of oxygen into a molecule. Foods are oxidised in the body to release their energy. Foods also go off because various enzymes pick up oxygen from the air and alter molecules within the food.

OXTAIL

The tailbone of the ox, stewed or made into soup. After long slow cooking, the tender flavoursome meat falls off the bones. The flesh is a good source of zinc and also contributes iron, protein and vitamins. Each 100 g of raw weight of oxtail contribute 710 kJ (170 Cals).

OYSTER
see Seafood.

OYSTER PLANT
see Vegetables, Salsify.

P

PABA

PABA (para-aminobenzoic acid) was once thought to be part of the vitamin B complex. Research showed that it was not a vitamin for humans. PABA is used in sunscreens but is not a necessary part of the diet. It is a growth factor for micro-organisms and is most undesirable in the case of bacterial infections in the intestine.

PAELLA

A Spanish dish based on rice, flavoured with saffron, onion, garlic and olive oil, cooked in chicken stock in a large heavy frying pan and topped with seafoods, chicken and a spicy sausage. The dish is served in the pan in which it is cooked and is often beautifully decorated.

PALM HEARTS
see Vegetables.

PALMITIC ACID

A saturated fatty acid containing 16 carbons, present in many foods. Palmitic acid accounts for over 40 per cent of the fat in palm oil and more than 30 per cent of the fat in icecream, biscuits, cakes and chocolate. It is also the major saturated fat in meat.

PALM KERNEL OIL
see Oils.

PALM SUGAR

Compressed cakes of richly-coloured brown

sugar extracted from several varieties of palm. Used in some Asian confectionery (especially in Malaysia) for its rich, sweet flavour.

PALOMINO
see Wine, Varieties.

PANCAKE

A thicker version of a French crepe, pancakes are made from milk, flour and eggs, and are cooked on a very hot greased pan until bubbles appear on the surface. The pancake is then flipped over and browned on the remaining side. Once cooked, you can reheat pancakes by covering them with foil and placing in a moderate oven for a few minutes. Alternatively, stack them on a plate, cover with a heatproof basin and place over a saucepan of boiling water for a few minutes. To make high-fibre pancakes, use wholemeal flour or a mixture of wholemeal flour and fine oat bran. An average-sized pancake (50 g) has 645 kJ (155 Cals).

PANCREAS

A large gland lying just under the stomach. Pancreatic juice contains the enzymes which carry out much of the digestion of proteins, fats and carbohydrates. The idea that foods containing these nutrients should not be eaten ignores the fact that the pancreatic juices provide all the enzymes in the 1 package. Pancreatic juices are alkaline and enter the first part of the small intestine, the duodenum. Together with bile and intestinal juices they neutralise the acid contents of the stomach as they enter the small intestine. About 1.5 l of pancreatic juice are produced each day.

The pancreas also secretes the hormones insulin and glucagon into the blood. These hormones control the level of glucose in the blood.

PANCREATITIS

Inflammation of the pancreas. This condition can occur in those who drink a lot of alcohol. The symptoms are pain, nausea and vomiting and an inability to digest fats or proteins. Diabetes may also occur. Pancreatitis can also arise as a complication of some types of hepatitis or from a blockage to the bile duct.

PANETTONE

An Italian yeasted cake, which also contains a high level of butter and eggs, as well as sultanas and candied citrus peel. Usually made at Christmas.

PANGAMIC ACID
see Vitamins, B_{15}.

PANTOTHENIC ACID
see Vitamins, B_5.

PAPAIN

An enzyme which can break down protein and is found in the flesh, stems and leaves of pawpaw. Can be used to tenderise meats, either by sprinkling meat with powdered papain or by wrapping the meat in a pawpaw leaf. Also used in some medications to relieve indigestion.

See also Enzymes.

PAPAW
see Fruits, Pawpaw.

PAPAYA
see Fruits, Pawpaw.

PAPPADAMS

Indian flat breads, traditionally made from lentil flour, rolled very thin and cooked by frying in hot oil until they curl up. They taste even more delicious if cooked quickly under a hot griller, with no added fat or a couple at a time in a microwave oven.

PAPRIKA
see Spices.

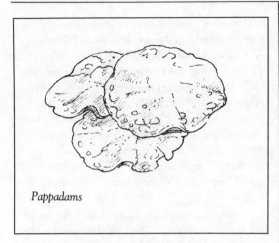

Pappadams

PARA-AMINOBENZOIC ACID
see PABA.

PARATHYROID GLAND

An endocrine gland near the thyroid gland. The parathyroid secretes a hormone called parathormone which regulates the level of calcium in the blood. This hormone plays a vital role since any drop in calcium level would affect nerves and muscles and produce muscular spasms known as tetany. If the level of calcium in the blood drops, parathyroid hormone causes some calcium to be withdrawn from the bones so that a normal blood level is maintained. The hormone also controls levels of phosphorus and magnesium.

PARBOIL

A process of partially cooking by boiling for a few minutes. Vegetables are usually parboiled before freezing. This kills enzymes which would otherwise cause discolouration of the products. Some vitamins are also destroyed by parboiling, but the quantity is small, usually less than are lost during a day or two in the home kitchen.

PARIETAL CELLS

Cells in the wall of the stomach which secrete gastric juices.

PARMESAN
see Cheese.

PARSLEY
see Herbs.

PARSNIPS
see Vegetables.

PARTRIDGE

A game bird native to Europe and related to the pheasant. Partridge are larger than quail. Most game birds do a lot more flying than domesticated birds. Their muscles are thus well supplied with oxygen and their meat has a higher content of iron and a colour darker than that of domestic birds. The flesh of partridge is very high in iron and protein and a good source of vitamins of the B complex. 100 g of roast partridge (without bone) have 880 kJ (210 Cals). When young, the birds can be roasted but older birds are best cooked in a clay pot or casserole.

PARTS PER MILLION
see PPM.

PASSIONFRUIT
see Fruit.

PASTA

Dough made from the endosperm of hard durum wheat mixed with water, cut into strips of various shapes and boiled until tender. Noodles may also have added egg and/or vegetable extracts. Hard wheat is used in making pasta as its endosperm has larger protein particles which give a strong dough. Pasta made from weaker flours breaks easily.

Legend has it that pasta originated in China and was brought to Italy by Marco Polo. Certainly noodles were a common part of the Chinese diet from the first century AD. Others claim that noodles were independently invented by many different people. There is evidence that sheets of flat pasta (similar to lasagne noodles) were used in Italy before Marco Polo's time. It is now commonly accepted that pasta was originally made by the Etruscans.

Whatever its origins, pasta is now enjoyed in many parts of the world. From the eighteenth century onwards, most pasta was machine-made. Over the last few years, there has been a trend for home-made or fresh pasta, although this still only accounts for a small quantity. Pasta is still most popular in Italy where the average consumption is about 30 kg/year — equivalent to 1 serve per person per day.

Pasta is cooked by adding it to a large quantity of rapidly boiling water. A small amount of oil will stop the pasta sticking together. As soon as the pasta is just tender ('al dente', meaning 'to the tooth'), it is drained. It should not be rinsed.

There are more than 600 named shapes of pasta, ranging from the broad lasagne sheets and cannelloni rolls to the finer tagliatelle or fettucine or the twisted fusilli or spirale or the many tubular or small shaped pastas, such as macaroni.

All have a common nutrient background, providing plenty of complex carbohydrate, some protein and dietary fibre and small quantities of vitamins and minerals. Wholemeal spaghetti and other pasta has a higher content of dietary fibre and other nutrients. 100 g of raw pasta have approximately 1425 kJ (340 Cals). 100 g of cooked pasta have approximately 375 kJ (90 Cals). The common view that pasta is fattening is only likely to be correct if a lot of oil, butter, cream, bacon or fatty meats are eaten with the pasta.

PASTEURISATION

A process of heating to destroy bacteria and so prolong the life of a product. Pasteurisation of

milk has virtually wiped out many milk-borne infections which caused widespread disease. The milk is heated briefly and then cooled. There is some loss of vitamin C and thiamin (B_1), but since milk is a very poor source of vitamin C and cannot be relied on to supply much thiamin in the diet, these losses are not really of great importance. The important nutrients such as protein, calcium and riboflavin are unaffected by pasteurisation. Some beer is also pasteurised to prevent further action of yeast.

Some cheesemakers claim that they cannot achieve the particular flavour they want if they use pasteurised milk. However, if milk for cheesemaking contains bacteria, it can be a source of food poisoning, especially with some of the soft cheeses. Processed cheeses are made from pasteurised milk but are also re-pasteurised after manufacture so that bacteria will not cause further ageing of the product.

In many countries, food laws prohibit the sale of certain products made from unprocessed cows' milk. Goats' milk is not always subject to the same restrictions and some unpasteurised goats' milk has been found to contain bacteria which are potentially harmful.

PASTRAMI

Cured meat which may be either beef, mutton, goat, pork or goose. In most Western countries,

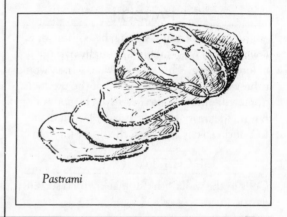

Pastrami

pastrami is made from beef. The meat is cured with a mixture of saltpetre, pepper, nutmeg, allspice, paprika and garlic and usually has a crust of these ingredients on top. It is high in salt.

PASTRY

Pastry doughs are made from flour and fat with added water. Some also contain eggs. They may have a dense biscuit-like structure, or be flaky and layered. Most pastries have a high fat content and the fat serves the purpose of holding the starch and protein apart. Lard is the ideal fat for making pastry because it forms large crystals and gives a 'shortness' to the pastry. These days, however, saturated animal or vegetable fats are used in preference to lard. They have no nutritional advantage, but do not turn rancid as quickly as lard.

In making pastry, the flour should not be stretched too much or the protein strands will become tough. The ingredients and cooking utensils should also be kept cool.

With the exception of filo pastry sheets, all pastry is high in fat.

- To make *shortcrust* pastry, the fat and flour are mixed together and then just enough liquid is added to hold the mass together. The pastry is chilled before being baked so that the gluten (protein) particles can relax and avoid shrinkage during baking. A normal-sized (20 cm) shortcrust pastry shell has 6565 kJ (1565 Cals) and will serve 6. Each serve of the pie shell (without filling) thus has 1090 kJ (260 Cals).
- *Puff* pastry is more difficult to prepare. The flour is mixed with iced water and the dough is placed onto a cool marble board. The shortening is placed on top, and the dough folded so that the shortening separates the dough layers. The dough is once again rolled out, more shortening added and the whole thing folded. This procedure is repeated to give anything from 100–250 layers. As the pastry bakes, the expanding air and steam puff the layers apart. An average serving of puff pastry has 1880 kJ (450 Cals).
- *Flaky* pastry also has layers of pastry dough and fat interleaved but has fewer layers than puff pastry. An average serve of flaky pastry has 1780 kJ (425 Cals). For frozen pastry, each 100 g have 1840 kJ (440 Cals).
- *Filo* pastry is made from very thin layers of flour and water dough. It has no fat, although some type of shortening is usually brushed between each layer. If you wish to avoid using fat, you can brush yoghurt between the layers of filo pastry. Each sheet of purchased filo pastry has 105 kJ (25 Cals), before adding any fat.
- *Choux* pastry is made by cooking a mixture of butter, flour and water until very thick and then adding egg yolks. The paste is allowed to cool and is then lightened with stiffly beaten egg whites to produce a soft pastry which is squeezed from a piping bag or shaped into mounds before being baked in a very hot oven. The pastry bakes into the familiar light puffs used in eclairs and cream puffs. Like most pastries, choux pastry is high in fat. An average serve (2 small puffs), without filling, has 1365 kJ (325 Cals). See also Tart.

PÂTÉ

Literally a paste, pâté originally referred to a meat or fish filling inside a pastry case. These days, pâté is usually taken to mean a liver paste, made from liver and seasonings cooked in butter and pureed with cream and stock or some form of alcohol. Most pâté has a high-fat content, although low-fat recipes can be prepared. An average pâté (60 g) has 770 kJ (185 Cals).

PATNA RICE
see Grains, Rice.

PAULING, LINUS

This eminent gentleman has won the Nobel Prize twice, for chemistry and peace. He has probably become best known among the general public, however, for his belief that the common cold can be prevented and cured by high doses of vitamin C. His theories concerning vitamin C also extend to its value in the prevention and treatment of cancer. Pauling's theories have not been verified by other researchers, many of whom are critical of the high doses of the vitamin which he recommends.

See also Vitamin C.

PAUPIETTE

A thin slice of veal or other meat, spread with a stuffing, rolled up, browned in a pan and then baked in wine or stock.

PAVLOVA

A meringue which is crisp on the edge and as soft as marshmallow in the centre. Usually served with whipped cream and passionfruit, the tartness of the latter balancing the sweetness of the meringue. There is great dispute as to who first made pavlova. Both the Australians and New Zealanders claim it as their own. The official story is that the dessert was created in the 1930s by Herbert Sachse, a West Australian chef. The dessert itself contains egg whites and sugar, flavoured with vanilla. It has no fat, although the cream which tops it destroys this advantage! An average serving of pavlova with cream and passionfruit has 1150 kJ (275 Cals).

PAWPAW
see Fruit.

PEACH
see Fruit.

PEANUT
see Nuts.

PEANUT BUTTER
Also known as peanut paste, this product is

made from ground peanuts. The peanuts are roasted and cooled and the husks or skins are removed by a gentle rubbing action. High-quality nuts are then ground to make peanut butter. Some manufacturers add salt, sugar, peanut oil and emulsifiers to keep the oil evenly distributed through the product. Others market a product which is just ground peanuts. Smaller health food stores may grind their own peanut butter. In such cases, the machinery used needs to be kept scrupulously clean since moulds which may form on peanuts can carry harmful toxins.

Nutritionally, peanut butter is an excellent source of niacin (one of the B vitamins) and a good source of vitamin E, protein and dietary fibre. It also provides iron, zinc, potassium and various B vitamins. With a total fat content of about 52 per cent, peanut butter is fairly high in kilojoules. A 50 g serve has 1300 kJ (310 Cals).

PEANUT OIL
see Oils.

PEANUT SAUCE
see Sauces, other.

PEAR
see Fruit.

PEARL BARLEY
see Grains, Barley.

PEAS, DRIED
see Legumes.

PEAS, FRESH
see Vegetables.

PECAN
see Nuts.

PECORINO ROMANO
see Cheese.

PECTIN

A form of soluble dietary fibre found in citrus peel, apples and other fruits and vegetables. The pectin in fruits helps jam to gel. There are different types of pectin; some have better gel-forming properties than others. Marmalade sets well (and is a good source of pectin) because of the type of pectin in citrus peel. In making jams from fruits with a low pectin level such as strawberries, pectin or lemon slices need to be added so that the jam will thicken.

Contrary to the popular image of dietary fibre as being stringy, pectin can be isolated as a fine white powder. Like other soluble dietary fibres, pectin is valuable in the diet. Researchers have shown that it delays the emptying of the stomach and helps lower blood cholesterol levels, presumably by removing cholesterol or its by-products from the body. It may well be the pectin in apples which has earned their reputation of 'an apple a day keeps the doctor away'.

As well as being used in jams, pectin is used in making some confectionery (such as fruit gums), desserts, icecream, mayonnaises and dressings and some sandwich spreads. It is listed as additive 440.

See also Jam.

PEDAH
see Fish.

PEEL

The skin of citrus peel is used to flavour foods and the very outside part of lemon or orange peel (without any pith) is called the zest. Citrus peel can also be boiled in a concentrated sugar solution to produce mixed or candied peel. 1 tablespoon of mixed peel has 190 kJ (45 Cals).

PELLAGRA

A condition caused by a lack of the vitamin niacin (B_3). It was once common in populations living mainly on corn as corn is naturally deficient in an amino acid, tryptophan, which is converted to niacin. New strains of corn now grown contain this amino acid and these have almost wiped out pellagra (see Corn). The early symptoms of pellagra include weakness, loss of appetite, irritability and depression. As the deficiency worsens, chronic dermatitis with thickened, scaly skin develops and mucous membranes throughout the body become inflamed. There is also delirium and dementia, and finally, death. The condition usually only occurs in chronic alcoholics.

PEMMICAN

A dried meat product made by some American Indians from strips of beef sun-dried to a leather-like consistency. Being so dry, pemmican does not contain enough moisture to support bacteria and so is a way of keeping meat without refrigeration. Many of the B vitamins will be lost but minerals and protein will still be present.

PENNE

Short tubes of pasta, usually cut with diagonal ends.

PENNYROYAL
see Herbs.

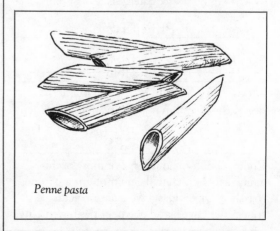

Penne pasta

PENTOSANS

One of the kinds of dietary fibre found in fruit, oats and rye. Pentosans are made up of long strings of 5 carbon sugars. They absorb water very well and that is why bread which has a high content of rye grain stays moist for so long. Pentosans are only slowly broken down by bacteria in the intestine. This makes them a valuable form of dietary fibre.

PENTOSE

A 5 carbon sugar (glucose is a 6 carbon sugar). Examples of pentoses are ribose (part of RNA, see page 290) and xylose (see page 405).

PEPINO
see Fruit.

PEPITAS
see Seeds.

PEPPER
see Spices.

PEPPERMINT
see Herbs, Mint.

PEPPERMINT CAMPHOR
see Menthol.

PEPPERONI
see Sausages.

PEPPERS
see Vegetables, Capsicum.

PEPSIN

An enzyme present in gastric juice which begins the digestion of proteins in the stomach.

PEPTIDES

Compounds formed when 2 or more of the amino acids which make up proteins are joined together. Dipeptides have 2 amino acids; tripeptides have 3 and polypeptides have many amino acids, forming proteins. Peptides are formed during the digestion of large protein molecules.

PERCH
see Fish.

PERIODONTAL DISEASE

A disease of the gums in which the gums separate from the teeth. If bacteria multiply in the space, the infection known as gingivitis develops. As periodontal disease advances, the teeth become loose and eventually fall out. Plaque on teeth and a lack of fibrous foods encourage periodontal disease.

PERIPHERAL NEUROPATHY

A disorder of the nerves supplying the limbs which may be due to a deficiency of thiamin (vitamin B_1) or vitamin B_6 (also called pyridoxine). The condition has recently been diagnosed in women who take large doses of vitamin B_6, usually as treatment for pre-menstrual syndrome (see page 278).

PERISTALSIS

The waves of contraction and relaxation which propel food along the intestine. Some types of dietary fibre produce acids when they are being broken down by bacteria in the large intestine. Researchers now suspect that one of these acids actually stimulates peristalsis. When the stomach is full, peristaltic waves are decreased and a high-fat meal can halt peristalsis for some hours.

PERNICIOUS ANAEMIA

An anaemia in which the bone marrow releases fewer red and white blood cells and platelets (see page 270). The condition arises from a lack of vitamin B_{12}. Usually it is not the vitamin itself which is deficient, but there is a lack of a substance known as 'intrinsic factor' which is essential for the absorption of B_{12}.

Taking extra vitamin B_{12} will not always cure pernicious anaemia since it is the absorption which is the problem; B_{12} may need to be given by intravenous injection (see also Vitamin B_{12}). Symptoms of pernicious anaemia include pale skin, weakness, loss of appetite, depression, loss of weight and abdominal discomfort.

PERNOD
see Drinks, Alcoholic.

PEROXIDES

Benzoyl peroxide is used as a bleaching agent to remove the slightly yellowish colour from flour used for making white bread. During the bleaching process, the benzoyl peroxide is converted to benzoic acid which most people can metabolise easily. However, the process of bleaching flour is purely cosmetic and is difficult to justify on any other grounds.

PERSIMMON
see Fruit.

PESTO

A sauce made from fresh basil, olive oil, pine nuts, garlic, Parmesan cheese and lemon. Served with pasta. A 60 g serve has 1030 kJ (245 Cals).

PH

A measure of acidity or alkalinity, ranging from 1 (extreme acidity) to 14 (extreme alkalinity).

PHEASANT

Game birds native to Asia. Their flesh is well flavoured, especially when roasted or braised. The hens are usually more tender than the cocks and the birds are often hung for several days to tenderise the meat. Like all game birds, the flesh of pheasant is darker than that of domesticated birds. This is due to a greater supply of oxygen to the muscles of the birds during physical activity. It also gives the flesh a very high quantity of iron. Pheasant is also rich in protein and is a good source of some of the B complex vitamins. 100 g of roast pheasant (weighed without bone) have 900 kJ (215 Cals).

PHENYLALANINE

An essential amino acid which is converted to tyrosine, another amino acid. Some people are born without the enzyme needed for this reaction and phenylalanine levels can build up to a high enough level to cause brain and nerve damage. These people suffer from the disorder known as phenylketonuria (PKU). If PKU is detected early in life, a synthetic diet containing known quantities of amino acids can be given. Without this treatment those with PKU suffer brain damage. In countries such as Australia, all babies are tested for PKU soon after birth.

Some artificial sweeteners contain phenylalanine. However, the quantities of these artificial sweeteners eaten would have to be enormous for anyone ever to develop high blood levels of phenylalanine. All protein foods contain phenylalanine.

See also Artificial sweeteners.

PHOSPHATES

Forms of phosphorus which are neded in the body in bones, teeth and many of the compounds involved in energy production.

See also Phosphorus.

PHOSPHOLIPID

A combination of phosphorus and a fat (or lipid). The best known phospholipid is probably lecithin (see page 203). These compounds are important in the structure of cell membranes.

See also Inositol; Myoinositol.

PHOSPHORUS

Present in the body as phosphate, this mineral is important in bones and teeth. It is also involved in the production of energy from fats, carbohydrates and proteins and assists the body in using some of the B complex vitamins.

Dietary deficiencies of phosphorus are very rare since it is widely distributed in foods and also comes in many food additives. A lack of phosphorus is only likely to occur in those whose kidneys are not functioning properly, or in people who take antacids over a long period. A deficiency of phosphorus is serious as it causes abnormalities in blood cells, muscular weakness and bone pains.

It is important that the quantity of phosphorus in the diet matches the intake of calcium. Excessive amounts of phosphorus decrease the amount of calcium which is absorbed into bones. Foods which contribute calcium with their phosphorus are useful. Milk, cheese and yoghurt fit this category.

There is no set recommended daily intake of phosphorus, but a level of 800 mg a day is usually considered desirable.

FOOD	PHOSPHORUS (mg)
Pasta, av. serve	160
Rolled oats, $\frac{1}{2}$ cup, raw	160
Wheat bran, 2 tablespoons	120
Bread, wholemeal, 2 slices	100
Wheat breakfast biscuits, 2	90
Rice, av. serve, 80 g, raw	85
Bread, white, 2 slices	50
Yoghurt, 200 g carton	320
Milk, any kind, 250 mL	250
Cheese, 30 g	160
Egg, 1	120
Chicken or turkey, lean, 120 g	380
Steak, av. serve (200 g, cooked)	360
Fish, av. fillet, grilled, 150 g	350
Shellfish, 100 g, flesh	350
Lamb chops, 2 av.	300
Pork steak, lean 120 g	240
Dried beans, 50 g, raw weight	160
Lentils, 50 g, raw weight	120
Sweetcorn, av.-sized cob	180
Mushrooms, 100 g	170
Peas, 100 g	100
Spinach, 100 g	95
Asparagus, 100 g	85
Cabbage, 100 g	70
Brussels sprouts, 100 g	65
Broccoli, 100 g	60
Potato, medium size (140 g)	55
Fruits, per serve	20−40
Brazil nuts, 50 g	295
Walnuts, 50 g	255
Almonds, 50 g	220
Peanuts, 50 g	185
Hazel nuts, 50 g	115
Coconut, 50 g, fresh	45
Chocolate, 100 g	240
Cola soft drinks, 370 mL can	55
Juices, 250 mL	35
Beer, 370 mL can	55
Yeast extract, av. serve, 3 g	50

PHOTOSYNTHESIS

The process whereby plants make carbohydrates from carbon dioxide and water. Ultimately all human life depends on this process.

PHYTIC ACID

A compound made up of myoinositol (see page 239) plus 6 phosphates. Phytic acid can trap minerals such as calcium, iron and zinc so that they are unavailable to the body. It is present in the outer layers of cereal grains but under normal circumstances, this is not a great problem in people eating a varied diet. The foods which contain phytic acid (cereal grain husks) are usually rich in the minerals to which it binds. This means that the zinc in, say, wheat bran, may not be of much use, but at least it takes up the phytic acid in the bran, thus making it less likely to attach to the zinc from other foods.

In wholegrain breads, phytic acid causes no problems since enzymes will break down the phytic acid during fermentation.

Problems may arise if wholegrain unleavened bread makes up a significant part of the diet.

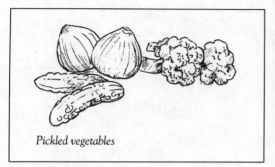

Pickled vegetables

This has occurred in some Middle Eastern countries and the high phytic acid content of the bread, combined with a total diet which is low in zinc, has produced zinc deficiency.

In Western countries, problems only arise when very large quantities of phytic acid are consumed. Some women, for example, eat several cups of unprocessed wheat bran a day in an attempt to lose weight. This is dangerous for several reasons (see Bran) and mineral deficiencies can occur. Taking 1–2 tablespoons of unprocessed wheat bran a day will not produce the same effect.

The phytic acid content of foods is as follows:

FOOD	PHYTIC ACID (g)
Bran cereal, 50 g serve	1.75
Rye bread, 2 slices	0.45
Rolled oats, $\frac{1}{2}$ cup raw	0.40
Muesli, av., 60 g serve	0.40
Wheatgerm, 1 tablespoon	0.40
Barley, av. serve, 60 g, raw weight	0.36
Wheat bran, 2 tablespoons, 10 g	0.34
Rice, av. serve (80 g, raw)	0.33
Wholemeal bread, 2 slices	0.30
Wholewheat breakfast biscuits, 2	0.15
White bread, 2 slices	0.02

PICA

A craving to eat items which are unusual. Examples of pica include eating dirt or chalk. Some pregnant women experience pica, often in the form of a craving for some out of season or particularly sour-tasting food. Whether pica represents a biological need for a particular nutrient has not been satisfactorily resolved.

PICCALILLI

A pickle made in the United States from green tomatoes, capsicum and onion pickled with vinegar, sugar and spices. In England, piccalilli is made from mixed vegetables and mustard seeds and served with cheese and bread.

PICKLES

Foods which are preserved by acid, usually vinegar. The high acidity level discourages the growth of most bacteria. Pickling can be done by two methods. The first, and simpler method, involves packing the food in acid so that bacteria cannot survive. The second method is more complicated. The food is first placed in brine and allowed to ferment. This kills most bacteria but allows those that produce lactic acid to survive. The acidity from these bacteria then make life too unpleasant for other bacteria to invade the food. Vegetables and fruits are used to make pickles.

PIES

Pastry filled with either a sweet or savoury mixture. Since pastry has a high content of fat, most pies are high in fat and kilojoules. Attempts to produce more nutritious wholemeal pies may increase the fibre but do not alter the fat and kilojoules. A slice of fruit pie (140 g) has 1540 kJ (370 Cals); an individual serve meat pie has 1720 kJ (410 Cals) and a small pork pie has 3225 kJ (770 Cals).

PIGEON

A bird which is found all over the world and, in some areas, eaten. The flesh is sometimes a little tough and needs long slow cooking. Nutritionally, pigeon is extremely high in iron and a good source of protein and vitamins of the B complex. 100 g of roast pigeon (including bones) have 420 kJ (100 Cals).

PIGNOLIAS
see Nuts, Pine nuts.

PIG'S TROTTERS

These are rich in a gelatinous substance which makes excellent stock or can be used as jelly around meats. They can also be boned and stuffed to make a dish known as 'head cheese'.

PIKE
see Fish.

PIKELETS

An Australian version of the griddle cake. Pikelets are made from a batter containing flour, a raising agent (or self-raising flour), milk and eggs. The batter is poured onto a hot greased frying pan to make pikelets about 8–10 cm in diameter. When one side is cooked, they are flipped to brown the other. An average sized pikelet has approximately 210 kJ (50 Cals).

PILAF

A Middle Eastern rice dish made by tossing rice grains and flavouring agents such as onion and herbs with some oil until the grains of rice are coated. Stock or water is then added and the mixture simmered until all the liquid has been absorbed by the rice. Generally 2 cups of liquid is used for each cup of rice. Other ingredients including seafoods, chicken and vegetables may also be added. Also called pilau.

PILCHARD
see Fish.

PILES
see Haemorrhoids.

PIMENTO
see Spices, Allspice.

PIMIENTO
see Vegetables, Capsicum.

PIMPLES
see Acne.

PINEAPPLE
see Fruit.

PINEAPPLE GUAVA
see Fruit, Feijoa.

PINE NUTS
see Nuts.

PINK BEANS
see Legumes.

PINOT NOIR
see Wine, Varieties.

PINTO BEANS
see Legumes.

PIPERADE

From the Basque region of France comes this mixture of beaten eggs and water, cooked in an omelette pan and topped with tomatoes, onions and capsicums.

PIPIS
see Seafood, Clams.

PIROSHKI

A Russian delicacy consisting of tiny pastry cases filled with cream cheese, fish or smoked meats and vegetables. The dough may be a yeasted dough or a pastry and the piroshki may be baked or fried. They are usually served with cocktails or soup.

PISTACHIO NUTS
see Nuts.

PISTOU

A mixture of basil and garlic, pounded together and used to flavour soups and stews.

PITA

A flatbread which puffs up during baking to form a pocket. Pita breads are made from white or wholemeal flour plus water and yeast. They contain virtually no fat and are good sources of complex carbohydrate and dietary fibre, the wholemeal varieties having about 2.5 times as much fibre as those made from white flour. The size of pita breads varies and this obviously affects the kilojoule value. A 50 g pita has 545 kJ (130 Cals). As they are mostly eaten with vegetables, dips or salads, these breads make suitable foods for those watching their weight or cholesterol levels.

PITANGA

see Fruit, Jambo.

PITH

The white material between the flesh of citrus fruit and the rind. Pith is an excellent source of dietary fibre, especially pectin. Its fibre content may be too high for some people who may find it produces flatulence.

PITUITARY GLAND

An endocrine gland at the back of the brain which secretes various hormones. In some instances, these hormones control the production of hormones from other glands. The thyroid gland, the production of milk during lactation, the control of blood pressure and the secretion of male and female sex hormones are all under the control of the pituitary. Endorphins, chemical substances which have an effect on the brain similar to that of morphine and are responsible for the well-known runner's 'high', are also under the control of the pituitary.

PIZZA

From its origins in Naples in Italy, this bread-based flat type of pie has spread to many countries, taking its part in the array of fast foods. A true pizza is baked in a special oven which quickly reaches high temperatures. Purists insist that the best pizzas are cooked in wood-fired ovens.

Pizzas usually have a topping of tomato paste, oregano, mozzarella cheese and olive oil. Ham, pepperoni, seafoods, ground beef, various vegetables (mushrooms, onions, capsicum), anchovies and olives may also be added.

In comparison with other commonly available fast foods, pizza probably has a better balance of nutrients. It certainly has less fat, although this will depend on the pizza being the genuine article and having a bread base. Some of the modern pizzas are substituting a pastry base; a few are even using fried pastry bases. These are high in fat, usually saturated fat derived from palm kernel oil.

Pizza has approximately 1000 kJ (240 Cals) and 8 g of fat per 100 g. Half a regular pizza has approximately 1800 kJ (430 Cals).

PLACEBO

A substance which has no pharmacological effect — in other words, a 'dummy pill'. A placebo often 'works' because the person taking the substance believes it will. The supposed wonders of many pills and supplements are due to the placebo effect. In controlled tests of drugs, food supplements and additives, either the real substance being tested or a placebo is given in identical packaging so that neither the researcher nor the persons being tested know which they are receiving. Once all effects are noted, the code is broken and it can be seen if the real substance had any significant difference in its effects from those of the placebo. Some studies using vitamin supplements, for example, have shown that both the group being given the vitamin and those on the placebo derive benefits but there is no difference between the two groups. This shows the value of taking substances which you expect to have some effect. It is the belief which works rather than the substance.

PLAICE

see Fish.

PLAKI

A Greek dish made by placing a whole fish on a bed of tomatoes, onions, olives and herbs, covering with wine and baking.

PLANKTON

Small organisms which live in fresh or salt water and are eaten by larger organisms. Plankton form the base for life in fresh and salt water. As yet, plankton soup does not appear on human menus although the possibility exists for plankton to form a very cheap form of human food. Certainly, the blue whale seems to grow well on a diet of plankton!

PLANTAIN

see Fruit.

PLAQUE

Deposits which form in parts of the body. Most of us are familiar with dental plaque which sticks to our teeth and provides an ideal residence for the bacteria which dissolve tooth enamel and cause caries. This plaque consists of sugar polymers built by enzymes from the *Streptococcus mutans* bacteria which live in the human mouth.

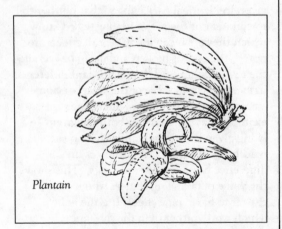

Plantain

Plaque also makes up the fatty deposits which lodge in the arteries and cause atherosclerosis. This plaque is made from calcium salts, cholesterol and fatty substances. See also Dental caries.

PLASMA

The light-yellow coloured portion of the blood after the red cells have been removed. The average person has 3−3.5 l of plasma in his or her body. This valuable liquid carries many substances to body cells.

PLATELETS

Small cells in the blood which are involved in blood clotting. Platelets will aggregate around an injury (such as a cut) and will then release substances which form a plug or clot. A blood clot which stops bleeding is good but one which blocks a vital artery obviously is not. With a fatty diet, platelets tend to be more sticky and form clots in arteries. With plenty of fish in the diet, platelets are much less sticky. Smoking shortens the life of platelets and increases their tendency to stick together.

PLUM

see Fruit.

PLUM PUDDING

Another term for Christmas pudding — a rich pudding made from dried fruits, eggs, suet (or butter), sugar, breadcrumbs, brandy or rum, nuts and a little flour. A medium-sized slice (100 g) of a typical plum pudding has 1445 kJ (345 Cals).

PLUM SAUCE

see Sauces, other.

POISONS, NATURAL

There are many perfectly 'natural' poisons or toxins ranging from the chemicals found in mushrooms or certain plants, to vitamins which are quite deadly in excess. In fact, it is fair to say that there is no safe substance, natural or manufactured; there are only safe quantities. Anything, even water, is toxic in excess.

Some naturally-occurring toxins are much more poisonous than others in the doses likely to be encountered. Various alkaloids and naturally-occurring substances called lathyrogens in some raw bean seeds, for example, are quite toxic in relatively small doses while the oxalic acid in spinach or celery leaves is much less so.

Some of the worst toxins in foods arise from mycotoxins produced by fungi (see page 239). Bacteria or the toxins they produce can also have devastating effects on human health.

The idea that only man-made substances in foods are harmful is not correct. Natural toxicants are a much greater threat to human health than substances used in preserving modern foodstuffs.

POLENTA

A yellow meal ground from Indian corn and made into a thick porridge which is eaten as is or can be fried. A typical serve of polenta provides complex carbohydrate and dietary fibre as well as iron and some protein and vitamins. 60 g of cornmeal made into a serve of porridge have 880 kJ (210 Cals).

POLISH SALAMI
see Sausages.

POLLACK
see Fish.

POLLEN

The part of a plant which joins with the ovule (small egg) to form the seed of a plant. Pollen gathers on the hairy body of a bee as it collects nectar from plants. The pollen is the main source of protein for bees and also supplies vitamins and minerals. It is stored in the cells in honeycomb and eaten by the worker bees while they are developing. Pollen is a good source of nutrients for a bee but has little relevance for humans since the quantities of nutrients required by humans are so much greater than for a tiny bee. There is no point in paying high prices for bee pollen; it contains nothing which cannot be obtained from other foods. It is useful mainly for bees.

POLYHYDRIC ALCOHOLS
see Artificial sweeteners.

POLYMER DRINKS

Glucose molecules can be joined in polymers, made up of thousands of glucose units. Unlike straight glucose solutions, these substances can empty from the stomach at almost the same rate as water. They are useful for endurance athletes who need to replace fluid and glucose but are unable to use regular glucose because it takes too long to empty from the stomach.

POLYNEURITIS

A disease involving many nerves, usually in the legs and feet. May be caused by a deficiency of several of the B complex vitamins, alcoholism or from poisoning with heavy metals.

POLYPEPTIDES

10 or more amino acids joined together. Proteins are large polypeptides. Polypeptides also form during the digestion of proteins.

POLYPHOSPHATE

Substances used in meat processing to hold water in the product. Used in making processed meats such as hams and bacon and some types of sausage. These additives are supposed to improve the texture of a product and reduce shrinkage. However, polyphosphates also improve profitability by enabling the food processor to sell more water! Additive number 450.

POLYSACCHARIDES

Carbohydrates containing many sugar units arranged in straight or branched structures. Complex carbohydrates found in grains, cereals and vegetables are polysaccharides. Most types of dietary fibre also fall into the category of being polysaccharides. Starches, glycogen, cellulose, the gummy fibre in oats and pectin are all polysaccharides. Some of these molecules can be broken down by digestive juices in the small intestine; others are digested by bacterial fermentation in the large bowel.

See Carbohydrates; Dietary fibre; Starch.

POLYUNSATURATED FATS
see Fats.

POME FRUITS

The apple, pear and quince are known as pome fruits. All belong to the rose family and have a compartmentalised core.

POMEGRANATE
see Fruit.

POMELO
see Fruit, Grapefruit.

POOR MAN'S CAVIAR

A dish made from the flesh of roasted eggplant, mixed with fried chopped onion and lemon juice.

POPCORN

Corn has both protein and starch. When heated, the small amount of moisture in a grain of corn starts to gelatinise the starch present. As the temperature increases inside the grain, the water expands and exerts too great a pressure on the protein of the grain and the kernel bursts open, allowing the centre section (the endosperm) to expand. At the same time, the gelatinised starch dries out, leaving a dry crisp popped piece of corn. To successfully pop corn, the corn should have about 12 per cent moisture.

Nutritionally, popcorn is an excellent alternative to high fat snacks. It has almost no fat and, without additives, is low in kilojoules. Popcorn also contributes some fibre as well as being a source of vitamin E. 1 cup of plain popcorn has 230 kJ (55 Cals). If the popcorn is candied, the sugar content more than doubles the kilojoules.

POPOVER

A batter mixture cooked in patty tins and served as soon as they are cooked. Savoury popovers taste a little like Yorkshire pudding. A slightly sweet batter may be served with butter and jam.

POPPYSEED OIL
see Oils.

POPPYSEEDS
see Seeds.

PORK
see Meat.

PORRIDGE

A mixture of ground or flaked cereal grains cooked in water (or milk and water) formed the porridge which once sustained people until lunch. With the current knowledge of the nutritional value of oats and other grains, there is a revival of interest in porridge.

The most commonly eaten porridges are made from oats, ground wheat, semolina (the endosperm of the wheat grain) and corn. In Asian countries a watery rice porridge is also eaten, along with its cooking water. Pease porridge is different from most other porridges in that it is made from dried peas soaked and then cooked to a thick puree.

The idea that porridge is 'fattening' is not correct. As so often occurs, some people have

NUTS

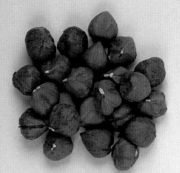

Hazelnuts

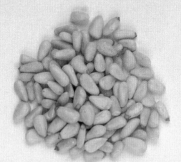

Pine nuts

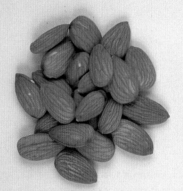

Almonds

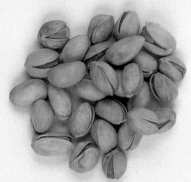

Pistachios

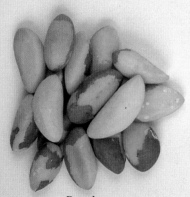

Brazils

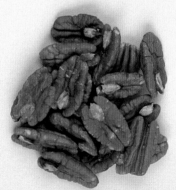

Pecans

SPICES

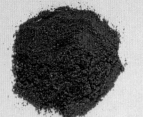

Garam masala

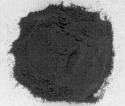

Paprika

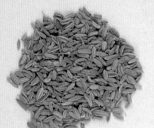

Fennel seeds

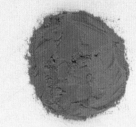

Turmeric

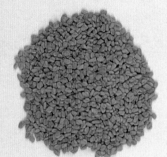

Fenugreek

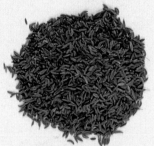

Carraway seeds

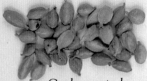

Cardamom pods

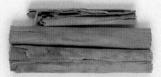

Cinnamon sticks

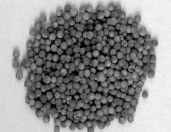

Coriander

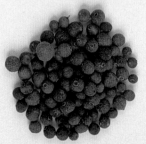

Pimento (allspice)

confused 'filling' with 'fattening'. Porridge is filling because of its high content of dietary fibre. An average-sized bowl of porridge has approximately 420 kJ (100 Cals) — about the same number as a bowl of cornflakes.

PORT
see Drinks, Alcoholic.

PORTERHOUSE STEAK

A sirloin steak cut from the back of the animal.

PORT SALUT
see Cheese.

POSTPRANDIAL

Following a meal. The postprandial glucose level is the amount of glucose in the blood after a meal.

POSTUM

A coffee substitute made from wheat, bran and molasses. Named after the American Charles W. Post, one of the first salesmen of health foods and a firm believer of the power of mind over body.

POTASSIUM

The major positively charged ion inside cells, especially muscle cells, potassium works with sodium to regulate the balance of water and acidity in the blood. Their action is controlled by the kidneys. Potassium also takes part in chemical reactions in the body and is vitally important for the transmission of impulses along the nerves which cause muscles, including the heart muscle, to contract. A deficiency of potassium can alter the rhythm of the heart.

When the levels of sodium and potassium change in the diet, water moves into or out of the cells. Too much sodium (from salt) can draw water out of the muscle cells. Since the modern diet tends to have much more sodium than potassium, the high concentration of sodium relative to potassium can draw water out of the muscle cells. For this reason, sportspeople need to increase their potassium intake.

The excess water which comes out of the cells into the blood can also lead to high blood pressure (see Hypertension, page 186).

Potassium is found in fruits and vegetables, meats, chicken, milk and grain foods. It is so widely distributed that a dietary deficiency is unlikely. Deficiency usually only occurs as a result of diarrhoea, vomiting, taking laxatives or diuretics. It may also occur during fasting. Symptoms include muscle weakness, fatigue and abnormal heart rhythm.

A dietary imbalance between sodium and potassium may occur. The more sodium consumed, the greater the body's need for potassium. Modern processing methods have disturbed the natural balance between sodium and potassium by depleting potassium and adding sodium in the form of salt. Foods which are rich in potassium should therefore be consumed in greater quantities to make up for some of the unavoidable salt in the food supply.

An excess of potassium in the body will only occur in kidney failure or as a result of shock after injury. The symptoms are similar to those of a deficiency — muscular weakness, mental apathy and altered heart rhythm.

Recommended daily intakes of potassium are as follows:

	mmol	mg
Infants up to 6 months	10−15	(400−600)
7−12 months	12−35	(480−1400)
Children, 1−3 years	25−70	(1000−2800)
4−7 years	40−100	(1600−4000)
8−18 years	50−140	(2000−5600)
Adults	50−140	(2000−5600)
Older adults	40−130	(1600−5200)
During pregnancy	50−140	(2000−5600)
lactation	65−140	(2600−5600)

Food sources of potassium

FOOD	POTASSIUM (mg)
Chickpeas, 100 g, raw weight	800
Steak, lean, 150 g	750
Baked beans, 200 g serve	600
Fish, av. fillet	580
Chicken, 150 g	415
Lamb chops, 2 av.	260
Milk, regular or low-fat, 250 mL	375
Egg, 1	85
Cheese, 30 g	40
Cereal, av. bowl, high-fibre type	200
Spaghetti, av. serve	140
Unprocessed bran, 10 g	120
Bread, wholemeal, 2 slices	110
Wheatgerm, 10 g	100
Rice, av. serve	90
Bread, white, 2 slices	50
Cereal, av. bowl, highly processed	30
Potato, 1 large, baked in jacket	990
Sweetcorn, 1 cob	640
Potato, 1 medium, 140 g	600
Spinach, 100 g	570
Jerusalem artichoke, 1	520
Kohlrabi, 100 g	510
Pumpkin, butternut, 100 g	470
Avocado, $\frac{1}{2}$	470
Mushrooms, 100 g	470
Snow peas, 100 g	420
Vegetables, 100 g, raw, av.	350
Vegetables, 100 g, cooked, av.	220
Parsley, 10 g	120
Prunes, 50 g	700
Tomato juice, 250 mL	650
Rhubarb, av. serve, stewed	540
Melon, 200 g	520
Dried fruits, 50 g, av.	450
Banana, medium	380
Apricots, 3	320
Average serve of most fresh fruits	250
Apple, medium	140
Nuts, 50 g	400
Cocoa powder, 10 g	150

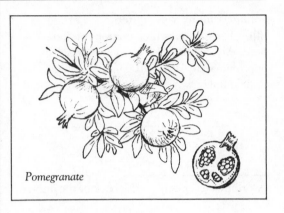

Pomegranate

POTATO
see Vegetables.

POTATO SALAD
see Salads.

POT ROAST

A piece of meat cooked by first frying quickly to 'seal' the meat and then braising in a small amount of liquid until tender. This method of cooking is more suitable for less tender cuts of meat.

POTTED MEAT

Traditionally served cold with slices of hot toast, potted meat is an Englishman's delight. It is made from a selection of meats (shin of beef, pig's trotters, veal shank) simmered with spices and herbs until extremely tender. The meat is then removed from the bones, the broth strained over it and the whole thing allowed to set.

POULTRY

The collective term for domestic fowl, usually including hens, turkeys and ducks as well as guinea fowl, geese and pigeons. The first jungle fowl, the ancestors of the modern hen, were used 4000 years ago. Throughout the world, hens have become popular both for their eggs and their flesh. Modern domesticated ducks are descendants of the mallard and the goose came from the graylag. Turkeys were first domesticated by the Aztecs of Mexico, taken to Spain and then back to America about 100 years ago. Turkey consumption in the United States is many times that of any other country.

Today, poultry are specifically bred as egg layers or for their flesh. With the exception of duck and goose, poultry flesh is fairly low in fat although the skin of all domestic poultry is high in fat. It can be roasted, grilled, barbecued, cooked in a microwave, stuffed and baked, braised, fried or stewed. Individual skinless cuts of chicken and turkey are now widely available and make a good choice for those who want to eat less fat.

In general, poultry is an excellent source of protein, has a good selection of minerals and vitamins and is relatively low in kilojoules. Fried chicken is an exception to this.

For nutritional values, see individual birds.

POUSSIN

A baby chicken, generally 4−6 weeks old and weighing about 900 g. Usually roasted or barbecued.

PPM

The abbreviation for parts per million. 1 ppm is equivalent to 1 mg per kilogram.

PRAHOC

A Cambodian fish paste made from cleaned fish which are pressed under banana leaves then mixed with coarse salt and left to dry in the sun. When dried, they are ground to a powder, mixed with a little water and allowed to ferment. Prahoc is a good source of calcium.

PRAIRIE OYSTER

see Drinks, Non-alcoholic.

PRALINE

A mixture of caramelised sugar and almonds, allowed to set and then broken into small pieces. The sweet praline is sprinkled over icecream or other desserts. In humid weather it may go soft. 25 g praline have 500 kJ (120 Cals).

PRAWN

see Seafood.

PREGNANCY

As a baby grows and develops, it takes its entire supply of nutrients from its mother. Ultimately, a baby depends entirely on her nutrition, and this, in turn, depends on what she eats and drinks.

The old idea that you should be eating for 2 during pregnancy certainly applies to the nutrients required but not necessarily to the kilojoules. This makes it important for the mother to eat foods with top quality nutritional value during pregnancy. A pregnant woman should follow the same sensible dietary guidelines advisable for everyone with special attention to foods which are good sources of calcium, iron and folacin — nutrients which are not always well supplied. Healthy meals and snacks, not too much fat, sugar, alcohol or salt, and plenty of complex carbohydrates and dietary fibre from fruits, vegetables, wholemeal bread and wholegrain cereals are the essentials. Lean meat (or legumes) and low-fat milk will supply extra iron and calcium.

Nature always protects the infant — it is the mother's diet which may need extra attention. A pregnant woman who neglects her diet will find she has fewer reserves after the pregnancy, a time when it is important to be in tip top condition.

Calcium is especially important to keep bones strong and healthy. The condition of fragile, porous bones of osteoporosis may not rear its head until after the menopause, but prevention involves having plenty of calcium in the daily diet during times of calcium withdrawal, such as during pregnancy.

Pregnant women are advised to increase their calcium intake from the usual recommended 800 mg/day to 1100 mg/day.

The foods which supply the most calcium are milk, yoghurt and cheese. Low-fat or skim milk and yoghurt and the lower fat hard cheeses have as much calcium as their full-cream equivalents. Some of the fortified or concentrated low-fat milks are especially rich in calcium.

Iron, folic acid, protein, vitamin C and most of the B complex vitamin needs also increase during pregnancy. For those women who do not feel like eating lean meat during pregnancy, iron can be supplied by chicken, seafoods, legumes, green leafy vegetables, wholegrain products, eggs and dried apricots (see page 192 for a list of iron content of foods). Plenty of vegetables will also increase folic acid and vitamin C intake. The B complex vitamins will be supplied by eating a range of wholegrain products, lean meat or fish, low-fat milk, nuts and seeds.

Teenage pregnancy creates special needs. A mother whose own body is still growing and developing needs to take special care to take in sufficient nutrients to meet her own needs as well the baby's. Protein, calcium and iron requirements need special attention.

As well as following the guidelines for a healthy diet and making sure the diet contains all the healthy foods the body needs, there are some other important considerations.

- Smoking — put simply, don't.
- Sleep — fatigue is much more commonly due to poor sleeping during pregnancy rather than a lack of vitamins. Relaxation techniques can improve sleep.
- *Exercise* — physical activity is important to keep muscles in good condition. Some types of vigorous exercise may become too difficult as pregnancy progresses, but walking, swimming, light gardening and general physical activities are suitable. Special pre-natal exercises are often available.

- Avoid alcohol — alcohol crosses the placenta into the baby's bloodstream, so whatever the mother drinks, the baby is drinking! Water or mineral or soda water are more suitable (see also Foetal alcohol syndrome).
- Cut down on sweet and fatty foods — this is important for everyone, but diet during pregnancy needs to be top quality. For those who crave something sweet, some beautiful fresh or dried fruits may satisfy. Raw vegetables, wholemeal bread or crispbread are also good snack foods.
- Avoid unnecessary vitamin supplements — large quantities of vitamins act more like drugs than nutrients. The effects of large doses of these substances during pregnancy is not fully known. However, some studies have shown that babies born to women taking large doses of vitamins begin life with much higher requirements for these vitamins. In theory, such a child eating a normal healthy diet (or being breast fed) could become vitamin deficient simply because his or her vitamin needs have been set at an artificially high level.

Weight gain during pregnancy

An ideal weight gain is at least 10 kg. Those who try to restrict their weight gain to less than this have a higher incidence of complications with the pregnancy and have babies of lower birth weights. Since small birth weight babies have more problems than those of normal weight, the restrictive weight gains of the past are no longer recommended.

On the other hand, some women find their appetite during pregnancy is greatly increased. An excessive weight gain should, in theory, be used during the period of breast feeding. In practice, however, many women find it difficult to lose a large amount of the extra weight gained during pregnancy.

A suitable compromise seems to be the weight gain of 10−11 kg. This is made up as follows:

	kg
Baby at birth	3.4
Placenta	0.5
Amniotic fluid	0.9
Increased weight of uterus	1.1
Increased weight of breasts	1.4
Increased blood volume	1.8
Fat on the mother	1.0−2.0

To gain this amount of weight, most women find they do not need to eat much extra food during pregnancy. In theory, around 320,000 extra kilojoules (about 76,000 Cals) should be needed during the whole pregnancy. In practice, most women decrease their physical activity as they grow larger and find that a mere 630 kJ (150 Cals) a day is all the extra they require. This is equal to the kilojoules in an extra glass of milk each day.

Cravings

Although cravings for particular foods are common during pregnancy, they are of some psychological origin rather than representing any physical need for the particular food. There is no harm in indulging cravings if they are for pickles, vegetables or even fruits. However, cravings for chocolates, icecreams or sweets can leave a lasting heritage on the hips!

Morning sickness

Also a common occurrence, morning sickness, a feeling of nausea, may occur early in the morning for the first 3 months of pregnancy. In some women it lasts longer and may also occur in the afternoon or evening. It is caused by the body's inability to handle the changed hormone levels and usually subsides after 10−12 weeks.

For morning sickness, it is best to eat small amounts of low-fat foods at frequent intervals throughout the day. Many women find that a carbohydrate snack (such as a slice of dry toast, a dry savoury biscuit or some fruit) before getting out of bed in the morning is a help. Some also report that they feel better if they drink plain water rather than tea or coffee, and avoid fatty foods. Sour-tasting foods are often more popular.

PREHISTORIC HUMAN'S DIET

Our earliest ancestors were gatherers and lived on whatever they could find. Berries, fruits, nuts, roots and young shoots, insects, birds' eggs, reptiles and any small mammals they could catch made up the diet. There is evidence that they were omnivores rather than herbivores.

Once early man learned how to make weapons, he began to hunt for larger animals. Gradually life changed, for a hunter has to have a base to which he can return. Fire introduced cooking and this made the meat easier to eat.

The diet changed little during this period and it was not until about 10,000 years ago with the beginnings of agriculture that significant changes occurred. Cereals and grains increased the carbohydrate content of the diet. Vegetables were grown and new varieties developed. Seeds and their oil became a regular part of the diet. Domestication of animals followed and the diet went through a relatively stable period until comparatively modern times.

In nutritional terms, the early human diet had only a fraction of the fat of the modern diet. Sugar was only available from fruits and salt was confined to that present naturally in meat, eggs, and some vegetables. Mineral and vitamin levels were quite high and there was plenty of fibre from fruits, vegetables, nuts and seeds.

PRE-MENSTRUAL SYNDROME (PMS)

This condition occurs in some women in the 5–7 days prior to menstruation. It is characterised by fluid retention with a bloated feeling in the abdomen and, sometimes, swollen ankles or fingers. Headache and irritability may also occur. Many women also report a craving for sweet foods. Others have no such symptoms.

Pre-menstrual syndrome seems to be due to a retention of sodium caused by changes in female hormones. The sodium then holds water in the tissues resulting in many of the symptoms.

Many women make PMS worse by drinking little or no fluid, wrongly believing it will increase their bloated feeling. Many also restrict their intake of carbohydrates to unnecessarily strict levels, again wrongly believing this is a healthy move (see page 398).

Treatment for PMS involves drinking lots of water to flush out the sodium which is causing the problem. A moderate increase in foods containing carbohydrate (such as bread, fruit or cereal products) may help to avert the craving for sweets.

Vitamin B$_6$ is frequently prescribed for PMS but recent studies have not found any improvement apart from the placebo effect (see page 384).

PRESERVATIVES

A class of compounds added to foods to prevent spoilage by bacteria, moulds and yeasts. Since some of these micro-organisms cause illness and death, the use of preservatives obviously has some advantage. Some preservatives have also proved safer than the traditional methods of preserving foods by smoking, salting or drying. Others have made possible a vast array of nutritionally inferior products.

Regulations in each country specify which preservatives may be used and specific quantities. Different preservatives are used depending on the likely type of micro-organism which would spoil the product. Some preservatives work best in acidic foods; others are better in foods which are less acidic.

Canned foods do not generally contain preservatives since the canning process destroys micro-organisms. Alcoholic and soft drinks, breads, cakes, biscuits, pastries, desserts, dried fruits, sausages and other processed meats all contain preservatives.

Some of the commonly used preservatives include:

- *Sulphur dioxide* (also added as sulphites — additives nos. 220, 221, 222, 223, 224) — permitted in soft drinks, beer, wines, fruit juices, juice drinks, potato chips, gelatine, sausage meat, vinegar, toppings and dried fruits
- *Benzoic acid* (or benzoates — additives nos. 210, 211, 212, 213) — permitted in fruit juices, cordials, soft drinks, flavour essences, flour, tomato juice (not canned)
- *Propionic acid* (or propionates — additives nos. 280, 281, 282, 283) — permitted in bread, cakes, biscuits, pastry and other flour products
- *Sorbic acid* (or sorbates — additives nos. 200, 201, 202, 203) — permitted in cakes, biscuits, bread, cheese, cordials, soft drink and juice drinks, low-kilojoule jams, Maraschino cherries, flavour essences, fruit yoghurt, imitation fruit, toppings, wine and flour
- *Nisin* (additive no. 234) — permitted in processed cheese, soups and canned tomato products

Not all of the foods in these categories

necessarily contain any of these preservatives. Some food manufacturers are producing foods without preservatives. For those with sensitivities to additives, this comes as a welcome relief.

There is no doubt that preservatives have given greater variety to the food supply. Whether we need or want some of the items which are now possible is another matter. Certainly those who are sensitive to particular preservatives have not fared well from the modern supply. For example, asthmatics are often sensitive to sulphur dioxide. The numbering system for food additives makes it easier for such people to avoid particular compounds.

PRESSOR AMINES

Also known as catecholamines, these substances raise blood pressure. Adrenalin is a pressor amine.

PRESSURE COOKING

Invented by Denis Papin in 1679, the pressure cooker is a sealed pot which produces steam and forces the temperature inside the vessel up to 130°C. This cooks food quickly and is especially useful at high altitudes where the boiling temperature may be too low to cook foods quickly. Pressure cookers are also useful for foods such as legumes since they reduce the cooking time dramatically. After soaking, beans take only 15–20 mins in the pressure cooker. Pressure regulators and safety locks are fitted to the modern pressure cooker. The nutritional value of foods cooked in a pressure cooker can be excellent as long as the timing is correct and foods are not overcooked.

PRETZEL

Thin sticks rather like a hollow biscuit about half the size of a drinking straw. Made from a stiff yeasted dough, pretzels are sprayed with sodium hydroxide or sodium carbonate which

has been treated so as to gelatinise the starch in the pretzel. Coarse salt is added and the pretzels baked in a very hot oven to a shiny hard finish. Pretzels are not rich in nutrients and have about 15 kJ (4 Cals) each.

PRICKLY PEAR
see Fruit.

PRITIKIN, NATHAN

The author of the 'Pritikin Programme', Nathan Pritikin was an engineer who found that his own and many other people's blood fats could be lowered with a strict low-fat diet. His Longevity Centre and Pritikin Research Foundation went on to show that his diet (very low in fat, pre-formed cholesterol and salt, relatively low in protein, no added sugar, caffeine or alcohol, but high in complex carbohydrate and dietary fibre) was of benefit for those with high blood fats, high blood pressure, diabetes, cardiovascular disease and excess weight.

Nathan Pritikin himself died of leukaemia, but his diet lives on and has many devotees among those who have found it has worked for them.

Critics of the Pritikin Programme maintain that it is too low in fat and is unattainable for the average person. Eating out in restaurants also becomes difficult.

PROCESSED FOODS

This broad range of products includes any food or beverage which is not in its original form. Almost everything we eat has been processed in some way: wheat is made into bread, specific cuts of meat are taken from animals, poultry is plucked of its feathers, fish is filleted and even nuts are usually removed from their shells. Only fruits and vegetables tend to come to us in a relatively unchanged state.

Processing is not necessarily undesirable. In some instances, it actually makes foods safer by removing toxic substances such as moulds.

Cooking, which is a form of processing, also makes many foods more easily digested as well as killing bacteria and increasing the availability of some nutrients for absorption.

Food processing is mainly a problem because it means that the types of foods available can produce an unbalanced diet. Many of the highly processed foods we eat have a surfeit of fat, sugar and salt while protective dietary fibre is often removed. With so many processed foods now available, people in Western countries need to know much more about what is in the foods available so that they can make an informed choice. At present, processed pet foods have more information on the label than foods intended for human use. For more information on processed foods, see Additives, food.

PROFITEROLES

Small puffs of choux pastry with a savoury or cream filling.

See also Choux pastry.

PROLAMINES

Proteins found in plants, especially cereals. These storage proteins have a low content of the amino acid lysine (see page 214).

PROLINE

An amino acid which can be made in the human body.

PROOF (OF ALCOHOL)

The term 'proof' has been used since the seventeenth century to show the absolute alcohol content of distilled liquors such as brandy or whisky.

Many years ago, the proof of a spirit was measured as the lowest concentration of alcohol which would allow gunpowder to be ignited. Some took the proof reading by burning the particular liquor. If the remaining liquid made up half the original volume,

the spirit was shown to contain 50 per cent alcohol and was 100 proof. More modern methods determine the specific gravity of the liquor (the weight per unit volume compared with that of water).

Each country can have a different method of expressing the proof of their spirits and some relate this to weight, while others prefer volume (1 g of alcohol = 1.2 mL). In the United Kingdom, proof spirits are 48.2 per cent alcohol by weight or 57 per cent by volume. In the United States, the proof number is almost twice the percentage of alcohol. This means that an American whisky marked 100 proof contains 50 per cent alcohol by volume. Underproof means that the alcohol content is less than the standard; overproof means that the liquor has a higher level of alcohol.

PROPIONIC ACID

A fatty acid formed when bacteria act on dietary fibre in the large intestine. Propionic acid also stimulates the nervous and muscular activity of the walls of the bowel and this helps to propel material through the intestine, preventing constipation.

PROPOLIS

A substance (containing waxes and resins) collected by bees to repair damage to their hives. Used as a food supplement because of its antioxidant properties.

PROSCIUTTO

Also known as Parma ham, this fine quality raw and very lean ham is cured at Langhirano, near Parma in Italy. The hams are rubbed with a mixture of salt, sugar, nitrates, and spices (including pepper, nutmeg, mustard and coriander) and are packed together for 10 days. The process is repeated and the hams are pressed and steamed. They have a very low fat content, an intense flavour and are usually served in paper-thin slices.

PROSTAGLANDINS

These are hormone-like substances which are produced when polyunsaturated fatty acids containing 20 carbon atoms are metabolised in the body.

There are three types of prostaglandins. The first type (sometimes called Series 1) are derived from gamma-linolenic acid, a fatty acid found in breast milk and in some seed oils (borage, blackcurrant and evening primrose). Usually formed during the breakdown of linoleic acid (see page 208). The second type (Series 2) come from arachidonic acid (see page 26) found in liver, kidney, beef and eggs and also formed during the break down of linoleic acid. Series 3 prostaglandin comes from eicosapentaenoic acid found in fish fats.

Prostaglandins regulate processes such as the maintenance of blood pressure, temperature control, the way blood clots, the movements of the intestine, uterine contractions during childbirth, pain, inflammatory responses and defence against infection.

The prostaglandins and two other groups of chemicals, prostacyclins and thromboxanes, occur in different forms, depending on their source. For example, thromboxane 2 (derived from the omega 6 fatty acids) causes blood cells to clump together while thromboxane 1 (from omega 3 fatty acids) has the opposite effect.

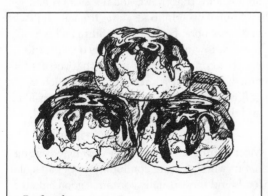

Profiteroles

Achieving a balance between the different types of prostaglandins produced from the omega 6 and omega 3 fatty acids is the subject of continuing research.

The products from the omega 3 fatty acids, in general, suppress blood clotting, inflammatory reactions and immune responses. These substances may therefore be useful in controlling or treating some aspects of coronary heart disease, organ transplants and certain types of arthritis, and, possibly, even cancer.

See also Fats, Essential fatty acids.

PROTAMINES

Small protein molecules with a high content of the amino acid arginine. Found in caviar. Some types of insulin are bound to protamine to delay their action.

PROTEASES

Enzymes which break down proteins. Found in pineapple and figs and will prevent these fruits setting in a jelly as the protease breaks down the protein in the gelatine. Cooking will destroy proteases.

See also Enzymes.

PROTEINS

The word protein means 'of first importance' and protein is a vital part of every cell in the body, including those in muscles, the heart, liver and kidneys, blood cells, skin, hair and nails, teeth and bones. Whenever growth is occurring, new cells are forming and protein requirements are increased. A child requires a higher percentage of protein than an adult. Protein needs also increase during pregnancy to provide for the needs of the growing baby.

Once growth stops, protein is used to replace cells which are lost through the wear and tear of normal living. Protein is also used by the body to make enzymes, antibodies which fight infection, haemoglobin (which carries oxygen in the blood) and hormones such as insulin.

Although protein is obviously important, there is no valid reason for the excessive enthusiasm exhibited for animal protein foods. These were once high status foods since many were expensive. However, in most Western countries, consumption of animal protein foods has become excessive. Many of these foods are high in fat and contribute to a high-fat diet. Protein's greatest problem thus concerns the company it keeps. Slabs of steak, hamburger patties, hearty helpings of meats in stews, cheeses, and breakfasts of sausages, bacon and eggs will contribute protein but also a lot of saturated fats.

Once the body has met its protein requirements, any excess protein is converted to body fat. Some protein can be used for energy, but the body prefers to use carbohydrates or fats.

There is also a common misconception that eating more protein benefits muscle development. Eating extra protein will not produce bigger biceps and triceps. Muscles develop when they are used, and the ideal fuel for the use of muscles is complex carbohydrate, not protein. The growth of muscles requires protein, but the quantities for this are quite modest. Ordinary physical activity does not increase protein requirements much since the muscles use carbohydrate or fat as fuel in preference to protein.

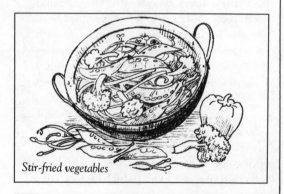

Stir-fried vegetables

Proteins are made up of smaller units called amino acids. After digestion, proteins are broken down to their separate amino acids. The body proteins are then synthesised from the appropriate amino acids. Foods contain a mixture of 23 amino acids. Provided the total amino acid pool is sufficient, most of our amino acids can be made in the body. However, 8, known as essential amino acids, must be supplied from the food we eat (see page 21).

See also Collagen.

Animal vs vegetable protein

Animal protein foods such as meats, fish, eggs, milk, yoghurt and cheese contain all the essential amino acids. Vegetable protein foods are usually low in 1 or 2. However, combinations of vegetable foods can easily supply the entire range of amino acids, including the essential amino acids.

Vegetarians rarely have a problem obtaining sufficient protein. However, anyone who tries to live on a very restricted diet, such as fruitarians (who eat nothing but fruit), can become deficient in protein. As with most things, it is only the extremes which produce problems.

Some vegetable proteins, such as those found in soya beans and wheatgerm, are almost as good as most animal proteins. Some animal proteins such as gelatine are so lacking in some amino acids that they could not sustain life.

Animal protein foods suffer from a total lack of dietary fibre. Since fibre is filling, a high-protein, low-fibre diet can easily deceive the appetite control mechanism so that you eat too much. Vegetable sources of protein, such as grains and legumes, have plenty of dietary fibre and thus are less likely to be overconsumed.

Complementary proteins

Most primitive cultures have developed eating habits which feature combinations of particular foods and these usually contain a good balance of the essential amino acids. Over a long period of time, it was probably noted that those who ate certain foods together were healthier than others. Such food combinations then became the accepted way to eat. The beans and corn eaten in Mexico, the rice and soya beans of Asia, and the couscous and chickpeas of North Africa, are examples of excellent food combinations where the essential amino acid missing from one food is well supplied by the other.

Many Western food combinations also provide an excellent balance of amino acids. Baked beans have a good protein level and contain plenty of the amino acid lysine but lack the amino acid called methionine. Bread happens to be a good source of methionine but is relatively low in lysine. Baked beans on toast therefore makes an excellent combination. A peanut butter sandwich, or spaghetti with cheese each combine to provide a complete set of essential amino acids.

Good protein combinations

cereals and legumes
wholemeal bread with baked beans
bread roll and pea or lentil soup
lentil burger
corn tacos and kidney beans
brown rice and chickpeas
peanut butter sandwich
rice and soya bean curd (tofu)

cereals and dairy products
pasta and cheese
muesli and milk

legumes and vegetables
soya beans with stir-fried vegetables
pumpkin stuffed with peas and nuts

cereals and vegetables
tabbouli (cracked wheat and parsley salad)
spinach pie (wholewheat pastry base)
vegetable or potato pies

seeds with legumes or cereals
lima beans with crunchy topping of sunflower seeds and wheatgerm
muesli (containing pepitas or sunflower seeds and oats)

The daily requirement of protein is estimated differently by various authorities. In countries such as Australia, the recommended daily intakes (RDIs) are at the higher end of the range of levels recommended by the World Health Organisation (WHO). The Australian levels have been adopted to reflect usual eating patterns in this country. The lower WHO figures would be perfectly adequate for most people.

The Australian RDI for protein is 1 g per kilogram of body weight. This figure takes into account variations in physical activity levels and will be adequate for even the most active people, including those involved in body building.

A level of 10–15 per cent of the day's energy coming from protein is desirable. An average man should aim for a protein intake of around 75 g a day while 60 g will be appropriate for most women. The World Health Organisation recommends a daily intake of 37 g for a 65 kg man and 29 g for a 55 kg woman to meet the body's needs for good health.

There is no harm in eating more protein, providing it does not come in foods which also provide fats and providing total kilojoule needs are not being exceeded.

Food sources of protein

FOOD	PROTEIN (g)
Large T-bone steak, with fat	75
Rump steak, 205 g, cooked	60
Chicken, take-away dinner box	50
Pork forequarter chop, with crackling	45
Roast leg of lamb, no fat, average serve	44
Veal chops, 2	42
·Turkey, av. serve	35
Lean fillet steak, small serve	35
Chicken breast, av. serve, no fat	34
Kidneys, av. serve	32
Lamb loin chops, 2, lean and fat	31
Hamburger	30
Liver, av. serve	26

Barbeque chicken, $\frac{1}{4}$	24
Bacon, 2 pieces, grilled	20
Salami, 60 g	13
Meat pie or sausage roll	12
Sausage, 1, grilled	12
Ham, 60 g, leg	11
Egg, 1	6
Fish, grilled, av. fillet	35
Prawns, 4 king size	27
Tuna or salmon, canned, 100 g	22
Cottage cheese, $\frac{1}{2}$ cup	23
Milk, 250 mL glass	9
Cheese, amount on sandwich	7
Icecream, regular, av. serve	2
Hot potato chips, av. serve	9
Peanuts, 25 g	7
Vegetables, av. serve	2
Bread, 2 slices	2
Fruits, av. piece	1

PROVING

In baking bread, the time allowed for the yeast to 'work' on the dough until it increases in size is called 'proving'. In general, the first rising of the dough takes longer than the second since there are more yeast cells present for the second fermentation.

PRO-VITAMIN

A substance which the body can convert into a vitamin. Examples include carotene which is converted to vitamin A in the body, the amino acid tryptophan which is converted to the B vitamin niacin and 7-dehydrocholesterol in the skin which sunlight converts to vitamin D.

PROVOLONE

see Cheese.

PRUNE

see Fruit.

PSORIASIS

A severe skin disorder with red patches covered with white scale-like lesions. The areas most commonly affected include the head, elbows, knees, chest and buttocks. The disorder affects about 1–2 per cent of the population and is often brought on by psychological upsets or it may follow other infection. In severe cases, the skin becomes highly inflamed and arthritis develops. Recent treatments using fish oil have proved beneficial to some sufferers. This is thought to be due to the omega 3 fatty acids found in fish oils which influence some inflammatory responses in the body (see Omega 3 fatty acids).

P:S RATIO

The ratio of polyunsaturated fats to saturated fats. A popular concept in the 1960s when the P:S ratio of the diet was thought to be important in the prevention of coronary heart disease. While it is still recognised that polyunsaturated fats have advantages over saturated fats, it is no longer considered wise or necessary to consume large quantities of any fat. The P:S ratio has thus fallen from favour.

See also Fats.

PSYLLIUM

A gummy type of dietary fibre obtained from the husk or seed of *Plantago psyllium*. Most of its fibre is of the soluble type (as found in oats and legumes) but it also contains a residue which does not seem to be fermented by bacteria in the large bowel. Used in bulking agents for the treatment of bowel disorders. There have been some reports of sensitivity to the substance.

PTARMIGAN

A game bird of Northern Europe related to the grouse.

PTYALIN

An enzyme (also known as alpha amylase) present in saliva which begins splitting complex carbohydrates into maltose. Its action is halted by the acidity of the stomach.

PUDDING

A pudding may be a dessert (as in chocolate pudding), a skin filled with seasoned meat (as in black pudding) or a hot savoury mixture (as in pease pudding). These days the word pudding used on its own signifies a cooked dessert — often a steamed pudding made in a round basin or a cereal-based dessert such as a rice pudding.

PUFF PASTRY
see Pastry.

PULSES
see Legumes.

PUMPERKNICKEL

A dark rye bread originally made in Germany in 1540 at a time of famine. Its strong flavour (from wholegrain rye and caraway seeds) was appreciated by those who had little other food. Pumperknickel became popular after World War II and is now made in many parts of Europe, the United States and Australia. It is a heavy bread but remains moist for many days. It is high in dietary fibre, supplies a good range of minerals and vitamins and has 480 kJ (115 Cals) in a 50 g slice.

PUMPKIN
see Vegetables.

PURINES

Substances such as adenine, guanine, xanthine and uric acid. In humans, all purines are broken down to uric acid and are excreted. In gout, uric acid levels in the blood increase and crystals of sodium urate accumulate in the big toe, causing swelling, redness and extreme pain. Foods high in purines include liver, sweetbreads, brains, kidneys, fish roe, beer, wine, sardines, wine, gravies and meat extracts. Meats, peas, lentils, some vegetables (cauliflower, beans, asparagus, mushrooms and spinach) and fish and chicken contain moderate quantities of purines. Fruits, other vegetables, dairy products, eggs, cereals, nuts, fats and sugar have negligible quantities.

PYRIDOXAL
see Vitamin B_6.

PYRIDOX AMINE
see Vitamin B_6.

PYRIDOXINE
see Vitamin B_6.

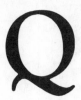

QUAHOG

A species of clam sold in the United States as 'littlenecks' or 'cherrystones'.
    See also Seafood, Clams.

QUAIL

Small game birds found in Africa, Southeast Asia and related to the pheasant. Those bred for eating are ready for the table at about 6 weeks of age. Quail eggs are also considered a delicacy and are used in Asian cookery as a garnish in soups.

    Quail are high in protein and provide an excellent source of iron. They also supply many of the B complex vitamins and have only about 3 g of fat per 100 g of edible flesh and skin. 100 g (flesh on 2 birds) have 505 kJ (120 Cals).

QUANDONG
see Fruit.

QUARK
see Cheese.

QUENELLE

A very light dumpling, usually served in soup or as an entree. The basic mixture, usually containing some type of seafood or poultry mixed with egg whites and cream, is formed into small pieces which are simmered in stock until they swell and are firm but light.

QUICHE

A pastry shell containing a rich custard mixture, often flavoured with herbs, bacon, cheese, seafood, spinach or another vegetable.

Although quiche has been taken as a lighter, healthier alternative to more traditional meat and vegetable meals, it is quite high in fat. One-quarter of a 20 cm quiche Lorraine — the most popular variety of quiche — has 3300 kJ (785 Cals). This calculation represents a quiche made with half milk, half cream. If made with cream only, it would be even higher.

QUINCE
see Fruit.

QUININE

A bitter alkaloid derived from the bark of the cinchona tree and used to treat malaria. Quinine is also added to tonic water to provide the characteristic slightly bitter contrast to the high sugar content. The amount added to tonic water has no therapeutic value.

R

RABBIT

Unlike other game, rabbit has never become a meat with much status. This probably reflects the wide (and free) availability of the animal to poorer people. The rabbit is native to Europe, Asia and Africa. Introduced to Australia, its prolific breeding habits have made it a pest.

The flesh of rabbit is tender and versatile, although it can become dry if overcooked. Rabbit is excellent when made into a casserole with red wine and herbs or, if young, marinaded and grilled.

Nutritionally, rabbit is an excellent meat. It is high in protein and niacin, very low in fat and has a good selection of minerals and vitamins. Of the fat present in rabbit, a high percentage is polyunsaturated and includes the omega 3 fatty acids not usually found in meats. 100 g of rabbit flesh have 1.5 g fat and 440 kJ (105 Cals).

RACLETTE
see Cheese.

RADDICHIO
see Vegetables.

RADISH
see Vegetables.

RAFFINOSE

A 3-unit sugar found in seeds. (See Oligosaccharides.)

RAGOUT

A French stew made from meat, poultry or seafood cooked with vegetables and stock.

RAGU

A rich Italian tomato and meat sauce served with pasta.

RAISIN

see Dried fruits; Fruit.

RAKI

A rice wine.

RAMBUTAN

see Fruit.

RANCIDITY

This is the process whereby fats become oxidised and develop off flavours and odour. It occurs at room temperature and is hastened by trace minerals, salt, light, bacteria and moulds and slowed down by vitamin E (natural or added), synthetic antioxidants and some herbs (including rosemary and sage). Cooking fats go rancid because of a chemical reaction between moisture in the food and the fat. Minerals such as iron (from iron cooking vessels) will accelerate the process. Rancid fats should be discarded.

RAPESEED OIL

see Oils.

RASPBERRY

see Fruit.

RATATOUILLE

A French dish made from eggplant, onion, capsicums, zucchini, tomatoes, olive oil and garlic. Can be served hot or cold and is delicious on thick slices of crusty bread. High in fibre and fairly low in kilojoules — the exact number depending on the amount of oil used.

RAVIOLI

A small pasta dumpling, usually filled with spinach and ricotta cheese or with a meat mixture, boiled and served with a sauce.

RDA

Recommended daily amount — used in some countries instead of the terminology RDI.

RDI

Recommended daily intake of nutrients. The RDIs represent the amount of each nutrient which will meet the nutritional needs of most people in a population. The levels for each nutrient are usually determined by looking at the physiological needs for the substance and adding a margin of safety. It is quite possible that some people may need a little more than the RDI for some nutrients; others may need less. The RDIs cover the needs of almost everyone. Those who take drugs which interact with specific nutrients and those with certain illnesses may need more or less of some nutrients than the RDIs.

If you do not meet the RDI for some specific nutrient, you should not assume you are deficient in it. Many people need much less than the set values.

For some nutrients, there is insufficient knowledge about physiological requirements. For these, a safe and adequate intake is set.

RECTUM

The last section of the intestine, from the colon to the anus. The rectum is 13−15 cm long. Food wastes accumulate in the colon and pass to the rectum when they are ready for excretion. The contents of the rectum exert pressure on the muscular walls which then send

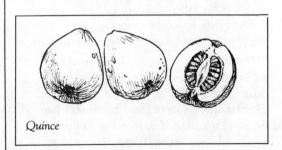

Quince

impulses to the anus, the muscles of the chest and abdomen and to the brain that defaecation is imminent.

Cancer of the rectum is thought to be related to a low-fibre/high-fat diet. Excess weight, and possibly a high protein intake, also increase the risk.

RED CURRANT
see Fruit.

REFRIGERATION

The biochemical activity of plant cells and also various micro-organisms slows down in cold temperatures. For this reason meats, poultry, seafoods, dairy products and many fruits and vegetables should be kept refrigerated to prolong their shelf life.

Some tropical fruits do not fare well under refrigeration. Bananas release enzymes which turn their skins black; avocados will not soften; citrus fruits can develop spotty skins; potatoes become sweet.

Vegetables should be kept in special crispers in the refrigerator where the humidity is a little higher to prevent the products drying out. Some foods, such as mushrooms, should be kept in the refrigerator in paper or cloth bags rather than in plastic so that they will not sweat.

Refrigeration has been a great step forward in reducing dependence on nitrates used to preserve meats. These additives are known to cause stomach cancer and, since refrigeration has become common, the incidence of this type of cancer has fallen dramatically.

There is some loss of vitamins during refrigeration but losses are much smaller than at room temperature.

REHEATING FOODS

There is always loss of some nutrients when foods are reheated. The major vitamins affected are C and some of the B complex vitamins.

Microwaves cause much less than other reheating methods.

RELIGION (AND DIET)

Many religions have taboos on certain foods. Some of these once had good reasons; others are simply part of the laws of the religion.

Jews are not supposed to eat any animal without a cloved hoof (pigs and rabbit are thus forbidden), or any seafood without fins and scales (which means no shellfish, shark or eel, or any reptile or amphibian). Animals and poultry must also be slaughtered in a ritual manner (see page 198) and meat and dairy products are kept separate. Strict Jews even have different cutlery and dishes and separate sinks for meat and milk and do not cook them at the same time.

Followers of the Islamic or Moslem religion do not consume any alcohol, many do not eat meat or fish and some avoid certain vegetables. Muhammad forbade Moslems to eat the flesh of animals found dead and they were not to eat any food which had been offered or sacrificed to idols. Moslems also refuse to eat pigs because of a belief that pigs are unclean. Other meats may only be eaten if they are killed according to a prescribed ritual. During the period of Ramadan (the ninth month of the lunar Moslem year), Moslems do not eat between sunrise and sunset. Young children, the aged, sick, pregnant women and travellers are exempt from this restriction.

Hindus consider the cow sacred and so do not eat beef or buffalo. Most would rather die of starvation than eat the flesh of cow or buffalo. Their food taboos also help to define their caste ranking. Brahmins, the highest caste, avoid meat and eat only foods prepared in the finest manner (pakka). Strict Brahmins do not eat onions and garlic. Lower castes eat the inferior foods (kacca). Pakka foods contain ghee which they believe promotes health and virility. Such foods can be offered to honoured guests. Hindus also avoid alcohol.

Buddhists from different faiths have a variety of food taboos. Some may eat meat but are not permitted to kill or butcher meat or take any interest in how the killing is done. Most are vegetarian, especially the monks. Others follow a vegetarian diet on certain days or during particular months of the year. At such times, all animal foods may be forbidden. Like many other groups, Buddhists do not drink alcohol.

Among Christian groups there are also some food taboos. Seventh Day Adventists do not drink tea, coffee or alcohol and most do not eat meat. Mormans have similar restrictions. Baptists avoid alcohol and use grape juice in place of Communion wine.

In many instances the religious taboos on certain foods have their basis in health considerations. Tea, coffee and alcoholic beverages all contain drugs. In parts of the world without refrigeration, meats often carry a heavy load of bacteria so it makes sense to avoid them.

It is also common for those of many religions to be vegetarian so that they do not need to kill. This usually stems from a desire to preserve nature and live in harmony rather than practise unnecessary destruction.

RELISH

A mixture of chopped or ground fruits and/or vegetables with vinegar and spices. Most relishes contain sugar. They are served with cold meats, curries and other dishes. One tablespoon of relish has about 70 kJ (17 Cals).

REMOULADE

A spicy mayonnaise served with fish or seafood. Made by mixing mayonnaise with pickles, capers, mustard and herbs.

RENAL CALCULI

Kidney stones which result from inadequate fluid intake, excess vitamin C (from supplements) or an excess of oxalic acid. Characterised by extreme pain.

RENNET

A substance used in cheesemaking to set the curd which forms after the milk has been acidified by bacteria. Rennet contains rennin (see below) and is made from the fourth stomach of the sheep. A legend has it that cheese was first made when a traveller carried some milk in a bag made from an animal's stomach. The heat of the day allowed bacteria to sour the milk and the rennin from the stomach firmed the curd. For vegetarians, a rennet can be made from plants.

RENNIN

The enzyme in rennet (see above) which curdles milk and turns it into a solid curd and some whey.

See also Junket.

RESINS

Gummy substances found in plants. The resins in hops are used to give bitterness to beer. Those from some trees are used in chewing gum while the resin from pine trees is used to give the Greek wine retsina its characteristic flavour. The quantities of resins consumed are too small to confer any nutritional advantages.

RETINAL

A form of retinol (vitamin A) which is involved in the formation of visual purple, a pigment in the rods of the retina of the eye and needed for vision in dim light.

RETINOIC ACID

An acid form of vitamin A.

RETINOL

see Vitamin A.

RHEUMATOID ARTHRITIS

An inflammation of the joints, especially those in the hands, arms and legs. Occurs 3 times as commonly in women as in men and has no apparent cause. Usually symmetrical so that each side of the body is equally affected. The joint pains and stiffness are worse in the morning.

Rheumatoid arthritis often comes and goes spontaneously. This has given rise to many 'cures' and it is easy to understand how the misconceptions arise. If you have rheumatoid arthritis and you go into remission on the day you have eaten lots of bananas, you may well assume that bananas have 'cured' your arthritis. In fact, the 2 events — the eating of bananas and the disappearance of the arthritis — are coincidental. Many stories exist about the wonderful effects of particular diets for arthritis.

Many people claim that their arthritis is much better on a meat-free diet. No controlled trials have been done to verify this common observation.

Current clinical trials are showing some improvement in stiffness from the known anti-inflammatory effects of fish oils but there are no vitamin supplements which will do wonders for rheumatoid (or any other) arthritis. Weight loss can be helpful for the overweight as it reduces the strain on joints.

RHINE RIESLING
see Wine, Varieties.

RHIZOME

An underground stem such as ginger root.

RHUBARB
see Fruit.

RIBOFLAVIN
see Vitamins, Vitamin B_2.

RIBONUCLEIC ACID (RNA)

A nucleic acid needed for making proteins in the body.
See also Nucleic Acids.

RICE
see Grains.

RICE BRAN OIL
see Oils.

RICE NOODLES

Pasta made from rice flour rather than wheat flour. Noodles are a symbol of longevity in China and are traditionally served at birthday celebrations. Nutritionally, rice noodles have little to offer apart from their complex carbohydrate and small quantities of minerals. 100 g of raw rice noodles have 1510 kJ (360 Cals). When cooked, this amount would make 3–4 serves.

RICE PAPER

A very fine paper made from the stem of a small shrub or tree related to the ginseng and native to China. Very thin sheets of the paper are used around sweet fillings. It is quite edible but the quantities used are so small that it does not contribute significant amounts of any nutrient.

RICKETS

A condition in which the developing bones do not have sufficient calcium and phosphorus and so become bent and misshapen. May occur from a lack of calcium or insufficient vitamin D which is essential for calcium to be used in bone. Common in Europe until fairly recently because of a lack of both calcium and vitamin D.

RICOTTA
see Cheese.

RILLETTES

A potted meat dish made from pork belly (or occasionally rabbit or goose) and seasonings which usually include garlic, thyme, pepper and spices such as cinnamon. The meat and its fat are simmered slowly with the seasonings until cooked. The mixture is then placed into small pots, weighted to press the mixture firmly and left in the refrigerator until firm. Rillettes are commonly served with bread. They are usually high in fat.

RIND

The outside edge of cheese or some fruits, such as citrus. The rind protects both the moisture content and the nutrients in the product.

Rinds on cheeses may form naturally or may be made of a wax coating or a fine material (cheesecloth). Cheeses with a high salt content form a thick rind while they are maturing. Swiss cheese (which has a lower salt content) forms a particularly hard rind. The natural rinds on cheese may be removed or eaten; the waxes and cloth are removed.

The rind on citrus fruits is quite bitter due to the volatile oils they contain. These intensely flavoured oils are quite flammable. In small quantities, finely grated citrus rind (known as zest) is used to impart a strong citrus flavour to sweet or savoury dishes.

RISOTTO

An Italian rice dish made by heating some rice with butter or oil until the grains are well coated and then adding wine and/or stock and allowing the rice to cook slowly until it has absorbed all the liquid. Served with grated

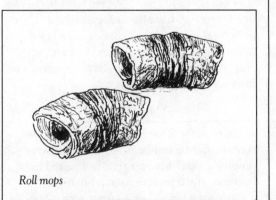

Roll mops

Parmesan cheese. An average serve of risotto has 1870 kJ (445 Cals).

RISSOLES

Originally rissoles consisted of a mixture of minced meat, fish or poultry wrapped in pastry and deep-fried. Today the term is used for a small patty made from minced meat, fish or chicken mixed with breadcrumbs and seasonings and shallow fried until crisp and brown. Most rissoles have a high fat content.

RNA
see Ribonucleic acid; Nucleic acids.

ROASTING

The term roasting is usually applied to the oven-baking of foods such as meats, poultry, vegetables or nuts. The cooking comes from infra-red radiation from the oven walls and on convection through the air inside the oven. For meats with a high degree of connective tissue, roasting may not be the best cooking method as the meat tends to dry out before it is tender. For muscle meats with little connective tissue, the roasting time needs to be relatively short and the temperature reasonably high (175°C). For slightly less tender cuts of meat, a lower temperature and a slower cooking time is more appropriate. Meats with a higher fat content also roast better than very lean meats.

Vegetables are roasted by placing them in fat or oil. Nuts are roasted without any additional fat since they have plenty of their own.

ROCK CAKES

Small slightly dry cakes containing dried fruit, cooked in individual patty tins. An average 60 g rock cake has 995 kJ (238 Cals).

ROCKET
see Vegetables, Arugula.

ROCKET CRESS
see Vegetables.

ROCKMELON
see Fruits.

ROCK SALT

Made from sea salt which has been boiled and allowed to crystallise to fairly large salt crystals. Rock salt has no nutritional advantages over regular salt. All salt is sodium chloride.

ROE

The eggs and spawn (or milt) of female and male fish. Roe is a source of most vitamins (including vitamin C) and also has some minerals. It is high in protein and low in fat. 10 g of cod roe has 40 kJ (10 Cals) and almost no fat. The same quantity of herring roe has 35 kJ (8 Cals) and, again, almost no fat. The roe of the sturgeon (caviar) has a high content of iron and protein and a little more fat. 10 g of caviar has 105 kJ (25 Cals) and 1.5 g of fat.

ROLLMOPS
see Fish.

ROMAN BEANS
see Legumes, Borlotti beans.

ROMANO
see Cheese.

ROOT BEER

A drink once flavoured with an oil extracted from the root of the sassafras tree. Since this oil has been shown to be toxic it is no longer used. Artificial flavouring is now added to root beer — a popular soft drink in the United States. Root beer is like most soft drinks and contains 10−11 per cent sugar and no nutritional value. A 250 mL glass has 440 kJ (105 Cals).

ROOT VEGETABLES

Vegetables which grow under the ground including beetroot, carrots, parsnips, radishes, swedes and turnips. Potatoes are really tubers but are often included with root vegetables. All root vegetables are good sources of dietary fibre.

For details, see individual entries under vegetables.

ROQUEFORT
see Cheese.

ROSE APPLE
see Fruit, Jambo.

ROSECOCO BEANS
see Legumes, Borlotti beans.

ROSE HIP
see Fruit.

ROSELLA
see Fruit.

ROSEMARY
see Herbs.

ROSEWATER

An essence made by steeping rose petals in water. Used as a flavouring for desserts in Middle Eastern and Indian cookery in much the same way that vanilla is used.

ROSTI

The national Swiss dish which looks like a crisp potato cake. To make rosti, potatoes are first boiled until almost tender. When cool enough, they are coarsely grated and packed into a cake in a frying pan (usually with melted bacon fat or butter). The cake is cooked over a gentle heat until crisp and brown and is then turned and browned on the other side. It is served cut into wedges.

ROUGHAGE

A old term for fibre. Since roughage implies that the fibre is indigestible, and since some types of dietary fibre are totally digested by bacteria, the term roughage is no longer considered a helpful or accurate term. The old measurements of crude fibre or roughage generally only measured the cellulose content of the food. As is explained under Dietary fibre, page 92, this under-represents the true fibre content of a food.

ROUILLE

A mixture of garlic, chilli, bread and olive oil pounded together to form a thick paste which is used to flavour soups in Southern France.

ROULADE

A roll, usually made from a light cake mixture, pastry, a vegetable or meat or fish mixture wrapped around a filling. The outer part of the roulade may be a thinly sliced piece of meat or it may be a souffle-type mixture (either sweet or savoury).

ROUX

A mixture of equal parts of butter and flour used to thicken sauces. The word 'roux' is the French word for 'red' and presumably signified that the flour being used had been allowed to brown. In making a roux, the butter and flour are heated together and cooked for a minute or two. For a brown sauce, the mixture can be allowed to brown; for a white sauce, it is heated more gently and does not brown. The darker the roux, the less thickening power it will have because the carbohydrate in the flour is altered during the browning.

ROWAN
see Fruit.

ROYAL JELLY

A thick white substance produced by bees and fed to worker and drone larvae until they are 3 days old and to queen bee larvae throughout their larval life. Royal jelly is rich in pantothenic acid and also contains vitamin B_6. The quantities present are significant for something the size of bee larvae but there is little point in humans eating royal jelly since the quantities required to provide significant quantities of nutrients would be very large. Most royal jelly preparations sold through health food shops do not contain substantial quantities of nutrients and do not justify the high prices charged. Claims of the rejuvenating properties of royal jelly have not been proved in properly controlled tests.

RUM
see Drinks, Alcoholic.

RUM BUTTER
see Hard sauce.

RUSKS

Slices or long thin pieces of bread which have been dried out in the oven until they are light and crisp. To make rusks: slice sweet or regular bread into any shape, place on an ungreased baking tray and leave in a slow oven until crisp and quite dry. Small thin rusks will take 15–20 mins; thicker pieces may take twice as long. Serve with drinks or soups or give to babies to suck.

Some of the B complex vitamins in the original bread will be lost during baking. The kilojoules will not alter per slice of bread used although the kilojoules per 100 g will be much higher in rusks compared with bread since the rusks have lost their water.

RUSTY NAIL
see Drinks, Alcoholic.

RUTABAGA
see Vegetables.

RUTIN
see Bioflavenoids.

RYE
see Grains.

S

SABAYON SAUCE

A sweet sauce made from egg yolks beaten with sugar and white wine or fruit juice. Served with fruit, cakes or desserts.

SACCHARIN
see Artificial sweeteners.

SAFFLOWER OIL
see Oils.

SAFFLOWER SEEDS
see Seeds.

SAFFRON
see Spices.

SAGE
see Herbs.

SAGO

The dried starchy granules from the pith of the sago and other palm trees native to Indonesia. The palms are cut down when a flower spike appears, as the pith or centre of the palm is full of a starchy material from which sago is produced. If the flower is allowed to develop, it will absorb the starchy pith for its own food.

The pith is grated to form a powder which is mixed with water and rubbed through a sieve with particular shaped holes to produce either pearl or bullet sago.

Sago has become a basic food for the South Pacific region where it is made into a thick dessert or used in cakes and soups. In other areas it is used mainly with milk and eggs in sago pudding or as a thickener in Scandinavian fruit soups.

Sago provides complex carbohydrate and a small amount of iron and other minerals. It is extremely low in protein and has no significant quantities of any vitamin. If it forms the major part of the diet, malnutrition is likely. 100 g of raw sago have 1485 kJ (355 Cals).

ST JOHN'S BREAD
see Carob.

SAINT PAULIN
see Cheese.

SAKE
see Drinks, Alcoholic.

SALAD BURNET
see Herbs.

SALADS

Salads were first served during the Middle Ages. Records of early salads served around AD 1390 gave great emphasis to onions and a variety of fresh herbs, dressed with oil, vinegar and salt.

By the second half of the eighteenth century, salads appear to have become quite popular and were heartily recommended by French 'hygienists' as the ideal way to end a meal.

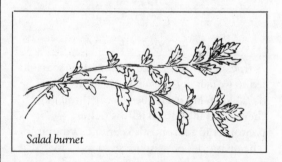

Salad burnet

A salad was described as something which 'moistens, refreshes, frees the stomach, encourages sleep, enlarges the appetite, tempers the ardours of Venus and appeases the thirst'. Some of our waist-watching citizens might agree that salads 'enlarge the appetite'!

Today a salad may include an incredible array of foods ranging from vegetables, fruits, nuts, seeds, legumes, poultry, fish or meat. Pasta, rice and wheat are also evident in salads. Dressings may range from mixtures of oils and vinegars or mayonnaises to straight lemon juice. Salads do not even have to be cold. A warm salad is now quite popular and German potato salad is served hot. It is therefore extremely difficult to define a salad.

A few common salads are:

- *Caesar* — crisp lettuce with a raw egg broken over the top, mixed well, dressed with olive oil mixed with lemon juice and pepper, tossed with bread cubes fried until crisp in garlic-flavoured oil. Anchovy fillets are often added. The salad was created by Alexander Cardini in honour of his brother, another chef named Caesar.
- *Coleslaw* — an American Salad of shredded red or green cabbage (often with celery, capsicum, carrot, shallots), dressed with a very thin mayonnaise.
- *Gado gado* — an Indonesian salad with rows of sliced or shredded vegetables (usually potatoes, bean sprouts, cabbage, carrots, snow peas, cucumber, watercress) and hard-boiled eggs served with a peanut sauce.
- *Greek* — cubes of tomatoes, cucumbers, black olives and fetta cheese dressed with olive oil and a little lemon juice.
- *Green* — various types of lettuce, tossed just before serving with an oil and vinegar dressing which may be flavoured with herbs or a little lemon.
- *Potato* — potatoes (or cubes) with mint, parsley and shallots, dressed with mayonnaise.
- *Tabbouli* — cracked wheat soaked and

drained and mixed with lots of chopped parsley, mint, shallots and tomato, dressed with olive oil and lemon juice. Tabbouli is highly nutritious and the large quantity of parsley used contributes to its value. It is a good source of dietary fibre, vitamin C, carotene, iron and complex carbohydrate. 1 cup of tabbouli has 1000 kJ (240 Cals). This will be reduced to half this level if the olive oil is omitted.

- *Waldorf* — chopped apple (with skin on), celery and walnuts with a creamy mayonnaise dressing. Invented for the opening of the Waldorf-Astoria Hotel in New York but now enjoyed in many countries. An average serve of Waldorf salad (1 cup) would have approximately 630 kJ (150 Cals).

SALAMI
see Sausages.

SALICYLATES

Aspirin-like substances found naturally in many fruits and vegetables, nuts, seeds, herbs, tea, honey and wines. Salicylates are also used in perfumes, toothpaste, medications and some toiletries. Some people are sensitive to salicylates, showing reactions of hyperactivity, skin rashes, gastrointestinal upsets or, occasionally, migraine.

Foods with high levels of salicylates are listed below. (Other foods also contain salicylates and anyone needing a diet very low in salicylates should seek the assistance of a dietitian.)

See also Aspirin.

- *Vegetables* — tomato products, gherkin, endive, button mushrooms, radishes, olives, capsicum, zucchini, chicory, eggplant, watercress, cucumber and alfalfa.
- *Fruits* — dried fruits, most berries, red and black currants, cherries, oranges, guavas, apricots, rockmelon, grapes, plums, pineapple, passionfruit, citrus fruits,

avocado, peaches, nectarines, Granny Smith and Jonathan apples, watermelon, lychees and kiwi fruit.

- *Nuts*— almonds and water chestnuts
- *Herbs* — all except parsley
- *Sweets* — honey, licorice, peppermints, chewing gum, mint-flavoured lollies or chocolates, biscuits and cakes which include dried fruit or spices.
- *Beverages* — tea: all varieties including herbal teas (camomile has the lowest level of salicylates), some cereal coffees, cider, beer, wine and liqueurs.

SALIVA

The liquid secreted by the three pairs of salivary glands in response to the thought, smell or taste of food. Saliva is very slightly acidic and contains an amylase which begins the break down of complex carbohydrates.

See also Amylases; Ptyalin.

SALMON

see Fish.

SALMONELLA

Bacteria which cause food poisoning if present in sufficient numbers. Salmonella live and grow in the intestines of humans, animals and household birds and are transmitted to foods by excreta, flies, pests and lack of hygiene. They are also found in some chickens and this can sometimes be a source of contamination to other foods. Salmonella are responsible for most cases of food poisoning.

Salmonella are easily killed by cooking but cooked foods can be recontaminated if they come into contact with raw foods or the knives or equipment used with raw foods. The bacteria multiply rapidly at room temperature but not in the refrigerator. All cooked foods or those to be served without further cooking should therefore be kept either hot or cold.

Food poisoning from salmonella appears in 12−36 hours and lasts a day or 2 with abdominal pain, diarrhoea, vomiting and fever.

SALMON TROUT

see Fish.

SALSIFY

see Vegetables.

SALT

Salt is made up of sodium and chlorine — both essential minerals. However, that does not mean that the more salt we eat, the better. Some salt is important but too much can be harmful.

Salt was once a highly prized commodity and was even traded for gold. It was valued because of its preservative action for meats, fish, fruits and vegetables and often made the difference between health and semi-starvation.

In some parts of the world where refrigeration is not available, salting is still used as a major food-processing technique. In such cases, the benefits of salt may well outweigh the disadvantages to health which have now been established from an excessive intake of salt. Wherever possible, however, salting has been replaced by refrigeration or other methods of food processing and this has reduced the incidence of stomach cancer.

Salt preserves food by altering the moisture content, drawing water out so that bacteria and moulds are unable to multiply. The food will then keep longer. With foods such as cheese or pickles, the addition of salt helps particular bacteria to grow and produce the fermentation which results in the final product. In making cheese, for example, salt controls the ripening, provides a firm texture, preserves the cheese and gives it flavour. Too much salt produces a dry, crumbly cheese while too little produces a soft, bland cheese which does not keep for long. Some cheeses, such as blue varieties, have a particularly high salt content so that undesirable bacteria won't survive but the blue mould, which is relatively salt-resistant, will be able to grow. On the other hand, a cheese such as Swiss, generally has very little salt so that a special bacteria can produce the characteristic sweet flavour and the holes in the texture.

The major problem with salt is its link with high blood pressure in many people. The current generation in countries such as Australia is consuming a diet with more salt than previous generations. Even though many people have stopped adding salt to their foods, the high intake of processed foods and fast foods items has raised the total salt intake in the average diet.

Now that it is not needed as a preservative, salt is added to foods for flavour. Modern processed and pre-cooked items often have less flavour than freshly prepared foods so salt is added. Since salty foods stimulate the body's thirst mechanism, it is likely that many fast foods contain a lot of salt so that consumers will also buy a drink!

The less foods are cooked, and the less water used in cooking, the greater the retention of the natural flavour in the food and the less need there is for the addition of salt. Compare different methods of cooking vegetables for example. Those cooked in a saucepan of water until they are quite soft will have lost a lot of their flavour to the water and will probably need salt for flavour. On the other hand, if vegetables are steamed or cooked without water in a microwave oven, there is much less loss of flavour and salt is unnecessary.

The greater the use of top quality food ingredients, and the more other foods such as herbs and spices are used, the less need there is for salt.

The liking for salt is learned. Babies do not like salt and have to learn to accept it. But having learned to want salt, most people maintain the desire for it. Salting foods also becomes a habit. Most people sprinkle salt on their meal even before they have tasted it! Once you are accustomed to the taste of salt, it can be difficult to give up. Taste buds which are overloaded with salt take time to adjust to foods without salt. But once the taste buds have

adjusted, the natural flavours of foods become more intense. One study found that it takes about 3 months for the average person's taste buds to become used to unsalted foods. Rather than enhancing the taste, salt simply gives everything a sameness of taste — salty.

See also Sodium.

Salt and high blood pressure

Early humans' diet contained very little salt — a situation which persists in some tribal and traditional societies who eat no salt apart from that present naturally in foods. High blood pressure is unknown in these people and even though some live in very hot climates, such as in parts of New Guinea, they do not suffer any symptoms of salt deficiency.

As they grow older, those who have eaten little salt throughout life continue to have low blood pressure. Strokes are unknown. However, if people live a Western lifestyle, and eat more salted foods as well as less potassium, blood pressure often rises and the incidence of strokes increases.

There are some lucky people who seem to be unaffected by large amounts of salt. However, if you are one of the fortunate few whose kidneys are not sensitive to added salt, you have no way of knowing. Neither do you know how much harm salt is doing to your body — until your blood pressure suddenly rises. There is little to gain by eating extra salt and a lot to lose by eating an excess.

Even though high blood pressure will fall when less salt is eaten, a person with normal or low blood pressure will find that eating less salt has no effect. Reducing salt normalises blood pressure.

See also Blood pressure.

Salt, sweating and cramps

Sweat contains salt, and many people assume that those who sweat a lot need extra salt or even salt tablets to help restore losses.

It is now known that a trained athlete loses less salt in sweat than someone who is only occasionally physically active. You also lose less salt in the urine after a heavy sweat. The body is basically very good at conserving the sodium from salt.

With any type of heavy work or exercise, much more water is lost than salt. It is vitally important to replace the water lost before replacing the salt. The salt naturally present in foods such as milk, meat and eggs, plus that added to breads and breakfast cereals, can easily replace sweating losses. Salt tablets are as unnecessary and harmful for sportspeople as they are for others. They cause too much water to pass into the intestine, causing nausea, vomiting and a feeling of weakness.

Many people believe that cramps are caused by a lack of salt and that extra salt will cure them. It is now known that cramps can occur for many reasons — the most common being a lack of appropriate warm-up for the muscle. A lack of water, or a temporary deficiency of magnesium, potassium or calcium, or the effect of female hormones on these minerals, may also be responsible for cramps. A lack of water is the major dietary suspect in cases of cramp.

Anyone who is experiencing cramps should make sure he or she is drinking sufficient water.

Requirements for salt

The body needs some salt to provide sodium and chlorine but most people in Western countries eat 10–20 times as much as they need. Sodium requirements are discussed on page 318. In general, a more than adequate intake of salt will be obtained from the natural salt in meats, poultry, seafoods, milk, eggs and vegetables plus that added to breads. Even the latter source is unnecessary for most people. Unsalted breads are not widely sold, however, partly because they are more difficult to make and partly because most people find them unpalatable.

You cannot always tell where the salt is in foods by the taste. Potato crisps, for example, taste salty whereas cornflakes do not. Yet a bowl of cornflakes has more salt than a small packet of potato crisps.

In general, it is highly-processed items, including fast foods, processed meats, frozen prepared foods, biscuits, snack foods, pies and some canned products which have high salt levels. As more unsalted processed foods are being made, it is becoming easier to follow a diet with a more moderate salt level. Unsalted canned vegetables, tuna and other fish, breakfast cereals, soups, stews, butter, margarine, sauces, peanut butter and crackers are now widely available. There are also many salt-reduced foods available with 30–50 per cent less salt than regular products. These include bread, processed turkey meats, hams, cheeses, soups and breakfast cereals.

SALUGGIA BEANS
see Legumes, Borlotti beans.

SAMBALS

Accompaniments to curry, generally designed to be either heating or cooling foods. The former include chopped or ground chillies with added onion, grated coconut, lemon juice, dried fish, fruit or vegetables. Cooling sambals have no chilli and may feature cucumber and/or yoghurt.

SAMBUCA
see Drinks, Alcoholic.

SAMOOSAS

Indian savoury pasties filled with lamb or vegetables seasoned with spices and herbs. The pastries are usually fried and are eaten as a first course. One fried Samoosa has 580 kJ (140 Cals).

SAMSOE
see Cheese.

SANDALWOOD

The dried bark of the sandalwood tree (native to India) contains an oil which can be extracted and used to flavour icecream or cakes.

SANDWICHES

One of the handiest meals to be found, sandwiches encompass any foods served between 2 slices of bread. The term 'sandwich' was not used until 1762 when Lord Montague, the fourth Earl of Sandwich, not wanting to interrupt a 24-hour gambling stint, asked for his meals to be placed between 2 slices of bread. Even though Captain Cook named the Sandwich Islands after him, Montague is remembered more for the snack which bears his name.

Before Lord Montague, people had often placed food into bread. The Arabs had been splitting their pocket (or pita) bread and filling it with spiced meat and salad vegetables for centuries. Strict Jews had kept their passover custom of eating sandwiches made from unleavened matzo bread filled with bitter herbs, nuts and apple. But it was not until Montague made the sandwich famous, that it really became popular.

Sandwiches vary between countries. Scandinavian sandwiches often have a slice of bread as their base and this is piled with an assortment of ingredients, artistically arranged. Sandwiches from a traditional New York delicatessen tend to have enormous fillings and are often served with chips and salad. Eating more than one such sandwich would indeed be a feat. In Europe and Australia, sandwiches have more modest fillings and an increasing variety of fillings are being used. Because of the differences in sandwiches, nutritional information about sandwiches is not always relevant in different parts of the world. Thus Americans tend to regard sandwiches as high-kilojoule 'fattening' foods — a description which is not appropriate to the sandwiches served elsewhere.

Basically, a sandwich can be a well-balanced meal, especially if the bread is wholegrain and the filling includes salad vegetables, fish, egg, chicken, turkey or lean meat.

SANTO DOMINGO APRICOT
see Fruit, Sapodilla.

SAPODILLA
see Fruit.

SAPONINS

Substances present in legumes and some vegetables which are sometimes included in the definition of dietary fibre since they pass through the intestine unchanged. Saponins have been shown to lower levels of cholesterol in the blood by helping fibre adsorb bile acids (see page 72). Soya beans, chickpeas, peanuts, broad beans, eggplant and alfalfa have the highest levels of saponins found in commonly eaten plants.

SAPOTE
see Fruit.

SAPSAGO
see Cheese.

SARDINE
see Fish.

SARSAPARILLA

A plant native to South America whose root provides a liquorice-flavoured extract used to flavour drinks, confectionery, cakes and desserts.

SASHIMI

A Japanese dish consisting of carefully prepared raw fish, usually served with hot horseradish known as wasabi and soya sauce. Fish used for sashimi must be very fresh and only sections selected from the back of the fish are generally used. The fish most prized for sashimi include tuna, kingfish, moonfish and salmon. Nutritionally, sashimi is an excellent meal, rich in protein, vitamins and minerals and containing only minimal quantities of fat.

SASSAFRAS

A North American tree whose bark and root produce an oil, saffrole, which was once used to flavour root beer. As the oil is known to be toxic, it is no longer permitted. Sassafras tea is used by some people as an alternative to regular tea. It is probably much more hazardous.

SATAY (OR SATE)

Satays have been served in Malaysia, Indonesia and other Asian countries for many years and have now become popular throughout many other countries. Pieces of meat, chicken, fish or other seafoods are threaded onto bamboo skewers, grilled and flavoured with various spices. To prevent the skewers burning, they are soaked in water before using. Satay is usually served with a spicy peanut sauce.

SATIETY

A feeling of satisfaction after eating. In general, high-fibre foods give a greater feeling of satiety than those which have little fibre. Foods such as rolled oats give a feeling of satiety because the particular type of fibre they contain forms a gel in the stomach.

There is also a psychological aspect to satiety. For example, if you are really longing for an icecream, you may not feel satiated until you actually eat one.

SAUCES

Traditionally, there have been 3 major types of sauces: white, brown and emulsion. However, various fruits and vegetables are also made into sauces to serve with savoury or sweet dishes.

The first written record of sauces being used comes from Roman times when the sauces consisted of various juices from meats or wine, flavoured with herbs and thickened with oil and pieces of bread beaten through them. They were used more as a condiment than to be poured over foods.

By about 1600, flour was used in place of bread as a thickening agent and spices were used with more delicacy and discrimination so that the sauce did not overpower the dish with which it was being served.

Many of the classic sauces have developed from French cuisine. Some of the common sauces include:

White sauces

- Bechamel — named after Louis de Bechameil, one of Louis XIV's courtiers: a white sauce made from butter, flour and milk flavoured with herbs and onion.
- Mornay sauce — basically a bechamel with added cheese.
- Veloute — similar to bechamel but with the milk replaced by fish or chicken stock.

Brown sauces

- Bordelaise sauce — a brown sauce with red wine and shallots for flavouring.
- Brown sauce (also known as espagnole sauce) — a basic sauce made from a brown roux (often flavoured with vegetables) and a well-flavoured meat stock. Peppercorns and herbs are added during the cooking and the final sauce is strained so as to be smooth.
- Piquante sauce — a brown sauce with white wine, vinegar and capers.

Emulsion sauces

- Hollandaise — a rich sauce, originally from Holland and made from egg yolks beaten. with lemon juice and thickened with butter
- Bearnaise — originally from Bearn, France, this sauce is made from egg yolks beaten with vinegar flavoured with peppercorns, bay leaf, tarragon and thyme, thickened with butter. High butter content makes it rich in kilojoules.
- Beurre blanc — reduced poaching liquid flavoured with lemon juice and shallots, thickened with butter.
- Beurre noir — a brown sauce (not black as its name would suggest) made by heating butter until it is brown and adding capers, vinegar and parsley.

- Beurre noisette — butter, gently heated until golden brown and usually flavoured with a little lemon juice.

Other sauces

Caramel sauce — another dessert sauce made by caramelising sugar and adding cream or butter. Some varieties are made from sweetened condensed milk.

- Chilli sauce — a fairly thick hot sauce made from chillies, garlic and vinegar, thickened with starch. Some varieties contain preservatives. Used as a condiment with many Chinese dishes.
- Custard sauce — made from eggs, milk and sugar, custard sauce is used over cakes or fruit (also known as creme Anglaise).
- Mint sauce — traditionally served with roast lamb, this sauce is made from chopped mint, vinegar and a little sugar.
- Peanut sauce — an Indonesian sauce made from ground peanuts, onion, garlic, chilli, shrimp paste, coconut milk and tamarind. A corruption of this sauce contains peanut butter, onion, tomato and soy sauce.
- Plum sauce — served with ham, pork or poultry, plum sauce is made from plums, onions, butter, wine, a little vinegar and sugar. It is often flavoured with cinnamon and pepper.
- Soy sauce — made from fermented soya beans, this dark, rich, salty sauce has minor differences in various Asian countries. In Japan, soy sauce is made from flakes of soya bean mixed with roasted wheat, and a particular strain of yeast and salt, and is allowed to ferment for a year. It is then filtered, pasteurised and bottled. It is also known as shoyu. Tamari is a soy sauce made from soya beans but has no wheat.
- Tabasco sauce — a famous hot sauce which uses two varieties of peppers (or capsicums) originally grown in Tabasco in Mexico. The peppers are ground to a pulp, packed into oak barrels with salt and left for 3 years. The mixture is then strained and mixed with vinegar and bottled as a thin, very hot sauce.
- Tomato sauce — fresh tomato sauce is made from tomatoes, onions, wine, herbs and a small amount of sugar. The ubiquitous bottled tomato sauce (or ketchup) is made from tomatoes, sugar, vinegar and herbs and spices. It has nothing like the flavour of fresh tomato sauce (see also page 197).
- Worcestershire sauce — A sweet-sour dark brown sauce made from an amazing collection of ingredients including vinegar, salt, walnuts, mushrooms, soy sauce, sugar, tamarind, pork liver, black and cayenne peppers, mace, coriander, anchovies, shallots, garlic, soy sauce and caramel. The sauce is left to mature for 6 months before being pasteurised and bottled. The final product contains some residue. Shake before use. It has an extremely long shelf life.

SAUERKRAUT

Made from fermented cabbage, sauerkraut was originally made in China and was brought across to Europe by early travellers. Sauerkraut has been an important way of preserving a vegetable to supply vitamin C through the winter months in cold climates when fresh vegetables were not available. Vitamin C is maintained in the acidity of the sauerkraut and may have helped prevent scurvy in many northern European countries.

To make sauerkraut, finely chopped or shredded cabbage is put into a brine solution strong enough to kill harmful bacteria but weak enough to allow some bacteria which produce lactic acid to survive. This process is controlled by allowing the cabbage to remain in the brine for a certain length of time so that the final acidity is a little less than 2 per cent.

Sauerkraut has the disadvantage of having a high salt content. However, it does retain vitamin C, even after canning. Sauerkraut is low in kilojoules and $\frac{1}{2}$ cup has only about 75 kJ (18 Cals).

SAUSAGES

A combination of finely chopped meat (or poultry or fish) seasoned with salt, pepper and spices and stuffed inside a casing. The word 'sausage' comes from the Latin 'salsus' meaning 'salted', and was used as a way of preserving meats. Dry sausages, made with less moisture, could be kept well without refrigeration.

The casings for sausages were once made from the internal organs of various animals. Nowadays, most casings are made of reconstituted collagen fibres from animals or are plastic. Skinless sausages are made by placing the ingredients into a cellulose casing, immersing the sausage into hot water, then dipping into cold water so that a protein film forms round the ingredients. The cellulose is then removed.

Throughout Europe, many areas have developed their special sausage, made from particular meats or with certain spices and herbs. They come in many different sizes and are known as salamis, wursts or saucisson. They may be fresh, smoked, salted or cooked and have a soft or hard texture. Some are dry, others are juicy. They are made from beef, pork, veal, chicken, rabbit or horse, with herbs, spices, garlic or breadcrumbs. Some include minced tripe. Most are high in fat. Some are discussed below.

Berliner

A sausage made from half veal and half pork. Mildly flavoured, seasoned with pepper and nutmeg, smoked and then simmered until cooked.

Bierwurst

A German smoked sausage usually made from pork, although sometimes from a mixture of beef and pork. Has flecks of fat throughout.

Black pudding

There are many versions of black pudding. The best known comes from the north of England and is made from pig's blood, fat, oatmeal, onions and spices. Usually served sliced and fried, making it a high fat meal. It is extremely high in iron and just 60 g will supply a woman's daily requirements for this mineral. A 60 g serve would supply 650 kJ (155 Cals) and 11 g of fat.

Bologna

One of the best known of all sausages, it is usually made from a mixture of smoked pork and beef. Another product, polony, is really the same as bologna. Fat content is usually about 20 per cent. 50 g of bologna have approximately 630 kJ (150 Cals).

Boudin blanc

A white sausage made with young veal, chicken or pork, often with added eggs, cream and spices. Can be boiled or grilled and is eaten hot.

Bratwurst

A long German sausage made of pork and veal, bacon, onion and milk and flavoured with mace, pepper and salt. Quite spicy.

Braunschweiger

A smoked liver sausage which also contains milk, eggs and pepper and brawn.

Cabanossi

Originally made in Russia, this smoked spicy sausage was traditionally made from pure pork but is now generally made from a mixture of pork and beef, seasoned with garlic, caraway and white pepper. Deeply smoked and needs to be refrigerated. 100 g have 1525 kJ (365 Cals) and supply 32 g of fat.

Cervelat

Although its name comes from the Latin word for brains, cervelat sausage is made from pork and beef. Available as a smoked sausage to cook or as a smoked salami type of sausage. Like all sausages, it is high in fat. The ready to cook sausage has 1300 kJ (310 Cals) per 100 g while the dry smoked variety has 1885 kJ (450 Cals) per 100 g.

Chorizo

A Spanish spicy, coarse-textured sausage made with pork and seasoned with cayenne pepper, chilli, red peppers, paprika, black pepper and salt. High in fat. Smoked for 15 hrs or sold fresh. The smoked dry sausage can be hung and its casing will wrinkle as it dries. It also becomes spicier.

Clobassy

A smoked Polish sausage made from pork (60—80 per cent) and beef and seasoned with garlic, pepper, cinnamon and coriander. Quite spicy and comes in a round or long shape. Can be eaten as it is or grilled.

Cotechino

An Italian pork sausage, usually cut into chunks and served hot with beans.

Crepinette

A general term for a small sausage, usually wrapped in a fine membrane.

Csabai

A spicy Hungarian sausage also known as kolbass. Coarsely textured and made from 90 per cent pork well-seasoned with paprika, red pepper, white pepper, coriander and red wine. Can be left hanging in a cool dry place indefinitely.

Devon

A bland luncheon meat sausage originally made in Australia as Fritz. After World War I, to show patriotism to the English, it was renamed Devon, after the English county of that name. Made from 80 per cent beef and 20 per cent pork, it is lightly seasoned with nutmeg, pepper and coriander and includes some soya protein, wheat flour and starch. Used on sandwiches. 50 g have 480 kJ (115 Cals) and 9 g of fat.

Frankfurt (or frankfurter)

A pork or pork and beef sausage which is smoked. Usually in a casing containing red dye to which some children are sensitive. High in fat. Each thin frankfurt (60 g) has 630—775 kJ (150—185 Cals) and 12—17 g of fat. Many frankfurts are larger than this and have more kilojoules and fat. Frankfurts can be boiled or grilled.

Haggis

A Scottish sausage made from oatmeal mixed with chopped heart and liver and suet, flavoured with onions and herbs and packed into a sheep's stomach before being boiled. 100 g of haggis have 1300 kJ (310 Cals) and 22 g of fat. It is high in iron and zinc, and a good source of protein and vitamins. Traditionally, a glass of whisky is drunk with haggis and it is served with 'neeps' (turnips).

Kabana

A long Polish smoked sausage made of minced beef (60 per cent) and coarsely minced pork, seasoned with pepper, nutmeg, salt and garlic. Does not require further cooking and is usually served with drinks.

Knoblauchwurst

A German sausage made with pork (plus pork fat), garlic and spices. Can be boiled or grilled.

Kolbass

see Csabai.

Kransky

A Yugoslavian sausage originally made in the

303

town of Kranj. Similar to the Russian sausage Ukrainska and the German Jagerwurst (reputedly carried by German huntsmen in their pockets to nibble while out hunting). A coarse-textured sausage made of 80 per cent pork and 20 per cent beef, seasoned with garlic, coriander, nutmeg and pepper. Smoked overnight and can either be refrigerated or hung to dry. Eaten hot or cold.

Liverwurst

A liver sausage mostly made with pork and calves' liver, often with added pork seasoned with onion, salt, pepper and marjoram. The mixture is finely ground and after filling into a casing it is simmered in water. Has a soft consistency to be used as a spread. Provides some iron although most commercial liverwursts have less than a home-made pâté which tends to have a higher percentage of liver. 50 g of liverwurst have 275 kJ (65 Cals).

Mettwurst

A German soft sausage which can be spread onto bread.

Mortadella

A large round Italian sausage with a fairly bland flavour. Made from pork and includes pieces of pork speck. Flavoured with garlic, pepper, cinnamon, cardamom, pistachio and marsala and deep smoked. Needs to be refrigerated. Served in thin slices on bread, pizza or as a snack. 50 g of this sausage have 670 kJ (160 Cals) and 15 g of fat.

Pepperone

Originally made in Spain, pepperone is now more familiar as the pepperoni which is made in Italy. It is a spicy sausage made of coarsely chopped pork with a small amount of beef and seasoned with pepper, paprika and garlic. Cold smoked and does not need to be refrigerated. Used on pizza or as an accompaniment to drinks. High in fat (about 36 per cent) but also supplies iron, zinc and protein. A 50 g serve has 890 kJ (210 Cals).

Polish salami

A fairly bland sausage with much more water than typical salamis. Made from pork (60 per cent) and beef seasoned with ground black pepper, cardamom, cinnamon and garlic. Smoked for a long period and must be refrigerated. 50 g have 500 kJ (120 Cals) and 9 g of fat.

Salami

Made from pork and beef mixtures with salt and spices, occasionally with added wine or spirits for flavour. After smoking, most salamis are hung in a cool dry place to allow their flavour to mature. Europeans prefer their salami to be quite dry and appear shrivelled and firm.

There are many types of salami. *Danish* is a mild salami with black pepper, coarse white pepper and salt. *Milano* is seasoned with marsala, fine black pepper, salt and coriander and has a mild flavour. *Budapest* is a spicy Hungarian salami seasoned with red wine, black whole pepper and nutmeg. *Calabrese* (from Calabria in Italy) is a very spicy, coarsely textured pure pork product seasoned with red peppers, red wine and coriander which goes well with beer or wine. *Hungarian* salami is mild, semi-coarse and seasoned with pepper, red wine, nutmeg, coriander and garlic.

Saveloy

A spiced frankfurt with a very high fat content.

Strassburg

A mildly flavoured sausage which is more like a Devon sausage than a salami. Used on sandwiches or served with drinks. 50 g have 525 kJ (125 Cals) and 10 g of fat.

Turkey Strassburg

Also called turkey salami, this is a sausage which looks and tastes like regular Strassburg but is made from lean turkey meat. Has much less fat and can be used in cooking as its higher content of lean meat does not melt. 50 g have 230 kJ (55 Cals) and 2 g of fat.

Weisswurst

A mildy spiced, soft textured German sausage, made from pork and veal. Boil or grill.

SAUTERNE
see Wine, Varieties.

SAUVIGNON
see Wine, Varieties.

SAVELOY
see Sausages.

SAVORY
see Herbs.

SCALLIONS
see Vegetables.

SCALLOPS
see Seafoods.

SCAMPI
see Seafoods.

SCARSDALE DIET

A popular American diet conceived by Dr Herman Tarnower. The diet is high in protein, low in carbohydrate and relatively low in fats. It is a rigid diet which claims to supply 4200 kJ (1000 Cals) a day although analysis shows it is much lower than this and will provide only about 3150 kJ (750 Cals). The strict diet lasts for 14 days, after which the would-be slimmer moves onto a 'keep trim eating plan' which has a little more variety, more protein and more fat but still very little carbohydrate. Like most low-carbohydrate diets, this one 'works' because of the loss of fluid which accompanies a curtailment of carbohydrate. It is not a diet which is recommended by most nutritionists.

SCHNAPPS
see Drinks, Alcoholic; Aquavit.

SCONES

Known as biscuits in the United States, scones are made from a soft dough of self-raising flour, milk and a little butter. They are best eaten soon after baking. A pot of tea, scones with jam

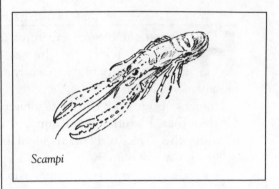

Scampi

and cream is popular in England and elsewhere as a Devonshire tea. An average scone has about 460 kJ (110 Cals).

SCREWDRIVER
see Drinks, Alcoholic.

SCURVY

A disease caused by a lack of Vitamin C. The connective tissues become inflamed. This is first apparent in the gums which bleed easily. Haemorrhages into the skin also occur and the body's defence against infection is lowered. Occurs after weaning when the diet does not contain fruits and vegetables. May also occur in babies born to women who took high doses of vitamin C during pregnancy causing their babies to be born with very high requirements for the vitamin which cannot be met from the normal content of breast milk.

SCUTELLUM

A small part of the wheat grain which absorbs, digests and takes food from the endosperm of the grain to the embryo or germ. The scutellum is thus rich in nutrients and contains about 60–70 per cent of the thiamin although it makes up only about 2 per cent of the wheat grain. Some of the scutellum is lost in making white flour.

SEA BREAM
see Fish, Morwong.

SEAFOOD

Humans resemble sea creatures in at least one respect. Both retain salt within the body. For the sea creatures, this ability is important; for humans, the inability to easily get rid of excess sodium from salt can be a nuisance (see Salt).

Humans also resemble at least some types of sea creatures in that each likes to eat the other. Fortunately for humans, only a few sea creatures are interested in us while the diversity of foods available from the sea is a constant source of delight for many humans.

Seafoods come in many shapes, sizes and flavours. Almost all have several features in common. They are excellent sources of protein, minerals and some vitamins and most are very low in fat. Even the idea that those with high cholesterol levels should not eat prawns has now been put into perspective (see Cholesterol). It is the low fat content of seafoods, as well as their delicious flavour, which makes them such a valued food. Added to that, even the tiny amount of fat found in many seafoods seems to be particularly valuable (see Omega 3 fatty acids).

Abalone

A large shellfish collected from the ocean floor by divers. The shell is used as mother-of-pearl and the flesh is greatly prized in Asian cuisine. The somewhat tough consistency of the flesh can be softened by pounding it before sautéeing briefly. Overcooking toughens it. Abalone has almost no fat but contributes iron and protein. 100 g have 420 kJ (100 Cals).

Calamari

see Squid.

Clam

A bivalve found in shallow waters. North American clams may be soft- or hard-shelled and are often quite large. In European countries, clams are somewhat smaller and are used in soups or sauces while in Australia, clams are available as pipis. The giant Pacific clam is large and may have a tough flesh which is best minced and used in soups. Clams should be well scrubbed and placed into fresh water to remove sand. They can be opened by inserting a knife between the 2 shells in front of the muscle which holds them together or by steaming them open. Those that do not open after steaming should be discarded as they are unlikely to be fresh.

Nutritionally, clams are rich in vitamin B_{12}, are a good source of iron and zinc and also supply protein. They have little fat. 100 g clam flesh have 335 kJ (80 Cals).

See also Molluscs.

Crab

Many varieties of these crustacea are eaten, after cooking in boiling water. The sweet flesh in the claws is especially prized.

Nutritionally, crab is low in fat, high in protein and has many minerals (especially copper) and vitamins. Contrary to popular belief, crab does not have a particularly high content of cholesterol. Since it has little fat, and most of that present is polyunsaturated fat, eating crab will not increase cholesterol levels. 100 g crab flesh have 525 kJ (125 Cals).

Crayfish

see Lobster.

Cuttlefish

A mollusc which is closely related to squid and

has an ink sac which should be removed before preparation. The body (or mantle) is thicker than that of a squid but like the latter they have 10 tentacles. The cuttlebone inside is used for small domestic birds to scratch their beaks. The flesh of their flaps and the mantle is prized by humans, especially the Japanese. The flaps are cut into strips for cooking while the mantle is often scored in a diamond pattern before cooking to tenderise it. They need fast cooking (2—3 mins) to prevent them becoming tough.

See also Molluscs.

Limpet

You may not fancy them, but limpets can be removed from their shells and eaten raw or added to soups.

Lobster

These saltwater crustaceans with sweet flesh in the tail and claws are sometimes called crayfish and vice versa. True lobsters have a large pair of claws on the first of their 3 pairs of legs. The crustacean known as a lobster in Australia has no nippers and is, technically, a crayfish. The European lobster has much larger claws with more flesh than the Australian rock lobster. Small sand lobsters, also known as 'bugs' are found in Australian waters, the Balmain Bug being found in southeastern Australia and the Moreton Bay Bug coming from northern Australia. The langouste is a rock lobster or crayfish.

The male lobster is larger and meatier than the female, but the female sometimes contains the coral (or eggs) which turn red when cooked and are delicious to eat.

Lobsters are generally a greenish colour on top with yellow, orange, red or blue colours underneath. After cooking, the shell turns a bright orange-red. Lobsters are often kept alive in water until ready to cook. Live lobsters should never be dropped into boiling water as this will toughen the flesh and cause the legs to fall off (to say nothing about the lobster's views

on the matter). It is better (though, again, not necessarily from the lobster's point of view) to drown them in fresh water or freeze them. To cook, place in cold water, bring slowly to the boil and simmer for 8 mins per 500 g. Lobster tails can also be grilled.

Lobster is a good source of protein, has little fat (and most of that is polyunsaturated) and supplies a variety of minerals and vitamins. It is low in kilojoules with 100 g of the flesh having 500 kJ (120 Cals). Served with a rich sauce, however, it becomes a high-fat, high-kilojoule meal. Contrary to popular fears, lobster is not particularly high in dietary cholesterol and has little saturated fat.

Marron

A variety of freshwater crayfish which is native to Western Australia and is now being farmed there and in other parts of Australia. The flesh in their tails is considered to be of excellent quality and they grow as large as 2 kg. Similar nutritional value to lobster.

Molluscs

see Molluscs.

Mussels

An edible mollusc found in clumps in estuaries and clinging to rocks, logs or piers. Although known as the 'poor man's oyster' mussels have their own distinctive flavour. The New Zealand green-lipped mussel is large and full-flavoured.

Mussels should only be used if the shells are tightly closed. Discard any with slightly open shells. They should be stored in a bucket of water and used soon after purchase. To prepare: scrub the mussel shells thoroughly using a small brush. Steam, boil, barbecue or microwave them until the shells open. Do not attempt to prise open any that do not open during cooking as these are usually stale. Mussels are also delicious served with a rich tomato and garlic sauce.

Like other molluscs, mussels are rich in minerals, especially iron and zinc. Because of their ability to concentrate minerals, it is important that mussels are only taken from clean waters. They also provide a variety of vitamins and have some protein; they are extremely low in fat and are quite suitable for those on cholesterol-lowering diets. Each 100 g of mussels (weighed with shells) have only 105 kJ (25 Cals).

See also Molluscs.

Octopus

An 8-legged variety of mollusc whose tentacles and body are delicious if grilled, braised or barbecued. Small octopuses can be cooked quickly; larger varieties need longer slower braising to become tender. To prepare octopus, cut out the beak and the ink sac (this can be used if desired). Either cut in halves, leave whole or, if large, remove tentacles and head to use separately. Some people maintain that octopus needs to be beaten and cooked for many hours to become tender. This is only necessary for large, old octopuses.

Nutritionally, octopus is high in protein and has almost no fat. 100 g of octopus flesh have 315 kJ (75 Cals). Octopus is reputed to have high levels of cholesterol. An average serving has only as much cholesterol as 2 fillets of fish and, since it has almost no fat, eating octopus will not raise the level of cholesterol in the blood (see page 72).

Oyster

Molluscs found in the Pacific, Atlantic and Mediterranean waters and used as food since ancient times. Oysters come in many varieties and many are farmed in cultivated oyster beds. Ideally, oysters are eaten straight from the shell but they can be grilled, poached or fried. Their flavour is best when they are not spawning. A fresh oyster should be plump, a natural creamy-grey colour with clear liquid surrounding it. Oysters which have been opened are referred to as being 'shucked'.

Nutritionally, oysters are one of the richest known sources of zinc and iron and also have plenty of other minerals. If they come from contaminated waters, they will also have a high concentration of undesirable minerals. They supply vitamins and protein.

A dozen regular-sized oysters will have just 295 kJ (70 Cals) and almost no fat. Contrary to popular belief, oysters are not high in cholesterol. Early measurements of the cholesterol content of some foods inadvertently measured some other sterols.

Pipi

see Clam.

Prawn

These crustaceans without claws are available in a range of sizes from small school prawns to the large king prawns. Small prawns are sometimes referred to as shrimp. In fact, shrimp have claws and, although they are very similar to prawns, shrimp are a different genus. However, what Australians call prawns are known as shrimp in the United States.

Prawns are a clear greyish colour when raw but turn pink when cooked. They are considered a delicacy in most countries of the world. Most people eat only the flesh of the prawn but in parts of Asia, the shell is also eaten and provides a valuable source of calcium.

When selecting prawns, they should be firm and unbroken and the flesh should appear translucent. They are cooked by boiling for a couple of minutes in fresh water. Do not add salt as it will toughen the flesh. Remove the head and, usually, the shell before eating.

Prawns have a higher content of pre-formed cholesterol than other seafoods. This fact has been used to damn them — somewhat unfairly, as it happens. The pre-formed cholesterol content of prawns is fairly unimportant since these crustaceans have almost no saturated fat — the major cause of high levels of cholesterol in the blood. However, if prawns are crumbed and deep-fried, the added fat plus the pre-formed cholesterol would make them unsuitable for those with high levels of blood cholesterol. Eaten as part of a low-fat diet, they cause no problems.

Banning prawns for those with high levels of blood cholesterol does not make sense, especially when fish are freely allowed. An average fillet of fish has about 100 mg of pre-formed cholesterol. An average serve of prawns (100 g of prawn flesh) has 200 mg of cholesterol. Yet many people claim that fish can be eaten as often as you like but prawns should be avoided. In fact, both fish and prawns are suitable for cholesterol-lowering diets since they have almost no saturated fats.

100 g of cooked prawn flesh (equivalent to about 300 g if weighed in their shells) have less than 2 g of fat and only 500 kJ (120 Cals). Prawns are a good source of protein and many minerals, including iodine.

Scallop

Shellfish found all over the world in sand or fine gravel in relatively clear water. Their distinctive fluted shell has 2 fan-shaped valves held together by a large muscle which forms the edible part of the mollusc. The animal swims by making clapping movements of its valves so that the ejected water propels it forward. Scallops are becoming scarce and consequently expensive in many parts of the world.

Scallops need only a minute or two in boiling water to cook; overcooking will toughen the beautiful flesh. In the United States, only the white part of the scallop is eaten. Elsewhere, the small pink-orange coral (or roe) is also enjoyed. After steaming they can be used with pasta, served with a sauce, used in a salad or enjoyed with bread.

Nutritionally, scallops are a good source of protein, iron and niacin. They have very little fat. 100 g of scallop flesh (about 4 scallops) have 440 kJ (105 Cals).

Scampi

Also known as the Dublin Bay prawn or the Norway lobster, these crustaceans are like small lobsters. The flesh from their tails is delicious and they are highly prized in Europe, Australia and New Zealand. Scampi live in burrows in the sand at the bottom of the ocean and reach an adult size of about 200 g. Their long slender claws are almost as long as their bodies. They are delicious grilled or sauteed with onion, tomato and garlic. Nutritionally, they are similar to lobster and have a high content of protein and little fat.

Sea urchin

Once the hard spiny shell of the sea urchin is cut open, its flesh can be eaten raw or cooked in a sauce. The most highly prized parts of the sea urchin are the sex glands. These are a delicacy in the Mediterranean region.

Shrimp

The name given to prawns in the United States and to small prawns in other countries. Technically, shrimps are a separate, but related, genus from the prawn. They are, however, remarkably similar and many people interchange the terms. Even in the United States, larger shrimps are called prawns. For nutritional information, see prawn.

Squid

Calamari is the Italian name for a variety of squid. Baby squid, known as calamaretti, are especially succulent. Found throughout the world, the squid is a cephalopod with a long tubular body, a short head and 10 long slender tentacles around its beak. Its backbone is made of a horny material. The squid has a sac of ink which it discharges if attacked. This ink is quite edible as is its body and tentacles. A variety of squid abound in different areas. One of the most popular is the southern calamari which has broad fins (or flaps) extending the length of its body. Its flesh is very tender.

To prepare squid, remove the head and tentacles from the hood and then slide the backbone out. Remove skin from the hood and the broad flaps by pulling firmly (it will not easily come off stale squid). The hood, flaps and tentacles can all be used, either pan fried, barbecued or steamed. The hood can also be stuffed or cut into rings, crumbed and fried. The ink can also be used in sauces to serve with squid.

Squid have almost no fat and provide a variety of minerals and vitamins as well as protein. 100 g of squid (before cooking) have 350 kJ (84 Cals).

Whelks

Spiral-shelled sea creatures which can be steamed and eaten. Popular in Europe. An excellent source of iron and zinc and a good source of protein. 50 g of whelks (flesh only) have 190 kJ (45 Cals) and less than 1 g of fat.

Winkles

Another shellfish with a round shell and edible flesh. Serve steamed. Extremely rich in iron. 50 g of winkles (flesh only) have 155 kJ (37 Cals) and almost no fat.

Yabbies

A freshwater crayfish, yabbies live in creeks, dams, lakes and even in swamps. They can reach a weight of 300 g and the meat in their tails and claws is sweet and succulent.

Yabbies can be cooked in boilng water for about 5 mins (until they turn pink) or are delicious barbecued. Use them like a small lobster or crayfish; they have similar nutritional value.

SEAL MEAT

The flesh of the seal is a staple part of the traditional Eskimo diet. The flesh is covered with a layer of fat which is high in omega 3 fatty acids. These are thought to have given the Eskimos protection from heart disease, in spite of their high-fat diet (see Eskimo diet, page 113).

SEA URCHIN

see Seafood.

SEAWEED

There are many edible seaweeds which grow throughout the world. They are used in some Asian diets, especially in Japan. Thickening substances, including agar-agar and carageenan have also been extracted from seaweeds and used in jellies, thickened cream and various desserts. Some of the types of seaweed used are listed below. They are rich in minerals, especially iodine. The ability of seaweeds to concentrate minerals may have been an advantage in the past, but it can now prove a health hazard in areas where there has been any industrial contamination. Heavy metals such as mercury and arsenic are concentrated in seaweeds, making some unfit for human consumption.

- *Carrageenan* — also known as Irish moss, this product is hand-raked in Northern Europe and parts of the United States. It can be steamed and used as a vegetable like spinach. Its main use is as a source of agar-agar gum which can be extracted from carrageenan and used as a thickener in foods such as cream, jellies, custards or other prepared desserts and salad dressing. This gum is also used to provide moisture in foods such as fruit cakes. Carrageenan can be a valuable form of dietary fibre. Food additive no. 407.
- *Dulse* — a red-coloured seaweed harvested in Britain, Iceland and parts of Canada. It is eaten fresh as a vegetable but is more often dried and consumed as a chewy snack or soaked and used in stir-fried dishes or soups.

- *Jellyfish seaweed* — this yellow-coloured product is sold as seaweed but is actually strips of jellyfish which are salted and dried. Used in China and Japan.
- *Kelp* — A seaweed often used as a supplementary source of iodine and other minerals. Unfortunately, kelp not only concentrates useful minerals but also undesirable metals such as arsenic or mercury. For this reason, other sources of iodine (such as fish, vegetables or milk) are preferable.

  Dried kelp is a good source of iron and iodine but its protein is not of a high quality. It is often a good source of arsenic! Kelp tablets are no longer permitted to be sold in many states of Australia since their arsenic level exceeds recommended levels. When dried, 20 g of kelp has 260 kJ (60 Cals).

  See also Food poisoning.
- *Kombu* — A dried kelp which is popular in Japan. After washing, it is used in soups and as a drink.
- *Laver* — another red-coloured seaweed gathered in Britain for many centuries. Sea lettuce is one type which is used in soups and salads. It is usually pressed into thin sheets and dried to form a product called nori which is used in Japanese cuisine for making sushi or as a garnish. Mashed and boiled, it forms a food called laverbread.
- *Mekabu* — another Japanese seaweed which is dried. Usually soaked to add to soups.
- *Wakame* — the main type of seaweed used in Japan. Broken into small pieces and added to soups.

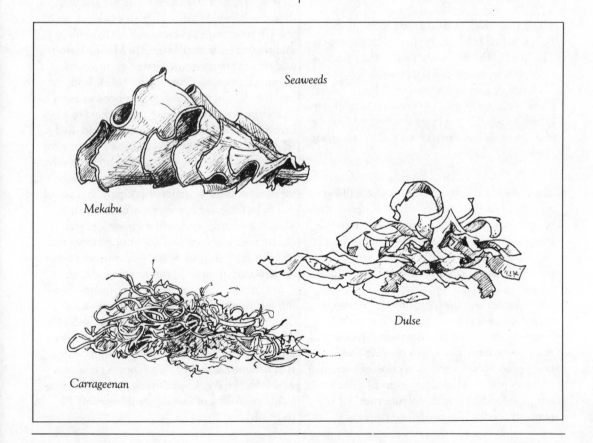

Seaweeds

Mekabu

Dulse

Carrageenan

SEEDS

Many fruits are eaten with their seeds. Some of the foods we call nuts are actually seeds. The seeds of some fruits contain toxic substances such as cyanide. This includes seeds from apples, apricots, peaches and plums. Other seeds, however, are excellent sources of nutrients and are delicious when roasted.

Pepitas

Green kernels from pumpkin seeds which can be eaten as they are or added to vegetarian dishes. Like most seeds, they are a good source of vitamin E and also provide iron, zinc, magnesium, potassium, protein, dietary fibre and some of the B complex vitamins. Of their fat, 48 per cent is polyunsaturated, 33 per cent is monounsaturated and only 20 per cent is saturated. A 25 g serve has 545 kJ (130 Cals).

Poppy

These tiny black or white seeds come from the opium poppy but have no narcotic properties. The fluid in the bud which forms the opium is only present before the poppy seeds form. White poppy seeds are used in Indian cooking; black seeds are popular in breads, cakes and in Jewish cuisine. The poppy is native to Greece and the seeds have been used since prehistoric times.

Safflower

These crunchy seeds come from the safflower, an annual flowering plant which is native to parts of Asia and Africa. Safflower is now grown in the United States, Australia, Israel and Canada for its seeds. From these the polyunsaturated safflower oil is extracted and used in polyunsaturated margarines and mayonnaises and the high-protein residue is used in stock feeds.

Eating the safflower seeds themselves would make more sense since they provide dietary fibre, protein and a good selection of minerals and vitamins (including vitamin E). The fat in safflower seeds is mainly polyunsaturated. 77 per cent is polyunsaturated, 13 per cent is monounsaturated and 10 per cent is saturated. 25 g of safflower seeds have 545 kJ (130 Cals) and 10 g fat.

Safflower seeds are delightful added to breads or biscuits and can be used in mueslis or various vegetable dishes.

Sesame

Sesame seeds come from a plant which is native to Asia and East Africa and is one of the world's oldest cultivated crops. There is evidence of the Chinese using sesame seeds 5000 years ago and they are also widely used in Middle Eastern and other Asian cuisines, often ground to a paste. Their oil has long been valued, both for making the finest Chinese ink blocks and as a flavouring for foods. They can be added to breads, biscuits and cakes or toasted and used with vegetable dishes, muesli or as a coating for various foods in place of (or with) breadcrumbs.

The sesame seed was once thought to have mystical powers — hence the 'Open Sesame' of Ali Baba fame. This was perpetuated in the idea that sesame seeds will increase virility. Sesame seed oil certainly does not go rancid as fast as other oils (due to its high content of the antioxidant vitamin E) but sesame seeds are simply a highly nutritious product rather than a miracle food. They are rich in vitamin E, dietary fibre, protein, zinc and iron as well as containing many other minerals and vitamins. However, their supposed high calcium content is of little use since they also contain oxalates which bind the calcium, making it unavailable to humans. 10 g of sesame seeds have 245 kJ (60 Cals) and 5 g of fat.

Sunflower

Native to North America, the sunflower was taken to Europe as a decorative plant. During the eighteenth century, sunflowers were being grown in France and parts of Germany for their seeds and the oil they contain. Today, the sunflower is widely cultivated so that its oil can be extracted and used as a vegetable oil and for making polyunsaturated margarine. The USSR is now the largest producer of sunflowers and they are also widely grown in the United States.

Like all seeds, sunflower seeds themselves make a very worthwhile addition to the diet. They are high in protein and dietary fibre and a good source of minerals, including iron. Their fat is largely polyunsaturated — 69 per cent polyunsaturated, 20 per cent saturated and 11 per cent monounsaturated. 25 g of sunflower seed kernels have 585 kJ (140 Cals) and 12 g fat.

SELENIUM

An essential trace element which is present in cereals and meat if the soil in the area contains sufficient selenium. Selenium has an antioxidant role and takes part in several enzymic reactions. In areas where the selenium content of the soil is low, such as in parts of China, there is a high incidence of cancer of the oesophagus and a defect in the heart muscle (Keshan's disease). There is also a suggestion that a lack of selenium may be involved in cardiovascular disease and the body's general immune response to infection and muscular disease.

Since selenium is quite toxic in excess, it is not permitted to be sold as a supplement in some areas. The first signs of selenium poisoning include a garlicky breath, loss of hair and nails and then skin lesions and disorders of the nervous system.

At present, not enough is known about selenium for a recommended daily intake to have been set. A safe and adequate level is estimated as 50–200 mg a day. As little as 5 times this upper limit has been found to be toxic.

The richest food sources (depending on the soil) are wholemeal flour and bread, mackerel, pork, cheese, egg, fish, rice, almonds and beef. Most fruits and vegetables and milk have little selenium. The normal concentration of selenium in the blood is 2.78 mmol/l of blood.

SEMILLON
see Wine, Varieties.

SEMOLINA

The inner part of the wheat grain, or endosperm. Used for making pasta or a porridge. Semolina is an excellent source of complex carbohydrate and provides some vitamins and minerals, protein and dietary fibre. 100 g of raw semolina have 1465 kJ (350 Cals).

SENNIT
see Fish, Pike.

SEREH POWDER
see Herbs, Lemongrass.

SERINE

An amino acid which is not essential as it can be made in the body.

SEROTONIN

A substance which is made in the body from the amino acid tryptophan. Serotonin functions as a neuro-transmitter and carries messages to nerve and brain cells. It appears to be involved in sleep. For this reason, tryptophan is sometimes given as a mild sleeping drug. Milk contains tryptophan and has been recommended as a hot drink before bed to aid sleep. Some malted milk products are higher in tryptophan. Serotonin also acts to constrict blood vessels and thus helps stop bleeding. Some drugs used in treating depression cause serotonin to be released from storage sites at nerve endings. The hallucinogenic drug LSD may inhibit the action of serotonin.

See also Mood, and food.

SESAME OIL
see Oils.

SESAME SEEDS
see Seeds.

SHALLOTS
see Vegetables.

SHARK
see Fish.

SHELLFISH

Any aquatic creature without a backbone but possessing a shell. Includes molluscs and crustaceans. Abalone, clams, crab, crayfish, limpets, lobster, oysters, mussels, prawns (or shrimp), scallops, scampi and whelks are commonly consumed shellfish.

SHERBET

Taking its name from the Persian 'sharbat', meaning an iced fruit drink, sherbet is a frozen dessert made with water, sugar, flavourings (often fruit) and some milk or cream. In the United States, sherbet must contain between 1 and 2 per cent butterfat. Sorbets do not need to contain any dairy products. No such laws apply in countries like Australia and New Zealand where sherbets are usually home-made desserts.

SHERRY
see Drinks, Alcoholic.

SHIRAZ
see Wine, Varieties.

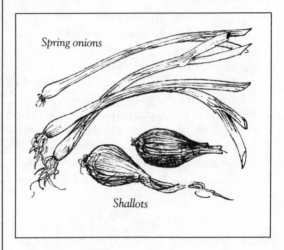

Spring onions

Shallots

SHISH KEBAB
see Kebab.

SHITAKE
see Vegetables, Mushroom.

SHORTBREAD

Crisp biscuits made from butter, sugar and plain flour. Traditionally eaten in Scotland at New Year. The dough is well kneaded until it becomes smooth and buttery. It is then pressed into a shallow tin and decorated before being baked in a moderate oven. Shortbread does not have the correct flavour if made with margarine. With its high content of butter, it is high in kilojoules. 1 piece (40 g) has 865 kJ (205 Cals).

SHORTCAKE

An American dessert made from butter, flour, sugar, baking powder and egg. The raw mixture is quite dry and patted into a baking tin then baked in a fairly hot oven. When cooked, it is split in halves and decorated with whipped cream and strawberries (or other fruit). It has a texture halfway between a soft cake and a biscuit and is served warm or cold. A typical piece of shortcake with cream and strawberries has about 1885 kJ (450 Cals).

SHORTCRUST PASTRY
see Pastry.

SHORTENING

Fats or oils which are added to flour-based pastries or cakes to 'shorten' the gluten fibres from the wheat protein which would otherwise produce a crusty cake.

In cakes, shortening acts more like a mechanical leavening agent, creating air cells when whipped with sugar.

In the home kitchen the most common shortenings used are butter or margarine. Commercial shortenings are made from hydrogenated vegetable oils (usually palm kernel oil), whipped and then allowed to form a soft substance. These shortenings contain a high percentage of saturated fats.

The ideal shortening for pastry is lard since it forms large crystals which will hold pastry layers apart.

SHORT SOUP

A Chinese soup also called wonton soup. The basic soup stock contains small dumplings consisting of a small square of pasta usually filled with minced pork, shallots, prawns, ginger and soy sauce.

SHOYU

Japanese soy sauce (see page 301) made from fermented soya beans, roasted wheat and salt.

SHRIMP
see Seafood, Prawn; Shrimp.

SIDEROSIS

A condition which develops from excessive amounts of iron which are deposited in the liver, pancreas and joints. Develops into the condition haemochromatosis (see page 175). Usually arises from taking excessive doses of iron or from regular cooking of acidic foods in iron pots. In some parts of Africa excess iron comes from the local beers which are brewed in iron pots.

SILICON

Possibly an essential mineral for humans. Silicon is thought to be involved in connective tissues and in minerals being deposited in bones. It is certainly dangerous in excess as has been shown by the hazards of silica dust in the lungs. Silicon is found in safe quantities in wholegrain cereals and citrus fruits. The exact amount required is not known.

SILVERBEET
see Vegetables, Spinach.

SILVERSIDE
see Meat.

SILVER WAREHOU
see Fish.

SIMPLE SUGARS
see Carbohydrates.

SKATE
see Fish.

SKATOLE

One of the products which results from a breakdown of the amino acid tryptophan. Partly responsible for the odour of human faeces.

SKIN

The largest organ in the human body, the skin can be a reflection of the adequacy of the diet. It really is a wonderful organ, keeping the flesh in and the water out, repairing itself when cut or bruised, and stretching or shrinking when we gain or lose weight.

Many factors can affect the skin, including sunlight (which ages the skin as well as causing freckles and other changes in pigmentation) and chemical agents in soaps and cosmetics. Diet can also affect the skin.

A deficiency or an excess of vitamin A can make the skin dry and rough. A lack of some of the B vitamins, especially riboflavin, can produce a waxy dermatitis. Too much niacin, from supplements, can cause a red rash on the skin, while a lack of the same vitamin causes a pustular dermatitis. A lack of essential polyunsaturated fatty acids can also produce a rough, reddish skin.

Basically, the skin is made of protein, but taking extra protein will not give you better skin. However, if a large amount of skin repair is required, for example, after burns or surgery, protein needs do increase significantly as the skin repairs itself.

Adequate fluid is also important for the whole body, including the skin. During dehydration, the skin becomes more wrinkled. Athletes and those who exercise should also remember that a great deal of water is lost from the skin. Whatever your level of fitness, the loss of water through the skin during exercise is related to your skin area. Large people lose more water through the skin than smaller people.

For a healthy skin, it is important that the general diet is good. This means including plenty of fresh fruits and vegetables, wholegrain breads and cereal products plus some foods such as fish, seeds or nuts to supply some essential fatty acids.

See also Acne.

SKINFOLD THICKNESS

Using calipers, the thickness of a fold of skin can be determined as a measure of subcutaneous body fat. The areas usually chosen for skinfold measurements include just under the shoulder blade, the underside of the upper arm, on the stomach, on the inside of the thigh and just above the hip bone. By totalling the sum of these skinfold measurements, an estimation of whether you are carrying too much fat can be made. The old method of relating the sum of skinfold measurement to a chart which gave a percentage body fat estimation is not considered valid.

SLIMMING
see Weight Reduction.

SLIPPERY ELM

The bark of this small North American tree is used as a laxative. Since it causes stomach cramps and is toxic, its use is inadvisable.

SLIVOVITZ
see Drinks, Alcoholic.

SMALL INTESTINE

The length of intestine from the end of the stomach to the beginning of the colon is called the small intestine. Most of the digestion and absorption of foods takes place in the small intestine. It consists of 3 sections: the duodenum, the jejunum and the ileum and has a total length of 6.5—7.5 m.

The duodenum is 25—30 cm long and most of the break down of proteins, fats and carbohydrates occurs here. The liver, pancreas and gallbladder provide juices containing enzymes which digest each of these nutrients. In spite of some fad diets, the digestion of proteins, fats and carbohydrates can proceed quite harmoniously together.

The jejunum extends to about half way down the small intestine and much of the absorption of nutrients occurs here. The ileum, in the lower part of the abdomen, is also involved in the absorption of some nutrients, especially some vitamins and minerals. Under normal circumstances, food remains in the small intestine from 3—6 hours before its residues pass through to the large intestine.

About 9 l of fluid enter the small intestine each day. This includes about 5 l from food, drinks, saliva and gastric juices, plus 4 l from bile, pancreatic juice and secretions from the small intestine. About 4 or 5 l of fluid is reabsorbed in the jejunum and an additional 3—4 l is absorbed in the ileum. The remaining 1.5 l goes through to the large intestine. Amino acids, sugars, vitamins and minerals are also broken down and absorbed from the small intestine each day.

SMELL

This sense is very important in our enjoyment of food. It also helps warn us of some foods being unfit to eat. There are some foods we smell before putting them in our mouths. But with others, what we think we are tasting is really what we smell as we swallow the food. During some blindfolded, olfactory-blocked tests, subjects were unable to distinguish the taste of foods normally thought to be strong-tasting including coffee, chocolate and garlic. It turns out that we really only smell these foods, and do not taste them at all. Other foods such as onion are tasted as well as being recognised by our sense of smell.

Our olfactory nerve cells have a direct line to the brain. Unlike other nerve cells, olfactory cells can be regenerated. They are replaced after about 6—8 weeks.

A loss of a sense of smell is sometimes due to a deficiency of zinc.

SMOKED FOODS

Smoking is one of the oldest methods of preserving foods. The smoke has the effect of drying the product and making it inhospitable to bacteria. Various chemical substances in wood smoke also act as preservatives. Some of these act by being toxic to bacteria while the phenolic compounds in smoke stop the fats in foods such as meats from oxidising and going off. The whole process of smoking also gives a characteristic flavour to the food. Since smoke does contain some cancer-causing substances, eating lots of smoked foods is not advisable.

SMOKING

Cigarette smoking not only makes it difficult

for the taste buds to work properly, but it actually decreases the appetite. In addition, smoking is a proven risk factor for heart disease. The nicotine in cigarettes also destroys vitamin C although the quantity could be replaced by eating 1 extra orange a day.

Ex-smokers often find they gain weight after stopping their smoking habit. This is due to increased appetite and increased flavour of foods and also to the fact that many people reach for food in place of a cigarette. Cigarette smoking also has the effect of increasing the number of kilojoules burned for basic metabolism.

For those who want to give up the unhealthy habit of cigarettes and do not want to gain weight, the following may be helpful:

- Divide the day's food into, say, 8 smaller portions rather than eating 3 meals a day. This has the effect of stimulating metabolic rate (to take over the effect of the cigarettes) and also gives you planned snacks rather than picking up any food which happens to be handy at those times when you would once have had a cigarette.
- Increase your exercise. This also stimulates the basic metabolic rate. It gives you something to do and allows you to experience the joy of physical activity with lungs which are not full of the aftermath of a cigarette.
- Eat slowly and enjoy every mouthful.
- Find a healthy habit to replace the cigarette which may have once signified the end of a meal. Some people go off and brush their teeth; some finish with a cup of tea; others get up and go for a walk or sit in a different spot and listen to a record. Meditation can also help.

SMOOTHIE
see Drinks, Non-alcoholic.

SNACKS

There is nothing inherently wrong with

snacking. Unfortunately many of the snack foods create their own problems by being high in fat, sugar and/or salt and lacking nutritional value. Many are harmful to teeth and the habit of eating frequently means that there are more acid attacks on teeth.

If snacks consist of healthy items such as fruit, vegetables, breads or cereal products, there is no harm in having smaller meals and between-meal snacks. For the overweight or those who have high blood cholesterol levels, such an eating pattern can be beneficial. Studies have shown that frequent healthy meals and snacks can stimulate the body's metabolism.

The reality is, however, that most people snack on biscuits, cakes, lollies, chocolates, potato crisps, doughnuts, soft drinks and pastries. None of these foods can be classed as nutritionally desirable for most people. Many people also find that any time they begin to eat, they overeat. For such people, 3 meals a day, in the more controlled situation of sitting at a table to eat, can help reduce their total food intake.

The common snack foods themselves are the major problem. Biscuits, cakes, pastries, chocolates, doughnuts and sweet snacks usually contain a high level of fat as well as sugar. Most have a low nutritional value and a high kilojoule level. They are damaging to teeth and are suitable only as occasional extras in the diet.

Potato crisps and savoury snack foods are high in fat and salt and have little nutritional value. The many extruded savoury snacks supply fat, salt and artificial colouring and flavouring. Again they are suitable only as occasional extras.

Lollies, sweets and chocolates also have a high kilojoule level and are harmful to teeth, chocolate being less harmful than other sweets. These foods should only be eaten occasionally, and only when teeth can be brushed soon afterwards.

Many children will not eat nutritious meals because they are still full of their snacks when mealtime arrives. Snack foods with a low fat content, such as fruits, muffins, bread or toast are more suitable since they fill the child at the time but are digested fast enough that hunger will have returned after a couple of hours.

SNAILS

Since the ancient Greeks pronounced them as a delicacy, snails have been considered a human food. Served in French restaurants, they are known as 'escargot' and are usually served hot with garlic and butter or placed in a spicy tomato stew. To cook snails, place some butter creamed with garlic in each snail shell, add the snail, top with more butter, place upright and bake for 6–7 mins.

SNAPPER
see Fish.

SNOW PEAS
see Vegetables, Peas.

SOBA

A popular Japanese noodle made from buckwheat. Usually presented in special bowls and accompanied by nori (Seaweed, Laver, see page 311) and Horseradish.

SODA WATER
see Water.

SODIUM

Sodium is the major electrolyte in the fluids which surround the body's cells, including the plasma portion of blood. Along with potassium, sodium balances the amount of water inside body cells and in the spaces around the cells. Sodium also looks after the balance between acidity and alkalinity and controls the pressure and volume of the blood.

Most of our sodium comes from salt. That is a problem in Western societies since most people eat far more salt than the body needs.

The kidneys control the amount of sodium in the body. When we eat too much salt, the kidneys excrete the excess sodium in the urine. After a salty meal, the kidneys need extra water to get rid of the sodium and so we feel thirsty. The kidneys also stop the body losing too much sodium. If the level of sodium in the body drops too low, the kidneys stop sodium being lost in the urine and return it to the blood.

Some sodium is also lost in sweat, although the body compensates for this and those who live in a hot climate or who exercise regularly lose little sodium by this route. With heavy sweating, the kidneys simply reabsorb a little more sodium. Except with kidney failure or after a period of vomiting or diarrhoea, sodium losses are easily controlled by the kidneys. Too much sodium is a much greater problem than too little.

During strenuous physical activity, water is needed *inside* the cells to allow for energy to be produced. Too much sodium (from salt) pulls the water *out* of the cells and the energy-producing reactions in the muscle cells cannot function efficiently.

After heavy sweating the *concentration* of sodium in the body fluids is *increased*. It is important to replace fluid losses *before* taking in extra salt. Salt tablets are particularly undesirable for sportspeople because they will further increase the concentration of salt in the body. They also draw too much water into the intestine, causing nausea and vomiting.

The kidneys do a good job of disposing of excess sodium from the body but after years of this, they sometimes start to retain too much sodium. This excess sodium then holds extra water in the blood, causing the blood vessels to become waterlogged. Once this occurs, the small blood vessels become overly sensitive to signals which cause them to contract and become tight. The heart then has to work harder to force blood through the narrowed, stiffer blood vessels — and the blood pressure rises.

Most people take in a lot of sodium from salt in processed and fast foods, as well as the salt they add to foods during cooking and at the table. The excessive amount of salt in the Western diet is a major factor in many of the cases of high blood pressure.

Sodium also has an indirect effect on bones. Strong bones require calcium but the more salt you eat, the greater the loss of calcium in urine. Those at risk of osteoporosis (see page 256) should therefore avoid eating too much salt.

See also Salt.

Food sources of sodium

FOOD	SODIUM (mg)
Fresh vegetables, av. serve	2–30
Beetroot, 100 g	54
Carrots, 100 g	47
Celery, 100 g	88
Endive, 100 g	76
Silverbeet, 100 g	200
Spinach, 100 g	21
Fruit, av. serve	2–10
Milk, regular or skim, 250 mL glass,	120
Yoghurt, 200 g carton	160
Cheese, 30 g	195
Cottage cheese, 75 g	305
Egg, 1	70
Steak, grilled, 150 g	80
Lamb chops, grilled, 2	90
Pork steak, cooked, 100 g	60
Chicken breast, cooked, 100 g	60
Fish, 150 g	130
Tuna, canned, 100 g	475
Tuna, canned in water, 100 g	80
Kidneys, lamb, cooked, 100 g	200
Liver, cooked, 100 g	100
Ham, leg, 100 g	1580
Steak and onions, canned, 200 g	900
Hamburger patty, pre-prepared, 120 g	850
Sausages, 2	1300
Luncheon meats, av. 50 g slice	385
Salami, av. 50 g slice	730
Baked beans in tomato sauce, 100 g	375
Hamburger, large	1080
Cheeseburger	815

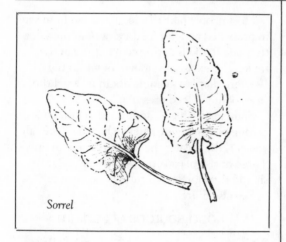

Sorrel

Barbecued chicken, $\frac{1}{4}$	180
Meat pie, 1	1030
Sausage roll, 1	840
Hot chips, av. serve	620
Fish in batter, 1 piece	685
Chinese take-away, av. meal	2350
Pizza, $\frac{1}{4}$ large pizza	1370
Potato crisps, 30 g	280
Salted nuts, 50 g	150
Pretzels, 30 g	590
Bread, 2 slices	240
Grains (eg. oats, rice), 100 g	3 – 30
Cornflakes, 30 g	330
Bran cereal, 50 g	255 – 740
Cracker biscuits, small, 6	200
Crispbread, 6	210
Shortbread biscuits, 2	200
Sweet biscuits, 2	120
Margarine or butter, 10 g	85
Yeast extract, amount on 1 slice bread	110
Peanut butter, 40 g	140
Salad dressings, 30 mL	235

SODIUM BICARBONATE
see Baking soda.

SOFT DRINKS

In making soft drinks, or carbonated beverages, water is first purified and mixed with sugar to form a syrup to which food acids, and a range of artificial colourings, flavourings and preservatives are added. More purified water is then put into the syrup and carbon dioxide is added under pressure to produce the familiar bubbles. Once the carbon dioxide has been added, the mixture is poured into bottles or canned. Artificially sweetened soft drinks do not use any sugar but use aspartame, saccharin or cyclamates instead (see page 27).

People in the United States, particularly children and teenagers, are the world's highest consumers of soft drinks. In countries like Australia, consumption is also high at about 80 l per person per year. Since many people do not drink any soft drinks, this average per capita consumption hides some very large intakes of soft drinks.

A 375 ml can of soft drink has 40 g of sugar — the equivalent of 10 cubes — an amount far greater than any person would ever add to other liquids. This large quantity of sugar is possible because the food acids take away what would otherwise be a somewhat sickly sweetness. Nutritionists often ask why the acid could not be removed and the sugar content reduced. The reply is usually that the drink would not have the right 'mouth feel'! Each can of soft drink has approximately 650 kJ (155 Cals). Soft drinks have no nutritional value.

Low-kilojoule soft drinks have virtually no kilojoules, and, presumably, no 'mouth feel'. They contain artificial sweeteners (saccharin, cyclamates or aspartame) in place of sugar.

Cola soft drinks dominate the soft drinks available throughout the world. They are flavoured with an extract from the kola nut and contain added caffeine.

See also Cola.

SOLANINE

A collection of glycosides which occur just under the skin and in the sprouts, stems and leaves of potato plants. Exposure of the potato to light increases the solanine concentration which appears as a green colour on the potato skin.

See also Food poisoning.

SOLE
see Fish.

SORBET

A flavoured ice made from fruit or vegetable juice, water and sugar. Some contain flavourings or egg whites. The juice mixture is frozen and then beaten to break up the ice crystals and re-frozen. A sorbet is sometimes served between courses at a formal dinner and is supposed to cleanse the palate. Sorbets are also served as a dessert. Half a cup of sorbet has 630 kJ (150 Cals) and no fat.

SORBIC ACID

A preservative added to cheese (especially processed cheese) to prevent mould forming. Also used in soft drinks, cakes and bread to prevent spoilage. Sorbic acid occurs naturally in berries but is usually manufactured. Additive no. 200.

SORBITOL

Sorbitol is a sugar alcohol which is used in some food products in place of sugar. This is of limited benefit since sorbitol contributes the same number of kilojoules as sugar. It was originally used because it is metabolised without involving insulin and this was thought to be a benefit for diabetics. Since most diabetics need to consider the total kilojoules they consume, sorbitol is of limited use.

Sorbitol can cause digestive upsets. A dose of 10 g of sorbitol — the amount in 4–5 sorbitol-containing mints or a tablespoon of some carbohydrate-modified jams — causes stomach cramps and diarrhoea.

It is a natural ingredient in apples and pears and excessive consumption of these fruits may increase flatus. In moderation, they cause no

problems. A variety of medicinal syrups, including multivitamins, expectorants and bronchodilators may also include sorbitol.

SORGHUM
see Grains.

SORREL
see Vegetables.

SOUFFLE

A very light baked dish, either sweet or savoury, whose airy lightness comes from beaten egg whites. The word 'souffle' comes from the French word 'souffler', meaning 'to blow' or 'to breathe'. Stiffly beaten egg whites are incorporated into a variety of base mixtures ranging from a sweetened fruit puree to a thick white sauce enriched with egg yolks.

When egg whites are beaten, the albumin traps air creating a foam. When this foam is cooked, the trapped air becomes hot and the foam expands. Normally such air would eventually burst out and the foam would collapse. However, the ovalbumin proteins in the egg white coagulate when heated and hold the foam stable. In making a souffle, the oven temperature must be hot enough to set the egg proteins before the foam has expanded to its maximum level but not so hot that the top burns before the inside is cooked. When the hot souffle is taken out of the oven, the trapped air cools and contracts so that the souffle soon collapses. Hence the cook's insistence that a souffle waits for no-one!

Salt should never be added to egg whites as it increases the time for beating the egg whites and reduces the stability of the foam. A very small amount of acid (a tiny pinch of cream of tartar) will increase the foam's stability but even a small excess of acid will make the souffle collapse faster.

A souffle made with a sauce of butter, flour and egg yolks appears as a light dish. However, an individual cheese souffle contains 1360 kJ

(325 Cals). Sweet souffles made from egg whites and sweetened fruit puree have approximately 335—420 kJ (80—100 Cals) and no fat.

SOUPS

Soups have long been a basic source of nourishment for humans. By adding various ingredients to water and cooking the mixture, small quantities of foods could be shared among many. It was also a good way to extract the flavour from bones and to soften otherwise tough cuts of meat.

Until recent times, soups were a meal in themselves. Hearty chunks of meat, legumes and vegetables all went into one big pot. The cooking was easy, the flavour was good and it was a simple meal to prepare for a large number of people. Any leftovers could be used at a later meal.

In many Western countries, soups have become part of a meal, usually being much lighter and served as a first course. With the relaxing of the social aspects of eating, hearty soups as the basis of a meal are enjoying something of a revival.

Canned soups, dehydrated soups in packets and ready to serve soups are available. Some of these suffer from being highly salted. Many have so little of the 'real' ingredients present that they cannot be made successfully without salt or the resulting product is tasteless. Apart from some of the newer ready-to-serve soups, a true soup still needs to be made from basic ingredients.

Stocks are the basis of soups and can be made by boiling up bones (chicken, beef, veal or fish) to extract their flavour. A variety of other ingredients can then be added (see page 330).

The nutritional value of soups will vary widely according to their ingredients. It can range from providing an excellent balance of nutrients to giving mainly a lot of salt and kilojoules derived from the starches used to thicken the mixture. In general, a serving of canned or reconstituted soup has about 295 kJ (70 Cals). A clear soup or consomme has only about 65 kJ (15 Cals) per serve.

SOURDOUGH

Famous in San Francisco, sourdough breads are made by using a different strain of yeast from that used in other breads. The yeast used, *Saccharomyces exiguus*, thrives in acidic conditions and does not make use of the maltose in the grain, as regular yeasts do. This means that the maltose is available for a group of bacteria which thrive on it and produce lactic and acetic acids when given a temperature of about 30°C and a pH of 3.8—4.5.

In regular breads, the maltose is used by the yeast and so such bacteria cannot grow. The pH level in a normal yeast dough is also closer to 5.5.

Sourdough breads can be made by allowing yeast to ferment before adding it to the flour and water mixture. Such breads do not achieve the unique flavour of the sourdoughs made in San Francisco.

SOURSOP
see Fruit.

SOUSE

Pieces of pork in a spicy jelly made of vinegar with dill, capsicum and bay leaves. Soused meat generally refers to meat which has been marinaded in vinegar with herbs and spices.

SOUTHERN COMFORT
see Drinks, Alcoholic.

SOYA BEAN
see Legumes.

SOYA BEAN MILK

Soya bean milk is made by soaking soya beans in water, draining them, grinding the beans, simmering them for an hour or 2 and then straining the liquid. It is widely used in China and is now available in cans, powdered or liquid form. As it is extracted, soya bean milk contains the same quantity of protein as cow's milk, has less than half the fat but only about one-fifth the calcium. Some commercial products are fortified with extra calcium to bring them to the same level as cow's milk. Some also have fat added to bring them to the same fat level as cow's milk. While some of this fat is polyunsaturated, it does contribute the same number of kilojoules as any other type of fat.

Soya bean milk is used in China because it can be prepared as required and thus does not need refrigeration. In Western countries, soya bean milk is mainly used by those with an allergy to cow's milk. Unfortunately, many infants who have a cow's milk allergy are also sensitive to soya bean milk.

100 mL of unfortified soya bean milk has 135 kJ (32 Cals), 1.5 g fat and 21 mg of calcium. 100 mL of fortified soya bean milk has 260 kJ (62 Cals), has 3.4 g fat and 117 mg calcium.

See also Legumes; Milk.

SOYA BEAN OIL
see Oils.

SOY SAUCE
see Sauces.

SPAGHETTI
see Pasta.

SPAGHETTI SQUASH
see Vegetables.

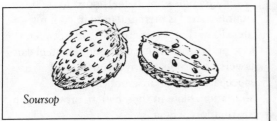
Soursop

SPARE RIBS

The rib bones of pigs or beef cattle, taken either from the belly of the animal or the actual rib bones themselves. They are usually barbecued or baked. Depending on the degree of trimming, spare ribs can be high in fat and kilojoules or moderately low. Usually served with a spicy barbecue sauce and eaten with the fingers.

SPECIFIC DYNAMIC ACTION (SDA)

The energy needed for the digestion, absorption and metabolism of foods can be measured and is known as the specific dynamic action of the food eaten. Pure protein requires more energy to digest and metabolise than pure fat which in turn takes a greater amount than pure carbohydrate. The effect of different nutrients was once considered to be important. However, in practice we rarely eat pure protein or pure fat. Egg white, for example, is one of the very few sources of pure protein which humans consume. Pure fat is available in butter, margarine or oil but it would be a bit hard to swallow. Almost as hard to swallow as some of the claims made for SDA! Even if we did eat lots of egg white, the effect on overall energy use would be minimal.

It is now known that the SDA for mixed nutrients is negligible but some of the literature available in health food shops still refers to the importance of SDA and the idea that protein is non-fattening has pervaded the thinking of many consumers and doctors for many years.

Specific dynamic action has also been used as the basis for some of the craziest slimming diets. A diet requiring its follower to eat 12 hard-boiled eggs a day, for example, maintained that the action of digesting the protein in the eggs would burn up more kilojoules than the eggs contributed. This is quite false, and, in any case, the fat present in the egg yolk would have ruined the supposed effect of the protein present.

SPHINGOMYELIN

A phospholipid (a combination of phosphorus and a fat) which also contains an alcohol called sphingosine. Both the brain and the nerves contain large quantities of sphingosine where it takes part in the transmission of signals in nerve cells.

SPICES

See following pages.

SPINACH

see Vegetables.

SPINKGANZ

German smoked goose. The breast of the goose is dry salted with salt and sodium nitrate and then smoked. The product is high in salt.

SPIRITS

see Drinks, Alcoholic, Proof (of alcohol).

SPIRULINA

A bluish-green algae which grows in some freshwater lakes. The algae can be dried and used as a food. It is high in protein, carotene and some of the B group vitamins, including small quantities of a substance which is similar to vitamin B_{12}. Unfortunately, the B_{12} look-alike in spirulina is of little use for humans. Spirulina also provides minerals so it has the potential to be a useful food. However, spirulina does not live up to many of the 'wonder food' claims made for it. It will not help you lose weight, it has no fat-dissolving properties, it will not provide instant energy, it does not help build muscle for sportspeople, it will not cure arthritis or any other disease.

SPLIT PEAS

see Legumes, Peas, Dried.

SPRAT

see Fish.

SPRING GREENS

see Vegetables.

SPRING ONIONS

see Vegetables, Shallots.

SPROUTS

see Vegetables, Bean; Brussels sprouts

SQUAB

A young pigeon, especially bred for eating. Usually only about 4 weeks old when killed and weighing about 400–700 g. Similar nutritional value to pigeon (see page 267).

SQUASH

see Vegetables.

SQUID

see Seafood.

STABILISERS

Substances added to foods to prevent parts of the item separating. For example, stabilisers are added to mayonnaise or various desserts to keep the fat evenly distributed throughout the food. Many stabilisers are derived from seaweeds or gums. They work in conjunction with emulsifiers in that the emulsifiers produce the consistency and the stabilisers maintain it.

STACHYOSE

A 4-unit sugar found in seeds.
    See also Oligosaccharides.

STAINLESS STEEL

An alloy material containing about 15 per cent chromium plus some nickel added to steel. Stainless steel is inert and used in cooking utensils so that no reaction occurs between the food and the utensil. Since stainless steel can develop hot spots, many stainless steel saucepans have an insert of copper or aluminium plate in their base to provide even distribution of heat.

SPICES

The history of spices would fill an entire book. In medieval times, spices were desirable for their unique flavours but also because they could be used to disguise foods which were no longer in prime condition. They were brought first from India and then from the Spice Islands, and there was great competition between nations to secure the highly profitable spice trade. Wars were fought and many lives lost and the triumphs of explorers such as Marco Polo, Vasco da Gama, Christopher Columbus, Ferdinand Magellan and Sir Francis Drake were due to their treasured cargoes of exotic Eastern spices. Indeed the history of the world owes a lot to the desire for spices.

Spices were expensive and a measure of status. Today many spices are still very expensive, with saffron and cardamom being amongst the most precious. Most, however, are affordable and add to our pleasure of eating.

Allspice

A spice ground from the dried unripe berry of a myrtle tree which grows in the West Indies and Central America. Sometimes called pimento. The flavour is rather like a mixture of cinnamon, nutmeg and cloves and can be used in pickles, cakes, biscuits and some meat dishes.

Anise

A herb whose fruit produces aniseed, used to flavour pastries, fish, meat and vegetable dishes and the liqueurs absinthe and pernod. Star anise is the dried fruit of an unrelated tree which grows in parts of Asia.

Caraway seeds

The seeds of a plant which grows wild all over Europe and parts of Asia. Originally eaten with apples, either raw or roasted, they are now mainly added to cakes, bread, cheese or cabbage dishes.

Cardamom

The seed pods of a plant which originated in India. The flavour is delicate and the ground seeds can be used in cakes and biscuits as well as in curry, pickles and chicken dishes. Cardamom-flavoured coffee is popular in Arab countries. After saffron and vanilla, cardamom is the next most expensive spice.

Cassia

Comes from the bark of a tree of the laurel family which is native to Burma. Also known as Chinese cinnamon and similar in flavour, cassia being a little harsher and more suited to curries than sweets. The easiest way to distinguish the two is by colour: cinnamon is brown; cassia is a darker reddish brown.

Cinnamon

The dried inner bark of a tree belonging to the laurel family and native to Sri Lanka. Widely grown in India, South America and the West Indies. Cinnamon was once valued more highly than gold and was the most valuable spice in the Dutch East India Company's trade. About 3000 BC, it played an important role in witchcraft, religious rites and embalming. Cinnamon is now used for flavouring baked goods, sweets, curries and drinks. Cassia is often substituted for true cinnamon. The latter is a tan colour in contrast to the reddish-brown of the stronger flavoured cassia.

Clove

The small dried bud of a tree which originated in the Molucca Islands in the East Indies. Its name comes from the Latin word for 'nail' which it resembles. Cloves have been used to sweeten the breath since about 300 BC. Most of the cloves sold throughout the world are now grown in Tanzania and half the total crop is used in Indonesia where it is smoked with tobacco. Oil of cloves contains a substance called eugenol which has local anaesthetic properties and has been used for centuries to alleviate toothache. In foods, cloves find a use in cakes and other baked goods, and in pickles, chutneys and curries.

Coriander

Used as both a herb (the leaves) and a spice (the ground seeds). Records from Egyptian papyrus show that coriander has been used for over 7000 years. In more recent times, it has been used in Thai cookery, in Indian curries and in some South American dishes.

Cumin

Sometimes known as cummin, this is an annual herb of the carrot family whose seeds are widely used to flavour curries and various legume dishes in Asian cookery, breads and cakes in Europe and sauces in South America (it provides the distinctive flavour of chilli con carne). Iran produces most of the world's cumin powder. Nutritionally, cumin is rich in iron, containing 66 mg per 100 g. Even as little as 5 g could thus provide a significant proportion of the daily needs.

The oil in cumin seeds is also used in perfumes and as an ingredient in some liqueurs.

Fennel seeds

The seeds of fennel are used in Asian and European cooking and have a slightly aniseed flavour. They are reputed to remove the smell of garlic from the breath.

Fenugreek

A spice made from slightly bitter, mustard-coloured seeds. Used in curry powders. Has a slightly 'raw' flavour and should be used sparingly. Best if roasted slightly before grinding.

Galangal

A root spice related to ginger but having a faint taste of camphor. Used in curries in Malaysia. Also used in bitters and some liqueurs.

Garam masala

A mixture of aromatic spices used in Asian and Middle Eastern cooking. There is no set recipe but the usual ingredients include cardamom, cinnamon, cumin, cloves, nutmeg and pepper. It is added just before the end of cooking a dish.

Ginger

The ground root of the ginger plant is used as a spice in both sweet and savoury dishes. The word ginger is derived from an old Sanskrit word meaning 'horn-shaped'.

The underground stem of the ginger plant is a rhizome which shoots and forms roots. It was first used as a food in China some 2500 years ago. It is still widely used in Chinese and Japanese cooking but has also found a place in the cuisine of Europe and North America. It contains small but insignificant quantities of nutrients. In the quantities eaten, its kilojoules can be ignored. A 5-g piece of ginger has less than 15 kJ (4 Cals.)

Juniper

Juniper berries are used in making gin but also delicious in dishes which include pork, veal and game meats. Juniper tea is used in some Scandinavian countries and is considered soothing.

Lengkuas

A member of the ginger family, lengkuas is widely used in powdered or dried form in Malaysian cooking. Also called laos. In the quantities consumed, lengkuas makes little nutritional contribution.

Mace

The outer covering layer of the nutmeg, an evergreen tree native to the Spice Islands.

Mace is separated from nutmeg by hand and allowed to dry before being cut into flakes or ground to a powder. Both mace and nutmeg were introduced to the Mediterranean region by Arab traders some 800 years ago and generated a high income. The Dutch became most aggressive in their efforts to win the spice trade and destroyed three-quarters of all the nutmeg trees to make the product a scarce and high-priced commodity. Mace has a slightly coarser flavour than nutmeg and is used in curries and pickles rather than desserts.

Mixed spice

Usually a mixture of cinnamon, nutmeg and cloves.

Mustard

see Mustard.

Nutmeg

The seed of an evergreen tree which grows in the Spice Islands. The oil of nutmeg contains a toxic substance called myristin which acts as a strong hallucinogen, causing headaches, vomiting and stomach cramps. Such symptoms would only occur if 1–2 whole nutmegs were consumed — a difficult task since large quantities of the spice have a strong bitter taste. Mainly used in small quantities in desserts, cakes, biscuits and curries.

Paprika

This powdered, dried sweet red pepper (or capsicum) is used in Eastern European cooking. Hungarian goulash relies on paprika for its flavour. Also used as a garnish on many dishes and in some cheese and potato dishes. Paprika should always be purchased in small quantities since it loses its flavour with storage.

Pepper

Both black and white pepper are the dried fruits of a tropical vine which grows in India and they represent the most commonly used spice throughout the world. To make black pepper, the fruits are picked green, allowed to mature in the sun to produce a stronger flavour and are then dried. For white pepper, the fruits are allowed to ripen to a red colour and are soaked in water, rubbed to remove the skins and then dried. The sharp bite of pepper comes from an alkaloid called piperine. This substance can irritate the lining of the stomach.

Pimento

see Allspice.

Saffron

The stigma of a type of crocus, saffron is the most expensive spice in the world. It must be harvested by hand and it takes over 1500 crocuses to provide 10 g of saffron. This valuable spice has been used for thousands of years and was introduced to Europe during the twelfth and thirteenth centuries. It is now used in Spanish and French cooking as well as having an important role in Indian and some Asian cuisines. Saffron is sometimes replaced with the cheaper yellow powder turmeric but the latter does not have the subtle and delightful flavour of the true saffron.

Star anise

The dried star-shaped fruit of a tree of the magnolia family, native to China. The seeds are contained in the pod and are ground to a powder to be used rubbed into the skin of chicken or duck. The aniseed flavour comes from an oil which is similar to that found in anise.

Turmeric

The dried ground stem of a plant found in Asia and the West Indies, turmeric is a bright yellow colour and is an ingredient of curry powders. It is also used as a fabric dye. Turmeric should be kept in a dark place since it loses its colour and flavour when exposed to sunlight.

STAPHYLOCOCCI
see Food poisoning.

STAR ANISE
see Spices.

STAR APPLE
see Fruit.

STARCH

The storage form of carbohydrate in plants. Starch consists of thousands of molecules of glucose arranged in straight and branched chains known as amylose and amylopectin (see page 22). Starches are found in grains and cereals, in vegetables (especially root vegetables and potatoes), legumes, nuts and seeds.

Modern dietary advice is that we should be eating more starch. However, since the term 'starch' had connotations of doughnuts, pies and sausage rolls for many people, the term 'complex carbohydrate' is now used in place of 'starch' to refer to the nutritionally desirable products such as grains, breads, cereals, legumes, nuts, seeds and vegetables.

The word 'starch' comes from a Germanic word meaning 'stiff' or 'strong'. Starches are useful because of their ability to thicken hot solutions. This occurs because the energy of hot liquid is sufficient to disrupt the starch granule which absorbs water, and it swells and forms gels. Cornflour or arrowroot are almost pure starch and so produce translucent thick gels. Wheat flour also contains some protein which packs the starch molecules more closely together so that they deflect light rays and do not give the translucency of pure starch.

As starch-thickened sauces cool, the amylose molecules form rather loose bonds between themselves and these take up water. Thus the sauce thickens as it cools. This is why a cook makes a sauce a little thinner than is desired at the stove, knowing that it will thicken when poured onto food.

Modified starches are used in many processed foods. These are basic starch molecules which have been oxidised, mixed into new cross linkages or pre-gelatinised (or pre-thickened). They are listed in the ingredients on food labels but have not been given additive numbers since they are regarded as forms of natural starch.

See also Amylopectin and Amylose.

STARCH BLOCKERS

There are substances in some legumes, especially raw kidney beans, which can interfere with the action of amylases, the enzymes which digest complex carbohydrates. These starch-blockers were isolated from kidney beans and sold as the latest weight reduction 'aid' in the United States. Unfortunately, they had several drawbacks including the fact that the undigested starch fermented and caused diarrhoea and stomach cramps, and also the fact that starches are not the major problems for the overweight — fats and alcohol have that role. These substances are not permitted for sale in Australia or New Zealand.

STAR FRUIT
see Fruit, Carambola.

STARVATION

Absence of food. Occurs in those who live in areas where there is insufficient food and also in Western society in those with anorexia nervosa who voluntarily starve (see page 24). As long as water is available, a person who is usually healthy can survive 6−7 weeks without food by using fat and breaking down muscle to supply energy for the vital organs. Exercise will not be possible and skin lesions will eventually develop due to vitamin deficiencies. A child, or someone who is already very thin, would not be expected to survive this long.

Terminal stages of starvation are usually accompanied by extreme weakness and diarrhoea. The kidneys cease to function and a build-up of nitrogenous waste products will cause a coma. Death usually occurs from disturbances to the heart muscle or from an infection in the lungs.

STEAKS
see Meat.

STEAMED FOODS

Foods can be cooked by placing in a container over boiling water. The steam from the water cooks the food without actually coming into contact with it. Steaming prevents some of the loss of vitamins into the water which accompanies boiling.

STEARIC ACID

A saturated fatty acid containing 18 carbons. Widely distributed in foods. Forms 11 per cent of the fat in milk, 9−10 per cent of that in human milk, 9 per cent of the fat in eggs, 27 per cent of the fat in suet, 15 per cent of the fat in beef, 6 per cent of that in chicken, 25 per cent of the fat in lamb, 27 per cent of the fat in chocolate and 11 per cent of the fat in Brazil nuts. Most other nuts and seafoods have little stearic acid.

STEATORRHOEA

The presence of fat in the faeces. Usually occurs because bile salts are not being produced or because pancreatic juices are not reaching the intestine to digest fats. Until the cause is remedied, a low-fat diet is advisable.

STERCULIA

The dried gum of an East Indian tree. Also known as karaya gum. The gum consists of several sugars (including rhamnose and galactose) and forms a mucilage in water. Used in faecal bulking agents in the treatment of constipation. Has also been shown to lower blood cholesterol levels and is used as a denture adhesive.

STERILISATION

Total destruction of all bacteria and their spores. Prolongs shelf life of a food, but usually the amount of heat required for the sterilisation destroys flavour, texture and colour. Nutritional value may also be altered.

STEROIDS
see Anabolic steroids.

STEROLS

Chemically, sterols are steroid alcohols. They are made up of a cyclic nucleus of 4 linked rings and an alcohol side chain. The most common sterol in foods is cholesterol. At one stage, some other sterols in oysters and other seafoods were inadvertently counted as cholesterol, giving these foods an apparently high level of cholesterol. Subsequent research showed that the sterols in these products did not have the same effect in the human body as cholesterol.

STEWS

Meats or other foods cooked in water or stock until tender. Since the gravy which forms around the ingredients of a stew is usually eaten, most of the vitamins which dissolve into it are also consumed. Stews are thus quite nutritious, depending on the basic ingredients.

STILTON
see Cheese.

STIR-FRYING

A method of cooking in which meats, fish, poultry and vegetables are placed in a wok over fairly high heat and tossed until cooked. Stir-frying can be done with a little oil or using a concentrated stock. Because the cooking period is brief, there is a good retention of vitamins and also the colour and texture in vegetables are retained. Many children who will not eat steamed or boiled vegetables are happy to have them stir-fried.

Originally a major cooking method in parts of China, stir-frying has now become common in countries such as the United States, Australia and New Zealand.

STOCK

The basis for most soups and sauces, stock is made by extracting the flavour from meats, bones and/or vegetables. For a brown stock, the meat or bones are browned in the oven or in a pot to produce a more intense flavour from the production of various amine compounds. White stocks are more subtle and the ingredients are not browned first. Veal and chicken bones are especially rich in collagen and so produce a 'sticky' stock which will set to a jelly when cooled or produce a thickened texture in a sauce when hot. See also page 322.

Stock cubes are made from dehydrated meat, yeast and vegetable extracts plus salt and some sugar and fat, usually beef fat. A stock cube has only 30 kJ (7 Cals) but has 309 mg of sodium.

STOLLEN

A German yeasted bread containing various dried fruits and nuts. The dough contains butter and eggs. Traditionally baked at Christmas. One slice (50 g) has 750 kJ (180 Cals).

STOMACH

The area between the oesophagus and the small intestine. The stomach has a strong muscular wall which secretes hydrochloric acid and gastric juices to begin the break down of the proteins in foods. In the stomach, food is mixed with the acid and passes to the small intestine as a thick creamy mass called chyme. Alcohol can be absorbed directly through the wall of the stomach. The primary function of the stomach is as a holding chamber for food before it passes to the small intestine where most digestion and absorption occurs.

STOMATITIS

Inflammation of the mouth. Usually only occurs from poor fitting dentures or from deficiencies of vitamins such as riboflavin or B_6. Severe iron deficiency may also cause stomatitis.

STONE FRUITS

see individual entries for apricots, nectarines, peaches, plums, under Fruit.

STOOL

Another term for faeces.

STOUT

see Drinks, Alcoholic.

STRASSBURG

see Sausages.

STRAWBERRY

see Fruit.

STRAW MUSHROOMS

see Vegetables, Mushrooms.

STREGA

see Drinks, Alcoholic.

STROKES

Strokes are the second most common cause of death in Australia, beaten only by coronary heart disease. A stroke (or cerebro-vascular

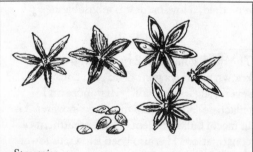

Star anise

accident) occurs when a blood clot forms in an artery leading to the brain. The harder or stiffer the arteries, and the more fatty deposits present, the more likely the chances of a stroke.

Strokes are caused by high blood pressure (or hypertension) and this is more likely when arteries are stiffened or partially clogged by fatty deposits. Excess weight or smoking cigarettes also increase blood pressure and the incidence of strokes.

STRUDEL

An Austrian pastry made from fine layers of delicate pastry filled with fruits, usually apples. The fine strudel pastry may also be wrapped around a savoury filling. An average serve has 1050 kJ (250 Cals).

SUCCOTASH

A traditional dish of American Indians, made by cooking corn and beans together. Although the Indians had no knowledge of modern biochemistry, succotash happens to contain a well-balanced mixture of amino acids.

See also Vegetarian diet.

SUCRASE

The enzyme which splits sucrose into its component sugars, glucose and fructose.

SUCROSE

The correct name for the sugar found principally in sugar cane and sugar beet. Made up of 1 molecule of glucose joined to 1 of fructose. Small amounts of sucrose are also found in some fruits and vegetables, especially in pineapples, peaches, apricots, sweetcorn and peas. However, these quantities are very small compared with the amounts added to foods.

See also Carbohydrates.

SUET

The fat around the kidneys of beef cattle and lambs. Bought as a solid lump of fat (usually from beef), it is grated and used in making puddings. 100 g have 3400 kJ (812 Cals).

SUGAR CANE

A member of the grass family, sugar cane originally grew in the South Pacific where its sweet sap was considered a delicacy. Sugar cane was taken to Asia many thousands of years ago, and was grown in India. Here, some time around 500 BC, the technique of pressing out the cane juice, boiling it down and allowing dark crystals to form was first developed.

By the sixth century AD, sugar cane was being grown and processed into crude brown crystals in North Africa, Spain and Syria. Consumption, however, was still very small.

In the fourteenth century, sugar crystals were being shipped from Africa and Spain to England to be used as a flavouring, mainly in medicines. The demand for sugar was growing but consumption was still small, amounting to only a few hundred grams per person per year.

By the early part of the sixteenth century, the Spanish had introduced sugar to the islands of the Caribbean in Central America where it flourished in the warmth and rain. Work on the sugar plantations was physically demanding and the Spanish were unwilling to do it themselves. The people of the Caribbean were coerced into working long and hard, but there were not enough of them to produce the amount of sugar which could be sold. And so the slave trade was born.

African slaves were brought across to work the sugar plantations and were forced to slave under inhuman conditions, growing and cutting the cane which provided enormous profits for the Portuguese and Spanish landowners. The first sugar factory opened in the Barbados in 1641, and, within a few years, the entire island was covered with sugar plantations. Other Caribbean islands followed.

The story of sugar cane is not a pleasant

episode in human history. Men and women lived and worked under appalling conditions to produce a substance of inferior nutritional value when compared with almost any other food. Sugar contains absolutely none of the vitamins, minerals, protein or dietary fibre needed for human health. It merely rots the teeth — and appeals to the taste buds.

It was not only sugar itself which contributed to the enormous profits to be made. Unwanted by-products from sugar refining could be used to make rum — a form of liquor which was cheap to produce since its raw material was otherwise regarded as waste.

The seventeenth century also saw an increasing popularity of coffee, tea and chocolate throughout Europe. Unlike the situation in the places where these drinks originated. Europeans preferred tea, coffee and chocolate to be sweetened with sugar. This increased the market for sugar still further. Sugar cane thus had a great effect on world trade and conditions and it is hard to think of any other food which could rival it for its influence on human affairs.

150 years ago, annual sugar consumption was of the order of 2 kg per person. Today, in most Western countries, annual sugar consumption is around 50 kg per person. In Australia, average consumption works out as 230 cubes of sugar (each weighing 4 g) per person per week. Most people are amazed that they could be consuming so much. More than 80 per cent of this sugar is present in processed foods and drinks.

Problems with sugar

Small quantities of sugar are unlikely to cause problems for most people. Even though it has no positive nutritional attributes, the average daily diet usually is not distorted by a small amount of sugar. Arguments between health professionals and the sugar industry usually centre on differing definitions of 'small'.

There is also no doubt that excess fats are a greater problem than excess sugar. However, it is often sugar which makes fats so palatable. Most people would not eat cakes, biscuits, icecream, desserts and chocolates if the sugar did not make them palatable. Those promoting sugar also argue that sugar makes other nutritious foods taste more palatable.

Sugar can become a problem when large quantities are eaten by people who are largely inactive. In Western populations, the majority of people are fairly inactive and need to curtail their kilojoule intake if they are to avoid obesity. However, the need for minerals, most vitamins, dietary fibre and protein remains. If a person needs to eat less, it makes good nutritional sense to cut back on foods which have little nutritional value and retain those which provide the essential nutrients. This is the chief reason why many countries have included advice to 'avoid eating too much sugar' in their dietary guidelines.

Sugar also plays a major role in dental decay unless the teeth are brushed immediately after eating sugar-containing foods. The effect on teeth is not confined to sugar, but refined sugar is recognised as the major culprit in this regard.

Sugar can also cause problems because it is not filling. A sugar-sweetened drink, for example, is no more filling than one without sugar. The sugar-sweetened beverage contributes kilojoules without necessarily satisfying the appetite.

Claims that sugar causes hyperactivity in children have not been proved by controlled tests. The reason for children's boisterous behaviour after a party cannot, at this stage, be blamed on sugar.

How much sugar?

It is not necessary to eat any sugar at all. However, a sugar-free life in most Western societies is difficult and also unnecessary. General recommendations are that sugar intake should not exceed 10 per cent of the day's kilojoules. Since sugar contributes 16 kJ/g

(4 Cals/g), a diet of 2000 Cals should not contain more than 50 g of sugar — less than half the typical intake in most Western countries.

Added sugar content of foods

FOOD	SUGAR (g)
1 level teaspoon	4
Typical sugar spoonful	8
Jam or honey (amount on 1 slice of bread or toast)	10
Fruit juice, sweetened, 250 mL	10
Thickshake, av.	25
Flavoured mineral water, 1 can	30
Soft drinks, 1 can	40
Egg custard, av. serve	10
Apple pie, 1 small	11
Icecream, av. serve	14
Iceblock on stick, av.	16
Jelly, av. serve	18
Chocolate flavouring, 2 tablespoons	26
Cake, iced, av. slice	30
Lollies, av., each	5
Biscuits, plain sweet, 2	6
Biscuits, chocolate, 2	9
Biscuits, cream-filled, 2	10
Health food bar, av. 50 g	11
Chocolate, 5 squares	20
Toffee, 30 g	20
Breakfast cereals, 30 g serve	0 – 14

See also Molasses.

SUGARS
see Carbohydrates.

SUKIYAKI

A Japanese dish made from thinly sliced beef, stir-fried at the table with vegetables and flavoured with soy sauce and sake. Each diner breaks a raw egg into a bowl, cooks some of the beef and vegetables in the central frying dish and dips it into the egg before eating. Served with rice.

SULPHITES

These food additives are used as sodium sulphite, sodium bisulphite, sodium metabisulphite and potassium metabisulphite (additives nos. 221, 222, 223, 224). They are added to products such as orange juice, dried fruits, frozen or prepared potato chips and wines to prevent the action of enzymes which cause browning.

SULPHUR

An essential element for making proteins, including those in enzymes, body cells, hair and nails. Also needed for the body to make the B vitamin biotin. Part of the amino acids methionine and cysteine. Widely distributed in foods, especially seafoods, eggs, meats, nuts, milk and some vegetables. There is no recommended daily intake of sulphur as it has been included when determining the amount of protein needed.

SULTANA
see Wine, Varieties.

SULTANAS
see Dried fruits.

SUMMER PUDDING

A pudding made by lining a mould with crustless bread, filling with berry fruits (which have been simmered for a few minutes with sugar) and placing more bread on top. A weight is then fitted onto the top of the pudding basin and the pudding left for at least 12 hours so that the bread soaks up the juices from the fruit. The pudding is then turned out. Summer pudding has no fat but is usually served with thick cream.

SUNDAE

A concoction of scoops of icecream, topped with syrups or sauces and decorated with fruits, cream and chocolate. The dish was created by

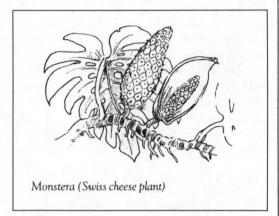

Monstera (Swiss cheese plant)

an American who sought a way around a law which prevented icecream sodas being served on Sunday. He omitted the soda and called the dish after its namesake. A typical sundae has about 2720 kJ (650 Cals).

SUNFISH

see Fish, Moonfish.

SUNFLOWER OIL

see Oils.

SUNFLOWER SEEDS

see Seeds.

SUNLIGHT

The action of sunlight on the skin is necessary for the formation of vitamin D (see page 391). Too much sunlight damages the skin. Once a tan develops on skin, vitamin D production decreases. This is a natural protection against excessive amounts of this vitamin being formed.

SUNSET YELLOW FCF

see Colourings.

SWEAT

The sweat glands are important for regulating the body's temperature. When the body's internal temperature rises, the sweat glands, under the control of the sympathetic nervous system, take water to the surface of the skin. As the water evaporates, heat is removed from the body and the internal temperature drops. Exercising without permitting sweat to evaporate (for example, by wearing garments which cover most of the skin) is hazardous as the body's internal temperature can rise to dangerous levels.

Other sweat glands are associated with hair follicles under the arms and in the pubic area. These glands produce a fatty sweat which is passed to the skin where bacteria break it down to fatty acids which have an odour considered unpleasant by many people.

During exercise, as much as a litre of fluid can be lost every hour. Dehydration is an ever-present threat to the success of athletes. It stresses the cardiovascular system and decreases the flow of blood to the skin and muscles, causing overheating and fatigue. Thirst is not a good indicator of fluid loss and it can take up to 72 hours for the thirst mechanism to replenish water lost after heavy sweating.

Sweat is mostly water and contains only small quantities of minerals. It has only about one-third the salt content of other body fluids. The idea that sweating causes large losses of sodium from the body is incorrect (see page 318). Sweat also contains small amounts of iron, potassium, magnesium, calcium, vitamins and amino acids. The quantities of these nutrients is small, with the possible exception of iron where losses in very heavy sweating can be 1−2 mg per day. This would increase the normal requirement of iron (which is 5−7 mg for men and 12−16 mg for women). All nutrient losses in sweat are easily made up from a normal healthy diet.

SWEDE

see Vegetables.

SWEETBREADS

The pancreas and thymus glands, usually of lamb. The thymus gland is located in the neck and is plump and round. The pancreas is near the stomach and is oblong in shape. They are traditionally eaten fried, with black butter sauce. Sweetbreads contain some vitamin C, some protein and a selection of minerals and vitamins. 100 g of sweetbreads (before cooking) have 545 kJ (130 Cals) and 8 g of fat.

SWEETCORN
see Vegetables.

SWEETNESS

A sweet taste is associated with pleasure for most humans. Honey and fruits are naturally sweet and some young vegetables also taste quite sweet. These foods are highly valued. Sugar itself is a fairly recent addition to the human diet. It is only during the last 150 years that sugar has become a commonplace item in the diet.

There are many other sweet-tasting substances besides sugars. Some combinations of amino acids in proteins taste sweet and there are sugar alcohols as well as intensely sweet-tasting substances in some berries and types of tea. Some of these are so sweet that they are never likely to be used by humans since an extremely small quantity would sweeten a huge vat of any food.

In some areas, naturally sweet substances have been used to disguise the taste of more bitter substances. This was the original use for sugar in medicines in Europe. In parts of tropical Africa, it was once a custom to use serendipity berries to disguise the taste of poison.

The following table sets out some of the different sweetening substances and compares their sweetness to that of sugar (sucrose). Sucrose is given a rating of 1. Substances sweeter than sugar score a higher rating (for example, aspartame is 200 times as sweet as sugar and so scores 200) while those less sweet have a lower rating (for example, lactose is less than half as sweet as sucrose and scores 0.4).

SUBSTANCE	RELATIVE SWEETNESS
Sucrose	1
Lactose (milk sugar)	0.4
Maltose	0.5
Glucose	0.7
Fructose (fruit sugar)	1.1
Sorbitol	0.5
Mannitol	0.7
Sodium cyclohexylsulphamate (cyclamate)	30
Chloroform	40
Acesulfame K	130
Aspartame	200
Saccharin	300
Serendipity berries	2,500
Some protein sweeteners in teas	4,000
Methyl diester of aspartyl amino-malonic acid, methyl, trans-2-methyl cyclohexylamine	33,000

See also Artificial sweeteners and Carbohydrates.

SWEET POTATOES
see Vegetables.

SWEETS
see Confectionery.

SWISS CHARD
see Vegetables.

SWISS CHEESE
see Cheese.

SWISS CHEESE PLANT
see Fruit, Monstera.

SWISS ROLL

A sponge cake, usually filled with jam or cream and rolled up.

SWORDFISH
see Fish.

SYRUPS

Syrups are concentrated solutions of sugar. At

different concentrations syrups behave quite differently and this is used in making different types of sweets including caramel, fudge, hard or soft lollies or candies. The weather will also affect syrups; with greater humidity a syrup will re-absorb water from the air and will thus become more dilute. Sugar syrups are used in making alcoholic cocktails since sugar does not dissolve easily in alcohol. See also Corn syrup, Golden syrup and Maple syrup.

T

TABASCO

see Sauces.

TABBOULI

see Salads.

TACO

A thin Mexican cornmeal pancake (a tortilla, see page 346), fried without browning or baked to a dry shell and filled with a mixture of spicy kidney beans (usually cooked with chilli, pepper and cumin), topped with lettuce, chopped tomato, grated cheese and sour cream. Cooked minced meat or chicken may also be included in the filling. Tacos are eaten frequently in Mexico and have become popular in countries such as Australia and the United States.

TAGLIATELLI

A pasta specialty of Bologna in Italy in the shape of ribbon-like noodles.

TAHINI

A paste made from ground sesame seeds. Used in Middle Eastern cookery and thought to be a good source of calcium. If made from sesame seeds which have not been dehusked, tahini will have a reasonably high calcium content. However, tahini also contains oxalic acid (from the husks on the sesame seeds) and this may 'tie up' the calcium so that it cannot be absorbed by the body. The calcium content of tahini ranges from 28 mg to 84 mg per 20 g. The same quantity of tahini has 10 g of fat and 495 kJ (118 Cals). Tahini does provide protein, dietary fibre, niacin, thiamine, vitamin E and a selection of minerals.

Tahini is used as a sauce on salads, fish, vegetables and kebabs, is a part of many Lebanese dips (such as hummus or baba ghannouj) and is also added to cakes.

TAKE-AWAY FOODS

see Fast Foods.

TAMALE

A steamed cake made from cornmeal and popular in Mexico for thousands of years. Cornmeal from dried corn is made into a thick paste, spread onto a corn husk, topped with a sweet or savoury filling and then wrapped in the corn husk and steamed. In some areas, banana leaves are used to wrap around the cornmeal and filling. Tamale meal can also be made into a pie crust.

TAMARI

See Sauces, soya.

TAMARILLO

see Fruit.

TAMARIND

see Fruit.

TANDOORI

An Indian method of cooking in a cylindrical clay oven (a tandoor) over a charcoal fire. The tandoor is thought to have originated in Persia. The oven is usually about a metre in height and is lit several hours before cooking. The intense heat cooks food quickly without burning it and produces tender succulent dishes. Most meats and fish are placed on long skewers, marinated in yoghurt and spices and then plunged into the oven. Naan, a small Indian yeasted loaf of bread is pressed against the inner neck of the oven and bakes quickly to produce a light puffy bread. The most famous tandoori dish is tandoori chicken in which a whole chicken is left to absorb the flavour of spices rubbed into it, placed on a spit and cooked in the tandoor.

See also Naan.

TANGELO
see Fruit.

TANGERINE
see Fruit.

TANNINS

Compounds found in some plants, especially those used for tea, including some herbal teas. Also found in wines. Tannins have an astringent taste and can prevent iron being absorbed. For this reason, tea is best consumed between meals rather than at meals.

See also Tea.

TAPIOCA

Known by millions of children as 'frog's eyes', tapioca is made from the root of the cassava or manioc plant, native to the West Indies and South America. The root itself tends to go stringy in water and so is processed into balls. This is done by shaking drops of a solution of the root onto a hot plate where they gelatinise and dry out into balls. The tapioca is cooked in water until the balls swell into pale translucent 'frog's eyes'. 100 g of raw tapioca have 1510 kJ (360 Cals). Alternatively, the tapioca can be ground and made into a thin pancake — a common food in Vietnam.

See also Vegetables, Cassava.

TARAMASALATA

A Greek dish of cod's roe mashed with lemon, garlic and potato or breadcrumbs. Served as an appetiser.

TARO
see Vegetables.

TARRAGON
see Herbs.

TART

A flan or open pastry crust. The term depends on nationality. English people refer to tarts, French to flans and Americans to an open pie. Tarts may be filled with jam, lemon butter, fruits, custard or savoury fillings. *Custard tarts* are popular in England and Australia. They should always be kept refrigerated as the combination of milk and eggs is very attractive to bacteria. A typical custard tart has 1260 kJ (300 Cals). *Neenish tarts* are filled with a mixture of icing sugar and butter and topped with icing, half white, half chocolate. One small neenish tart has 435 kJ (200 Cals). *Bakewell tart* is a pastry shell covered with raspberry jam and topped with a mixture of butter, sugar, flour and ground almonds.

See also Pastry.

TARTARE SAUCE

Mayonnaise with finely chopped chives, gherkins and, sometimes, olives added.

TARTARIC ACID

An acid which is found in many plants. Most commonly used as 'cream of tartar' — an ingredient in baking powder. Tartaric acid is also added to many foods, including soft drinks, jellies and jams. Tartaric acid is used to stop fruits turning brown and to prevent rancidity in fats. Additive no. 334.

TARTRAZINE

see Colourings.

TASTE BUDS

There are taste cells in the tongue which react when hit by salty, sweet, bitter or acid foods. Some people maintain that soapy and metallic tastes are also basic taste sensations. The front tip of the tongue is most sensitive to sweet flavours, the sides react mostly to sour tastes, saltiness is perceived near the front and bitterness at the back of the tongue.

Between 40 and 60 taste cells are clustered in each taste bud in small projections on the surface of the tongue. We start life with our greatest supply of taste buds but they gradually decrease with age. That is why children often do not like chilli or hot mustards — to them they taste much hotter. Most adults still have several thousand taste buds, about half of them at the back of the tongue. These are rejuvenated about every 10 days.

The actual taste of a food is a combination of the sensation on the taste buds and the aroma of the food. Some flavours are detected only by their smell, and the sensory apparatus for this is located near the back of the mouth. We also detect the odours of foods as they are being swallowed.

TAURINE

An amino acid which is found only in animal tissues. Humans have no specific requirement for it because we can make our own supplies. However, animals such as cats must have taurine in their diet as they cannot make their own. Thus cats cannot be vegetarians.

TEA

See following pages.

TEACAKE

A sweet yeasted bun, often containing dried fruit or apple. The top of the bun is usually glazed with sugar, sprinkled with icing sugar or iced. Teacakes are eaten in England, as their name suggests, to accompany tea. An average piece of teacake, without butter, has 735 kJ (175 Cals).

TEETH

The first, or deciduous, teeth usually begin to appear around the age of 6 months and all 20 should be through the gums by about 2 years of age. These teeth are important for the structure of the jaw and face as well as playing a vital role in chewing foods. It is important that they do not decay.

The secondary teeth begin to erupt at about 6 years of age and the deciduous teeth gradually loosen and fall out to allow room for the permanent set. 'Wisdom' teeth can appear later, or, in some people, never exist.

Tooth decay is a common but entirely preventable disease. It occurs when decay-causing bacteria use carbohydrates and produce acids which damage the enamel surfaces on the teeth. The factors involved include the:

- Presence of bacteria on teeth
- Presence of sugars around teeth
- Length of time sugars remain around teeth
- Strength of tooth enamel

Each of these points can be remedied to reduce the incidence of dental decay.

The bacteria live in plaque — a polysaccharide material which forms on teeth. Plaque can be removed by thorough cleaning of the teeth.

Sugars can be restricted in the diet. Sucrose, or cane sugar, is the most widely eaten sugar and is the most common cause of tooth decay. However, other sugars can also play a part. It is best to restrict sugary foods, especially those which stick in the teeth, to times when the teeth can be brushed immediately after eating.

There will be times when almost everyone

eats some form of sugar. If these sugar-eating occasions can be minimised, or if the teeth can be brushed immediately after eating sugar-containing foods, there will be less chances of dental decay.

Tooth enamel can be strengthened by fluoride. In some parts of the world, the fluoride concentration of the water or the fluoride in the normal diet is higher than in other areas. If the fluoride is present at too high a concentration, mottling of the teeth occurs. Where the natural fluoride in the diet and drinking water is low, tooth enamel tends to be weaker. For these reasons, carefully controlled levels of flouride are added to drinking water in many areas. In parts of Australia where the drinking water is fluoridated, dental decay has been drastically reduced. Over 100 studies from many parts of the world have also proved this point (see also page 133).

In general, the diet which is good for health is also the best one for the teeth. Plenty of fibrous foods help keep the teeth clean — wholemeal bread and wholegrain cereals, fruits and vegetables are excellent. Very little sugar also helps the body and the teeth.

The minerals in teeth include calcium and phosphorus. These need to be well supplied in the diet, especially the diet of young children. When calcium supply is limited in older children and adults, the body will withdraw calcium from bones rather than teeth. However, a protein in milk (known as an alpha s casein) has been shown to inhibit dental decay on the tooth surface and to have some ability to repair damage to tooth enamel.

Incidentally, if you have a passion for sweets, chocolate is less damaging to teeth than other lollies and sweets. However, chocolate is probably more damaging to the waistline and its high fat content is undesirable for many people.

TEA

On a world scale, tea is the most popular drink. It comes from an evergreen camellia which is related to the shrub and grows in high regions or in damp areas in the tropics. There is only one tea plant and the differences in various teas depend on the climate, soil, freshness of the leaf, flavour additives and size of the leaf.

Tea originated in India but soon was taken to China to become the national drink. The earliest mention of tea in China is in writings from 350 BC but it is thought to have been used much earlier than that. Tea was first brought to Europe by the Dutch in 1610 and reached England by 1644. Most of the world's tea is grown in China, India, Japan, Sri Lanka and throughout southeast Asia. Tea is also being grown in parts of Australia. It is drunk widely throughout Asia and is the most common beverage in Britain (after water). It is popular in Australia, although more coffee than tea is now consumed (1.6 kg of coffee/head/ year compared with 1.3 kg of tea). Throughout the United States and Europe, tea consumption is much less than coffee and most tea is used in the form of tea bags. Iced tea is a popular summer drink in the United States.

The two major types of tea are green and black. Green tea is made from leaves which have not been fermented. Black tea is made from fermented tea leaves.

Oolong tea, grown in China, is half fermented and is usually flavoured with jasmine flowers.

The best part of the tea bush is the bud followed by the two leaves which enclose it. It takes about 2 kg of leaves to make 500 g of black tea leaves. The leaves are hand-picked and, in some areas, picking for top quality teas is done only at certain times of the year.

After picking, the leaves are spread out to dry, losing about 50 per cent of their moisture in this process. They are then rolled by machine to release fermenting enzymes. The leaves are left to ferment at 27°C, the fermentation time differing for various types of tea.

Fermentation is followed by 'firing' in which a hot current of air passes over the leaves. They are then sorted into different grades — leaf teas and small leaf or broken leaf teas. In general, the larger the leaf, the better the quality. Smaller leaves give stronger darker teas.

For tea bags, the leaves are cut by machine so that they will infuse more quickly into the liquid.

In England, tea leaves are placed in a hot teapot and have boiling water poured over them. The resulting brew is left for 3—5 mins to allow the caffeine and tannins to be extracted, and is stirred to distribute the flavour of the leaves. It is then strained and served with lemon, milk and/or sugar. In North Africa, tea is usually infused with mint leaves and served with sugar. In Nepal, tea has added yak butter and salt.

Tea contains both caffeine and tannins. The caffeine content varies with the strength of the tea (see page 50). In general, average strength tea has about half the caffeine of brewed coffee. Weak tea has much less caffeine. The tannins in tea are extracted from the leaves during infusion. The longer the leaves sit in the water, the greater the tannin content. Tea poured out quickly after being made has little tannin but after 5 mins brewing in the pot, the tannin content is much higher. Tannins can interfere with the absorption of iron (see page 192). Adding milk to tea binds the tannins and reduces their astringency.

Tea leaves contain fluoride, potassium, iron, niacin, protein and a range of minerals. The infusion, however, contains few of these nutrients with the exception of fluoride. Tea leaves contain 460 kJ (110 Cals) per 100. The infusion which we drink has 5 kJ (less than 2 Cals) per cup.

In excessive quantities, fermented tea will contribute caffeine and tannin. In moderation (4—5 cups/day of average strength or more of weak tea), it is quite safe.

Assam
A variety of tea from the Assam province in northeastern India, grown at a little lower altitude than Darjeeling. Has a strong full flavour and a reddish colour.

Ceylon
High quality tea grown at very high altitudes. Has a delicate and fragrant flavour. Excellent for making iced tea since it does not go cloudy.

Darjeeling

Generally considered the top quality Indian tea. Darjeeling is a black tea with a rich and almost fruity taste. As its name suggests, it is grown in Darjeeling, on the lower slopes of the Himalayas.

Earl Grey

A blend of teas flavoured with bergamot. The tea was first presented to Charles, the second Earl Grey, by an envoy returning from China in the early part of the nineteenth century.

Fan Yong

An unscented black tea from China with a mild flavour. Very low in tannin.

Green

An unfermented tea served in China, Japan and other areas of Asia. Its taste is delicate and its levels of tannins and caffeine are low. No milk or sugar is added.

Jasmine

Green tea leaves blended with jasmine flowers. The tea is highly scented and is always served on its own, without milk or sugar.

Kanoy

A black tea with very small leaves which comes from Sri Lanka. Makes a golden coloured tea.

Keemum

A large-leafed black tea from northern China with a smoky 'orchid-like' flavour. Generally considered excellent to serve (without milk) with meals. English breakfast tea was traditionally made from keemum but now is often a blend.

Lapsang souchang

A fermented black tea with very brittle leaves. The tea comes from Taiwan and the province of Fukien and has a smoky flavour.

Oolong

A semi-fermented tea from Taiwan with a flavour half way between regular and green teas. A large-leafed tea, oolong has a scent which is a little like peaches. Tea made from these leaves is a pale yellow-green in colour.

Orange pekoe

This term represents a grading of tea rather than a flavour. Orange pekoe is the finest Indian tea made from the bud and 2 top leaves of the bush. Delicate clean flavour. Also available scented with jasmine.

Herbal

These products are made from the leaves, roots, seeds or bark of various shrubs and trees. They are used in many parts of the world because they grow there; in other areas they are used in place of regular tea or coffee, often by those who are trying to avoid caffeine or tannins.

Herbal teas are no more 'natural' than regular tea. Most do not contain caffeine; many do contain tannins — sometimes more than regular tea. A few may even be dangerous.

Uva ursi tea has 15–20 per cent tannin content; blackberry tea has 14 per cent; peppermint has 3.5–12 per cent; lady's mantle has 8 per cent.

Some herbal teas have also been found to have a stimulant action on the uterus and should not be used during pregnancy. These include juniper, mugwort, pennyroyal, raspberry, sage and yarrow teas.

Other herbal teas contain alkaloids which can damage the liver and possibly lead to liver cancer. These include comfrey, larkspur and pennyroyal.

Senna tea contains a potent drug which can cause diarrhoea and stomach cramps. Sassafras tea contains saffrole, once used as a food additive but now banned because it has been shown to cause liver cancer. Ginseng tea and licorice root may increase blood pressure while mistletoe can cause blood pressure to drop dangerously low.

Some herbal teas, however, are quite safe and are good alternatives for those who want to avoid the caffeine and tannin of regular tea.

Chamomile tea, linden and red bush appear to be quite safe. Hibiscus tea (made from the flowers) is unlikely to do any harm in the quantities used and rosehip seems safe, although it does contain some tannins. Rosehip tea also has valuable pectins and vitamin C.

TEFLON

A polymer containing carbon and fluorine which is used to coat cooking utensils. Teflon is fairly inert and has a surface characterised by very low friction. This means that foods do not stick to teflon-coated surfaces.

TEMPEH

A tofu-like product made from fermented soya beans. Made by inoculating soya beans with a mould and then proceeding as for tofu (see page 345).

Tempeh is a good source of protein and iron and also supplies B complex vitamins and some calcium. It has about 4 per cent fat and 100 g have 630 kJ (150 Cals).

TEMPURA

A Japanese dish consisting of vegetables or seafood dipped in a light batter and fried. Usually served with soya sauce for dipping. Tempura is one of the few Japanese dishes with a relatively high fat content.

TENDERLOIN

The muscle running along the back of an animal. As this muscle is not used very much it is usually very tender.

TEQUILA.
see Drinks, Alcoholic.

TERAGLIN
see Fish.

TERATOGEN

Any substance which causes malformation in a foetus. Some nutrients may be teratogens if given in excessive doses or if insufficient amounts are available to the foetus. Excess vitamin A, excess alcohol or insufficient folate are all teratogens.

TERIYAKI

A Japanese style of cooking in which meat, fish or chicken pieces are marinaded in a mixture of

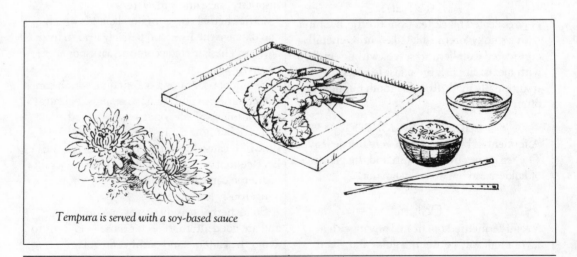

Tempura is served with a soy-based sauce

soya sauce, garlic, sake and sugar and then grilled. Ginger may also be added. The food takes on a glazed appearance from the use of the marinading sauce. Teriyaki sauce (a flavoured soya sauce) is now used in many Western countries to flavour foods. One tablespoon (20 mL) teriyaki sauce has 85 kJ (20 Cals).

TERRINE

A mixture of chopped meat, fish or vegetables with butter (or some other fat), seasonings and egg, placed in a clay or earthenware dish, often lined with overlapping rashers of bacon. The terrine is placed in a pan of water and cooked in a moderate oven until firm. Terrines are often served with salad or as a first course. Their nutritional value varies according to the ingredients. Those with a high content of bacon and fatty meats are high in kilojoules.

TEXTURED VEGETABLE PROTEIN
see TVP.

THEOBROMINE

A substance known as a methylxanthine (a type of alkaloid), present in coffee and chocolate. Unlike caffeine (also an alkaloid), theobromine does not seem to stimulate the central nervous system.

THEOPHYLLINE

A xanthine (see page 404) substance found in tea. Theophylline belongs to the same family as caffeine but has less potent effects.

THERMOGENESIS

The release of energy in the form of heat. Thermogenesis helps us maintain a constant body temperature. In cold weather, shivering generates extra heat. It is also thought that some people have more 'brown fat' which generates heat when it is burned. More research is required to determine the importance of brown fat in humans.

THERMOGENIC EFFECT OF FOOD

After eating food, we feel warm. Whether the food is hot or cold, it increases the body's metabolic rate and this produces heat. The increase in metabolic rate can range from 5–30 per cent for several hours after eating. In theory, proteins will have the greatest effect. In practice, since almost all foods contain mixtures of protein, fat and carbohydrate, the specific effect of certain nutrients is irrelevant (see Specific dynamic action).

THIAMIN
see Vitamin B.

THICKENERS

Food additives used to produce a thicker texture or consistency in foods. Includes gelatine, starches and vegetable gums which are used to thicken soups, desserts, gravies and sauces, jellies, cream and icecream. Most starch thickeners have not been given additive numbers. Vegetable gums have additive numbers from 400 to 416.

THIRST

A sensation which tells us the body needs water. Thirst is probably initiated by an increase in the concentration of sodium in the blood (which is why you feel thirsty after a salty meal). However, thirst is not always a good indicator of water loss in the short term. After a heavy sweat (during extended strenuous exercise) it may take up to 72 hours for the thirst response to be sufficient to restore water losses. For those who sweat heavily and regularly, such as athletes, it is often necessary to drink more water than thirst dictates to avoid dehydration.

THREONINE

An essential amino acid found in almost all foods.

THROMBIN

An enzyme in the blood which helps it to clot.

THROMBOSIS

Blockage of a blood vessel by a blood clot. Blood clots are more likely to occur with a high-fat diet, especially if the fats are saturated. Omega 3 fatty acids (see page 254) prevent thrombosis.

THROMBOXANES

Chemical substances formed in the body from both the omega 3 and omega 6 polyunsaturated fatty acids (see page 254). One of the thromboxanes causes blood fats to stick together increasing the chances of blood clots; another type has no effect on blood clots. Thromboxanes work in balance with prostaglandins (see page 281). Together these substances influence blood clotting times, blood pressure and coronary heart disease. They are balanced according to whether the diet has an excess of omega 3 or omega 6 fatty acids. In the Eskimo diet, for example, the omega 3 fatty acids predominate. This means that the Eskimos produce a lot of thromboxane 3 — a chemical which does not cause the blood to clot in the same way that thromboxane 2 (from a different fatty acid) does. The fats in the Eskimo diet also produce a lot of prostacyclin 3, which has definite anti-clotting properties. These factors explain why Eskimos have few blood clots and little heart disease, but bleed a lot if cut.

THYME
see Herbs.

THYROID GLAND

A gland in the neck which secretes a hormone called thyroxine which controls the body's rate of metabolism. The thyroid gland needs iodine to produce its hormones. If there is insufficient iodine in the diet, the gland enlarges and can be seen as a very large lump in the neck. See also Goitre, Endocrine glands, and Food poisoning.

THYROTOXICOSIS

Over-production of thyroid hormone caused by an excessive intake of iodine or by an over-production of a hormone called thyrotropin (which stimulates the thyroid to produce thyroxine).

THYROXINE

A hormone produced by the thyroid gland.

TIA MARIA
see Drinks, Alcoholic.

TILSIT
see Cheese.

TIMBALE

A deep round mould with straight or sloping sides used to cook a mixture of a savoury custard with fish or other seafood, poultry, meat, vegetables or a cereal. Timbales are unmoulded before serving. They are light and make an ideal first course or a good accompaniment to other dishes. Their nutritional value varies according to the ingredients. Many contain cream and butter and so are high in kilojoules; others are lightened with egg whites and have fewer kilojoules.

TIMNODONIC ACID

Another name for EPA, eicosapentaenoic acid (see page 110).

See also Omega 3 fatty acids.

TIN

A trace mineral which is known to be essential for growth in animals and is probably essential for humans. Very small quantities of tin are likely to be required and will be found in

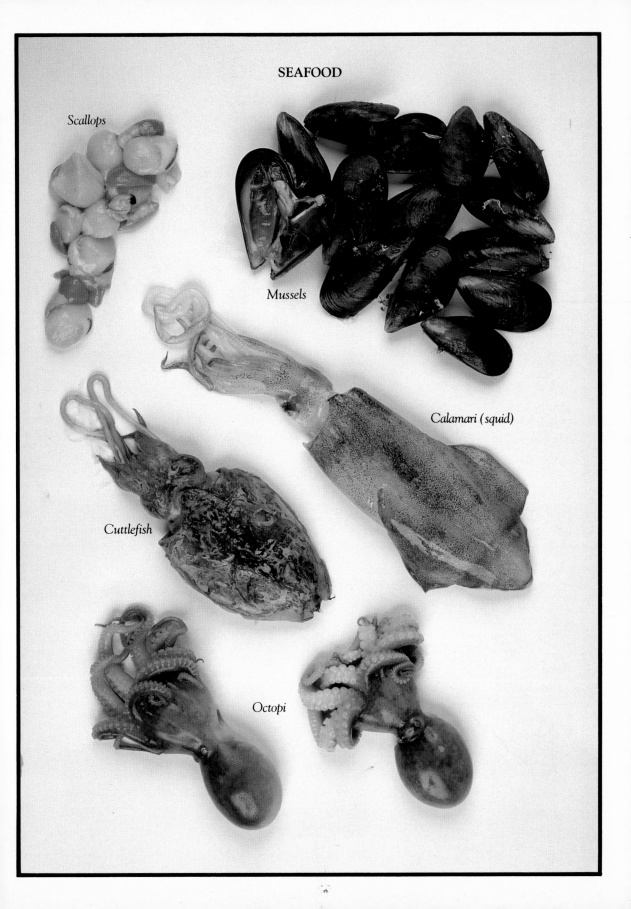

SEAFOOD

Scallops

Mussels

Calamari (squid)

Cuttlefish

Octopi

SEAFOOD

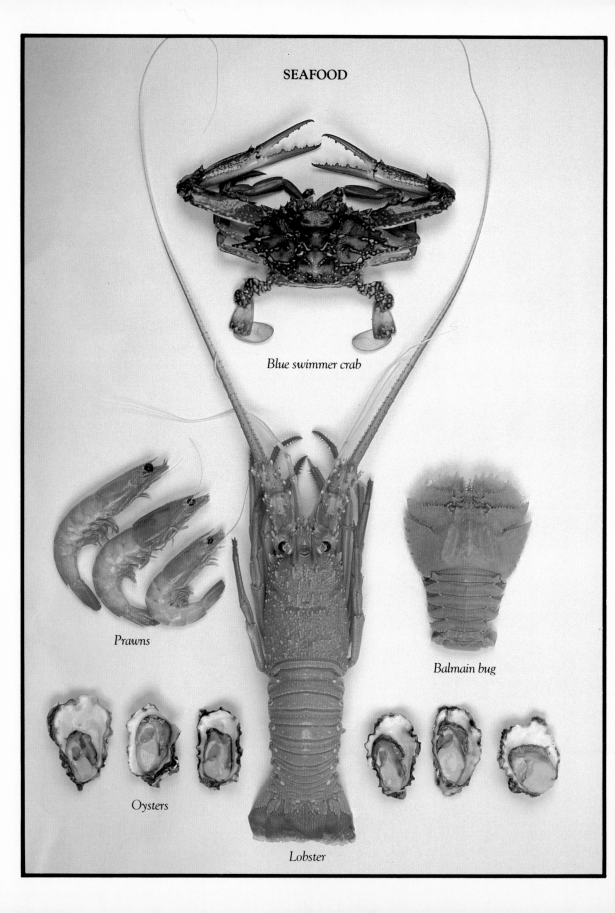

Blue swimmer crab

Prawns

Balmain bug

Oysters

Lobster

cereals, meat and vegetables. Some tin can also enter the body from tin cans, although this is likely to be excreted in the faeces. The quantity of tin required by humans is not known. The dose known to be toxic ranges from 350—500 mg for a 70 kg person. A lower dose than this would be toxic for children.

TIREDNESS
see Fatigue.

TIROPITAS

Small Greek pastries made from filo pastry filled with a mixture of feta and ricotta cheeses and parsley. Usually baked in the oven until golden brown. One small tiropita has 400 kJ (95 Cals).

TOAD-IN-THE-HOLE

A dish made by pouring batter over cooked sausages and baking until the batter is golden brown. A high fat dish.

TOCOPHEROL
see Vitamins, Vitamin E.

TOFFEE

Also known as taffy, toffee comes from a Creole word meaning a mixture of sugar and molasses. It is made by boiling sugar and water to a syrup (without stirring) until golden brown. Butter is added plus condensed milk if desired. The mixture is poured into appropriate containers until firm.

Toffee is harmful to the teeth. It is also high in fat and kilojoules. 50 g of toffee contain 9 g of fat and 945 kJ (225 Cals).

Toffee apples are apples pushed onto a wooden skewer and dipped in a thick syrup with added red colouring. The normal kilojoule value for an apple 285 kJ (68 Cals) increases to 1320 kJ (315 Cals) for a toffee apple.

TOFU

A curd product made from soya beans and used as a source of protein in China for thousands of years, tofu is widely used in China, Japan and throughout Asia. Occasionally called soya cheese, it is made by soaking dried soya beans in water, crushing the mixture, boiling it and straining it to separate the solid pulp from the milk. Coagulants (either an acid such as lemon juice, calcium chloride or magnesium chloride) are then added to curdle the mixture into curds and whey. The curdled mixture is then strained and the curds are allowed to set into a soft block.

Tofu has a bland flavour and can be used in spreads, stir-fried, roasted, added to casseroles, deep fried, made into noodles, eaten plain or used in various desserts. It is often used as an icecream substitute. Fermented tofu products are also common in Asian countries.

Nutritionally, tofu supplies protein, has very little fat (around 2 per cent, mostly polyunsaturated), small quantities of vitamins and iron and is a source of calcium (120 mg/100 g). 100 g of tofu has 140 kJ (33 Cals). If the tofu has been drained to produce a denser product, it will have approximately 265 kJ (63 Cals). Fermented tofu has from 420—715 kJ (100—170 Cals) per 100 g.

TOKAY
see Wine, Varieties.

TOMATO
see Vegetables.

TOMATO SAUCE
see Sauces, other; Ketchup.

TOM COLLINS
see Drinks, Alcoholic.

TONGUE

Veal, ox or lamb tongues are sold fresh, salted, smoked or canned. To cook fresh tongue, simmer in water with herbs and spices for 1—3 hrs depending on the size of the tongue. The tongue is cooked when the small bones near the root end can be easily pulled out. The skin is generally removed before eating the tongue. Nutritionally, tongue is a good source of iron, zinc and niacin and also supplies protein and other vitamins of the B group. It is fairly high in fat with 100 g of cooked tongue having 18—20 g of fat. The same quantity has 1215 kJ (290 Cals).

TOOTH DECAY
see Dental caries.

TORTE

A rich German or Austrian cake or pastry usually having several layers joined with cream or a butter cream. In some tortes the flour usually present is replaced with ground nuts. All tortes are high in kilojoules. A typical slice of torte with butter cream filling would have about 2930 kJ (700 Cals).

TORTELLINI

Small stuffed pasta dumplings, usually shaped in half-moons. Legend has it that the shape of the tortellini was modelled on Venus's navel. The stuffing in most tortellini is made from meat, chicken or vegetables.

TORTILLA

A flat Mexican bread made from ground white cornmeal. Tortillas are cooked on a hot plate without browning and are quite soft. Sometimes they are deep fried until crisp. The nutritional value will vary with the size of the tortilla. A small 60 g tortilla would have approximately 630 kJ (150 Cals). Tortillas are served with most Mexican dishes and are used to scoop up sauces, beans or meats. Often the food is placed on the tortilla which is rolled around it, forming a taco. Tortillas made from wheat flour and wrapped around a filling are called burritos.
　　See also Taco.

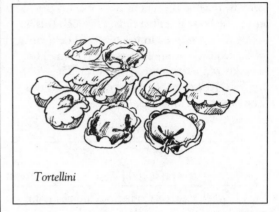

Tortellini

TOSTADO

A tortilla fried until crisp and topped with a filling of meat, beans, cheese, lettuce, tomato and chilli.

TOURNEDOS

A small thick fillet steak trimmed to a neat circular shape, pan fried and served on a piece of fried bread to catch its juices. A sauce is often added.

TOXINS
see Food poisoning.

TRACE ELEMENTS

Essential minerals which are required in very small amounts, generally less than 100 mg per day.

TRAGACANTH

A small Asian shrub which produces a gum once used in chewing gum and various lozenges.

TRAMINER
see Wine, Varieties.

TRANQUILLISERS

Some tranquillisers can affect nutrition (see Monoamine oxidase). They can also affect behaviour and this may be reflected in changes in eating or exercise behaviour. For example, someone who has been very active and agitated may alter with tranquillisers so that physical activity is greatly reduced. Unless that person begins eating less food than previously, excess weight may become an added problem.

TRANSAMINATION

The process whereby one amino acid is changed to another. It is because of transamination that only 8 of the 22 known amino acids must be eaten 'ready-made'. By transamination, the other amino acids can be produced within the body.

TRANS FATTY ACIDS
see Fats.

TRANSFERRIN

A protein which carries iron in the blood plasma. Each molecule of transferrin can hold 2 molecules of iron. It is responsible for transferring large quantities of iron to the placenta during pregnancy. Zinc can also be attached to transferrin.

TRANSIT TIME

As well as being the time when one waits for airline connections, transit time refers to the time it takes food to pass through the intestine. In general, transit time ranges from 36–72 hrs and is faster on a high-fibre diet. A relatively short transit time is considered desirable so that any harmful substances are excreted and do not stay too long in contact with the intestine.

TRASSI

A dried shrimp paste made from shrimp mixed with 10–15 per cent salt. The mixture is dried in the sun and kneaded with a red dye until sticky and thick. Keeps indefinitely.

TREACLE

A thick black liquid which is a by-product of sugar refining and closely resembles molasses (see page 232). Treacle can be used in cake, bean or sauce recipes which call for molasses. Light treacle often refers to golden syrup (see page 167). Dark treacle is high in minerals, especially iron and potassium, and contains some calcium. In spite of claims to the contrary, treacle or molasses are in no way superior sources of these nutrients to meat, vegetables or milk. 1 tablespoon of treacle has 220 kJ (52 Cals). It is just as harmful to teeth as any other sugar.

TREBBIANO
see Wine, Varieties.

TREHALOSE

A sugar found in mushrooms, other fungi and yeasts. Trehalose is made of 2 glucose sugars joined in an unusual fashion. The sugar is broken down in the small intestine by an enzyme known as trehalase.

TREVALLA
see Fish.

TREVALLY
see Fish.

TRICHINOSIS

An infectious parasite present in pork in some countries. Thorough cooking of the pork is necessary to kill the parasite or its larvae can migrate to the muscles and cause inflammation. The larvae are destroyed when pork reaches a temperature of 60°C or more. Trichinosis does not occur in countries such as Australia.

TRIFLE

An old English dessert composed of sponge cake soaked in sherry (or other sweet wine) topped with a jam, an egg custard and whipped cream. Fruits, nuts and jelly are also used to decorate trifle. An average serve has 1350 kJ (322 Cals).

TRIGLYCERIDES

A class of chemical compounds which includes fats and oils. Triglycerides consist of glycerol (an alcohol) with three fatty acids attached. If the fatty acids are saturated with hydrogen atoms (see Fats, page 118), the fat is solid; if the fatty acids are not saturated with hydrogen atoms, the fat is liquid (or an oil).

Animals, including humans, have stores of triglycerides in case food is not available. Plants store their triglycerides in seeds. Triglycerides are a compact way of storing energy. If we eat more proteins, fats or carbohydrates than we need, the excess is converted into triglycerides and stored for future energy use. More than twice as much energy can be stored in triglycerides than in proteins or carbohydrates. Triglycerides also contain very little water. For storage this is much more efficient than if energy is kept in the form of glycogen (a storage form of carbohydrate) since every gram of glycogen will hold approximately 3 g of water.

The level of triglycerides in the blood is normally kept within a range of 0.4−1.7 mmol/L. After a meal, the triglyceride level will be much higher but the fats will be removed from the blood and either used for energy or stored in fat depots. If levels of triglycerides are still high after fasting, it indicates that the body is not clearing fats. The resulting blood is fatty and makes the heart work harder, leading to an increased risk of heart disease.

The high level of triglycerides may be due to a high level of fats in the diet, but may also be present because the body is converting alcohol or sugars to fats.

There is still some dispute regarding the relative risk of high levels of triglycerides in the blood. Most medical researchers rate high levels of cholesterol as a greater risk than high levels of triglycerides. However, there is no doubt that high levels of triglycerides are also undesirable and may indicate an increased risk of diabetes.

To reduce high levels of triglycerides in the blood, it is necessary to eat less fat, less sugar and to drink less alcohol.

Compounds known as medium chain triglycerides (MCT) contain 8 to 10 carbon atoms and are easier to digest than other triglycerides. They are derived from coconut oil and are sometimes used to supply fat to people who have difficulty digesting other fats. Coconut oil itself, without modification, also contains long chain triglycerides.

TRIPE

The lining of the stomach of cows or sheep, usually from the first or the second stomach. The first is smooth while the lining from the second stomach has a honeycombed appearance. Tripe is cleaned and blanched before being sold. It is best prepared by long, slow cooking.

Those who are not fond of the taste of tripe will be pleased to know that there is no special nutritional reason for eating it. It has far less iron and vitamins than other meats and almost twice the level of pre-formed cholesterol. 100 g of cooked tripe have 420 kJ (100 Cals).

TRITICALE
see Grains.

TROUT
see Fish.

TRUFFLE, CHOCOLATE

A rich ball of cream and chocolate, flavoured with rum or brandy. Very high in kilojoules and fat.

TRUFFLES

An edible fungus which grows underground, usually in the roots of oak trees. The world's best truffles come from Perigord, in France. Truffles from the Piedmont area of northern Italy are also highly esteemed.

Truffles are harvested in autumn using specially trained pigs or dogs to sniff out the delicate little fungi in their underground homes. Once the pig has detected the truffle, it is carefully removed. It has been found that truffles produce a chemical which is secreted in a male pig's saliva and attracts the sow.

The flavour of truffles is so intense that a single sliver of a top quality truffle can flavour an entire basket of eggs. Small pieces are used with chicken, turkey or pheasant or in pâtés, terrines or egg dishes. Canned truffles are also available. They are expensive and truffles are probably the world's most expensive food product.

The intensity of the flavour of truffles comes from their high content of glutamic acid, an amino acid which is used to make monosodium glutamate. Such small quantities of truffles are used in cooking that their nutritional value is insignificant.

TRUSS

A method of securing poultry with string or skewers so that it holds its shape while cooking.

TRYPSIN

An enzyme in pancreatic juice which breaks down proteins into their component amino acids.

TRYPTOPHAN

An essential amino acid which is made into the vitamin niacin in the body. Vitamin B_6 is required for this chemical reaction. 60 mg of tryptophan produces 1 mg of niacin. Tryptophan is also important to produce serotonin, which affects alertness. For this reason, tryptophan is sometimes used as a mild sedative.

Tryptophan is not found in gelatin and is missing from a few cereals.

See also Amino acids.

TSAMPA

see Barley.

TUBERS

Starchy root vegetables including cassava, potatoes, sweet potatoes, taro and yams. Most tubers are excellent sources of complex carbohydrates and provide a good quantity of dietary fibre as well as a selection of minerals and vitamins. (See also individual entries under Vegetables.)

TUNA

see Fish.

TURBOT

see Fish.

TURKEY

The turkeys we eat are descendants of the wild turkey of Mexico. This bird was domesticated by the Aztecs and taken to Spain, to England and then back to America. In some countries, turkey has been considered as a traditional Christmas dish. In the United States, and, increasingly in Australia, turkey is being used throughout the year. Smaller birds are being bred and different cuts of turkey which cook quickly are becoming available.

Turkey breast can be roasted, microwaved or cut into steaks or strips for grilling or stir-frying. It is very low in fat, having less than 2 per cent. Turkey thighs need longer, slower cooking to break down the large amount of connective tissue in their darker flesh. Without the skin, turkey thighs are also low in fat.

Turkey is a very good source of protein and niacin and also supplies other B complex vitamins and minerals such as iron and zinc. The dark turkey meat is richer in minerals than the lighter breast meat. 100 g of cooked turkey meat have 585 kJ (140 Cals).

See also Poultry.

TURKEY STRASSBURG
see Sausages.

TURKISH COFFEE

A pulverised coffee traditionally made from Mocca beans. Usually made very strong and served in small cups.

TURKISH DELIGHT

A jellied sweet which is popular in Middle Eastern countries. It is made from a thickened, boiled syrup to which are added gelatine, citrus juices, colouring (pink or light green) and flavouring (usually rose water, lemon essence or peppermint). It has no fat. Each square has approximately 295 kJ (70 Cals).

TURMERIC
see Spices.

TURNIP
see Vegetables.

TURTLE

Turtle flesh can be eaten, cut into steaks or strips. Turtle eggs are also used in some parts of the world.

Turtle flesh has very little fat (only about 1 per cent). It is high in protein and supplies iron and some calcium. 100 g have 335 kJ (80 Cals).

Turtle eggs have a very similar composition to hen eggs, but have slightly less iron. 100 g of turtle egg have 630 kJ (150 Cals).

TVP (TEXTURED VEGETABLE PROTEIN)

Textured vegetable protein was produced during the 1950s and marketed extensively during the 1960s as a meat substitute. It is made by removing the oil from soya beans, then taking out the carbohydrate. The remaining protein slurry is then forced through a spinning device with small holes. The protein comes out of the holes in fibres which are washed, flavoured, coloured and spun into different textures.

Chunks of TVP can also be made from defatted soya bean concentrate. This is mixed with water, flavourings and colourings, heated and forced through holes of varying shapes. The resulting products are then cooked, canned or dried. Other oil seeds, including peanut, cottonseed, sunflower and safflower, can also be used to make TVP.

TVP is low in fat and high in protein, yet it has not become popular with the health-conscious section of society. This may well be due to its high salt content and the presence of artificial colourings and flavourings. 100 g of TVP have 1425 kJ (340 Cals).

TYRAMINE

An amine which is made from tyrosine. Tyramines are found in cheese, chocolates, fish and beans and may produce a sensitivity response in some people. It is essential for those taking monoamine oxidases to avoid tyramine-containing foods. Tyramine can raise blood pressure.

See also Monoamine oxidase inhibitors.

TYROSINE

Another amino acid which is not essential as it can be made from other amino acids. Tyramine is a precursor of melanin, the brown pigment in the skin and also of the thyroid hormone, thyroxine.

TZATZIKI

A Greek dish of cucumbers and yoghurt flavoured with garlic and mint. Half a cup has 290 kJ (70 Cals).

U

UDON

Japanese thin white wheat noodles served in hot soups. Nutritional value is similar to other noodles.

UGLI

see Fruit.

ULCERS, INTESTINAL

Ulcers occur when the acidic gastric juices eat into the lining of the intestine. They may occur at the lower end of the oesophagus where it joins the stomach (known as gastric ulcer) or at the other end of the stomach where it joins the duodenum (duodenal ulcer).

Ulcers are related to secretion of excessive amounts of acid, stress, smoking, excessive consumption of alcohol or regular intake of aspirin on an empty stomach. Treatment is rest and relaxation, regular small meals, elimination of smoking, alcohol and coffee (which stimulates acid production in the stomach).

Contrary to popular belief, those with an ulcer do not need to eat soft food, drink large quantities of milk, avoid certain vegetables or acidic fruits. Any food which upsets an individual can be omitted, but severe or restrictive diets are unnecessary.

Milk does have some ability to neutralise stomach acid, but it also stimulates the secretion of extra acid. It may give short-term relief, but has no long-term benefits.

ULCERS, MOUTH

Small, painful ulcers can occur in the mouth, usually as a result of a knock to the gum. On their own, they are not necessarily the sign of a nutrient deficiency and heal spontaneously.

There is no evidence that large doses of vitamin C will heal mouth ulcers.

ULTRA HIGH TEMPERATURE TREATMENT (UHT)

Sterilisation of milk by heating to a high temperature for a few seconds to kill all bacteria. UHT treatment results in less loss of vitamins and minerals from milk than occurs under normal pasteurisation. UHT milk can be stored at room temperature for many months, since it is a sterile product. Once opened, however, it must be placed in the refrigerator. UHT milk has a slightly different flavour due to the effect of the rapid heating.

ULTRAVIOLET RADIATION

Foods can be sterilised using ultraviolet radiation. This type of radiation from the sun is also useful in converting a substance in skin (7-dehydrocholesterol) to vitamin D. The skin tans from ultraviolet radiation, and burns if the dose is too high. Irradiation of foods is from gamma rays (see page 193).

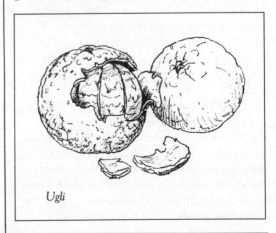

Ugli

351

UNDERNUTRITION

A state of having insufficient kilojoules of energy, protein, minerals and vitamins. Occurs in third world countries at times of famine. In Western society, undernutrition only occurs in those with anorexia nervosa or bulimia nervosa. Undernutrition during the early part of life damages brain cells and children who have suffered such a fate never fully recover their likely level of achievement had they been well nourished.

See also Anorexia nervosa; Bulimia nervosa; Malnutrition.

UNDERWEIGHT

Too little body fat can lead to underweight. While it is desirable not to be overweight, being underweight is not without hazards. Those who are extremely thin have a higher mortality rate at a younger age than those whose weight is within the healthy weight range (see page 40).

Underweight usually occurs from a lack of food or, more commonly in Western society, from a desire to be very slim. The underweight body generally lacks strength and becomes chilled or fatigued more easily. Those who are underweight also may have less resistance to infections.

Some people are underweight by nature. Most are underweight because they eat too little. Smoking is frequently associated with underweight because it reduces the appetite. A lack of sufficient exercise to stimulate a normal appetite may also be involved or there may be a general restlessness.

For the underweight to gain weight, they need to eat more and refrain from smoking. Relaxation exercises may also help. It is usually easiest to persuade very thin people to eat small amounts often than it is to encourage them to eat large meals. Nuts and milk are useful foods; nuts can be nibbled without producing a feeling of fullness and milk slips down effortlessly.

In general, the major barrier to underweight people gaining weight is their unwillingness to eat more food.

The occasional person who does not smoke, exercises regularly and eats well but is still underweight may simply have to accept their genetically inherited tendency to be very thin.

UNLEAVENED BREAD

Bread made without yeast. In a mixed diet, unleavened bread causes no problems. In some Middle Eastern countries where the diet is low in minerals such as zinc, the use of unleavened bread has caused zinc deficiency. This is because the phytic acid in the wholemeal flour forms a complex with the zinc, making it unavailable to the body. The use of yeast in leavened breads breaks down the phytic acid so that this binding of minerals does not occur.

URAD

The name given to the whole black gram bean in India. When split, the black gram is called urad dahl.

UREA

The major product used for excreting spare nitrogen from proteins. When proteins are digested to amino acids, the amino acids not needed for the synthesis of the body's own protein are used for energy or are converted to body fat. The nitrogen from the amino acids is made into ammonia — a highly toxic substance. The body converts this ammonia to urea in the liver, releases it into the blood, from where it goes to the kidneys and is excreted in the urine. About 80–90 per cent of the nitrogen which is excreted from the body is in the form of urea.

If urine stands, the urea reverts to ammonia — the familiar odour on a baby's wet nappy.

URIC ACID

An acid which forms when purines are broken

down. Purines are found in offal meats, sardines, other meats, alcoholic drinks, gravies, meat extracts and some vegetables (see page 285). High levels of uric acid in the blood usually accompany a high-fat diet. Uric acid is normally excreted via the kidneys. However, when a lot of alcohol is consumed, the level of lactic acid rises and the kidneys excrete this in preference to uric acid. Crystals of uric acid can then form in the joints, especially the joint of the big toe (see also Gout). Reptiles and birds excrete the waste nitrogen from the break down of protein as uric acid crystals rather than as urine.

To reduce uric acid, the first step is to lose weight (if overweight). Fatty foods, foods high in purines and alcohol should be avoided.

URINE

The liquid produced by the kidneys and excreted. About 1500 mL of urine are passed each day, containing any soluble waste products from the body, including excess vitamins and minerals. If there is insufficient water to form plenty of urine, the level of solids in urine increases. This can lead to kidney stones. The urine is fairly concentrated in the morning. At other times it should be almost clear. If urine continues to be yellow throughout the day, it means that insufficient water is being consumed.

USZKA

Small Polish dumplings made from a dough containing eggs and stuffed with mushrooms.

VACHERIN

A dessert usually consisting of a meringue case filled with whipped cream or icecream and fruits. Depending on its filling, a vacherin is high in fat and kilojoules.

VAGUS NERVE

A nerve which goes from the brain to the stomach and influences the production of acid in the stomach. This nerve represents one of the ways in which emotions can sometimes make it difficult to eat. For example, a child who is being scolded and is upset finds it difficult to digest foods.

VALINE

One of the essential amino acids. Rarely a problem since almost all foods contain valine.

VANADIUM

A mineral which is known to be essential for chickens and may also be needed by humans. The richest known food sources are radishes (with 79 mcg/100 g) and dill (14 mcg/100 g). Much smaller quantities are found in wheat, liver, fish and meat. No recommended daily intake has been set and quantities up to 4500 mcg/day have not been found to be toxic.

VANILLA

The pod of a climbing orchid native to South America, vanilla was used to flavour drinks in South America long before Europeans discovered it. Vanilla has little flavour until the unripe pods are put out in the sun each day for 10–20 days and then allowed to dry slowly for several months. This time delay allows

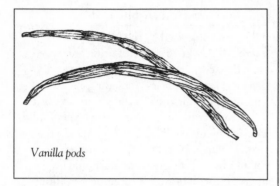

Vanilla pods

enzymes in the pod to free its essential flavour, vanillin, from its chemical links to glucose. The best quality pods have tiny crystals of vanillin covering them, providing the rich, sweet aroma of vanilla.

Early attempts to grow the vanilla vine in other parts of the world failed until it was realised that a particular type of bee and a species of hummingbird were responsible for pollinating the flowers of the vine. By introducing the bee to other areas and using hand pollination with a long wooden needle, vanilla vines can now be grown in other areas. Madagascar, the Comoro Islands, Mexico, Uganda and French Polynesia supply most of the world's vanilla beans.

Vanilla extract is made by crushing the cured dried beans and extracting the vanillin with alcohol.

Vanilla flavouring is made from vanilla extract, alcohol and water. Imitation vanilla is commercially synthesised from oil of cloves or from the lignin in wood. It does not have the complexity of flavour of true vanilla.

The full vanilla flavour comes from using the vanilla bean rather than the extract. For milk-based custards or icecreams, the vanilla bean is placed into hot milk and left for a few minutes. It can then be removed, washed and dried ready to use again. Many people store their vanilla bean in a jar of sugar. Gradually the sugar takes on the wonderful aroma and flavour of vanilla.

VARICOSE VEINS

Twisted or tortured veins which can occur in the legs and the oesophagus. Haemorrhoids are also a form of varicose veins. Varicose veins in the legs are the most common type and are related to being overweight, standing in the one place for long periods and possibly also to constipation. Straining to pass faeces exerts great pressure on the blood vessels and can force blood back down the leg veins, stretching them so that the valves do not function properly. The unsupported weight of the blood then distorts the veins.

In countries where people eat a lot of dietary fibre, varicose veins do not occur.

VEAL
see Meat.

VEGAN DIET

A diet containing no animal products at all. Milk, cheese, yoghurt and eggs are forbidden, as well as fish, poultry, gelatine and meat.

A vegan diet can still meet all the body's nutritional needs. However, this is not easy, especially for those with high nutrient requirements such as children, pregnant women and athletes. These people, especially children, may find it difficult to eat enough of the bulky vegetable food to provide their nutrient needs. Malnutrition is sometimes seen in vegan children, particularly if their diet is also low in fat or if there are some foods the children do not like eating.

The various amino acids which make up protein, and must be supplied in the diet, are all present in animal foods. No single vegetable food contains them all. This means that vegetable foods need to be eaten in combinations such as seeds with grains, or legumes with particular nuts or vegetables. (Appropriate combinations are on page 374.)

Calcium, iron and zinc can also be in short supply in a vegan diet (see individual entries for food sources).

The only vitamin likely to be in short supply if no animal products are consumed is Vitamin B_{12}. In spite of frequent medical warnings about the dangers of B_{12} deficiency, a few cases are reported regularly in children fed a vegan diet. Vitamin B_{12} has been found in mushrooms (it comes from the compost in which they are grown) and may also occur in fermented soya bean products (produced by the bacteria present in such foods) and in some drinking water. Some B_{12} may also be produced by bacteria in the intestine. The body normally keeps several years' supply of the vitamin, so deficiencies may take a long time to show up.

VEGEMITE

A yeast extract originally made by Fred Walker, a young Australian entrepreneur and developed by Dr C. P. Callister in 1923. Callister blended yeasts from different breweries and added celery, onion and salt. The name 'Vegemite' came from a competition among consumers. The Fred Walker company became the Kraft Walker Cheese Co Pty Ltd in 1926 and then Kraft Foods in 1950.

At one stage, early in the marketing of Vegemite, sales were falling and seemed slow so Walker introduced an additional product called Parwill, in direct opposition to Marmite, Vegemite's main competitor. Parwill was not a success and Walker returned to promoting Vegemite.

Vegemite was so rich in B complex vitamins that it was used by those in the army and in hospitals during World War II. Ordinary citizens had their supplies rationed.

The yeast from which Vegemite is made is one of the richest known sources of many of the B complex vitamins, especially thiamin, riboflavin, niacin and folacin. The vitamins are retained in the concentrated yeast extract. A thin spread of Vegemite (the amount on a single slice of bread) will supply the following

percentages of daily vitamin needs.

	A 7-YEAR-OLD	AN ADULT
• Thiamin	64 %	42 %
• Niacin	32 %	24 %
• Riboflavin	51 %	40 %
• Folacin	66 %	33 %

Vegemite also contains salt, although the present level of 8 per cent is less than the original 11 per cent. The present salt level equates to 3.2 grams of sodium per 100 g of Vegemite or, in a typical spread of Vegemite (3.5 g), 112 mg sodium — less than the sodium in the slice of bread on which Vegemite is spread. (1 slice of bread contains 132 mg sodium; butter or margarine adds a further 85 mg of sodium).

The daily recommended intake of sodium is 920−2300 mg a day. An average spread of Vegemite, with its 112 mg sodium, contributes 5−12% of the RDI. Yet this quantity of Vegemite provides a very substantial percentage of the day's vitamin B requirements. So Vegemite is not quite as black as it is sometimes painted.

See also Marmite; Yeast.

VEGETABLE GUMS

Vegetable gums are a valuable source of soluble dietary fibre and have been shown to lower blood cholesterol levels. They consist of methylcellulose or various polysaccharides which are not digested until they reach the bacteria in the large intestine. These polysaccharides are made up of glucose, xylose, galactose, rhamnose, arabinose, mannose and uronic acids. Other vegetable gums include guar gum, locust bean gum, gum arabic and tragacanth (see under individual entries). Alginic acid present in agar-agar and carrageenan from seaweeds is also a gum.

Gums are used to thicken foods such as salad dressings, desserts, icecreams, flavoured milk and some soft drinks. They help give body to these foods. Vegetable gums are listed as additives 400 to 416. See also Gums.

VEGETABLES

There are hundreds of foods cultivated throughout the world and known as vegetables. They include roots such as onions, parsnips and radishes; stems such as spinach; leaves such as spinach, cabbage or lettuce; fruits such as tomatoes or eggplant; and flowers such as cauliflower or French artichokes.

Most vegetables are highly nutritious with a useful content of minerals, vitamins and dietary fibre. They are mostly low in kilojoules and protein. They are especially valuable in the diet as a source of vitamin C, carotene, folacin and some of the tocopherols (vitamin E).

Many children are reluctant to eat vegetables. This is usually a method of arresting their mother's attention. It may also be a reflection on the way in which vegetables are prepared in some Western countries.

Alfalfa

A legume which is also known as lucerne. Often grown to be ploughed back into the soil to supply nitrogen. As a food, alfalfa is usually eaten in the form of alfalfa sprouts. Since the quantities consumed are usually quite small, alfalfa sprouts provide only small quantities of most nutrients. Part of their dietary fibre consists of substances called saponins which can remove cholesterol from the blood and thus reduce high levels of blood cholesterol.

Amaranth

A green leafy vegetable (sometimes with red veins) usually sold with its roots attached. To eat, the roots are discarded and the leaves are steamed or stir-fried. Also called Chinese spinach.

Nutritionally, amaranth is an excellent source of vitamin C and a good source of carotene, folacin (one of the B vitamins), calcium, iron and dietary fibre. A 50 g serve has 55 kJ (13 Cals).

Anise

see Fennel.

Arrowhead

A water plant with arrow-shaped leaves. Both the leaves and the root can be steamed or stir-fried. Arrowhead is an excellent source of potassium but has only small quantities of other minerals and vitamins. A 50 g serve has 210 kJ (50 Cals).

Artichoke

A large edible thistle which is native to the Mediterranean region and is variously called the globe, common or French artichoke. After steaming, the fleshy part of the leaves is scraped off with the teeth; once the leaves have been pulled off, the tender heart is eaten. The artichoke contains a unique organic acid which alters the taste of both water and wine for most people. After eating an artichoke, many people find water tastes sweet and the true flavour of wine is masked.

Nutritionally, the artichoke is an excellent source of dietary fibre and vitamin C and also provides potassium and small quantities of other minerals and vitamins. One bud has 105 kJ (25 Cals).

The Jerusalem artichoke is quite different, being a knobbly-shaped tuber looking rather like a small sweet potato. It has fewer nutrients than the globe artichoke and provides 80 kJ (19 Cals) per 100 g.

Arugula

Also known as rocket, this green salad vegetable has a slightly mustardy flavour and is popular in salads in Italy. It grows best in the spring.

Asparagus

A member of the lily family whose stalks are much prized as a food. Asparagus is usually green but may be grown underground to produce tender, delicate white stalks. Young stalks can be eaten raw but it is usually steamed until barely tender, or canned.

Nutritionally, asparagus is an excellent source of vitamin C, a good source of dietary fibre and also supplies the B group vitamins thiamin and riboflavin as well as potassium and iron. A 100-g serving has 70 kJ (17 Cals).

Aubergine

see Eggplant.

Bamboo shoots

The young shoots of bamboo can be eaten as a vegetable. They should always be cooked before eating or canning to destroy the cyanogens they contain and thus avoid cyanide poisoning. Nutritionally, bamboo shoots are a good source of potassium, free of fat and the cooked shoots have just 50 kJ (12 Cals) per 100 g.

Beans (green, French or string)

One of the most popular vegetables, the green bean originally came from Central America and records show it was used in 5000 BC. Many types of beans are available, including the purple bean (which turns green when cooked) and a variety of dried beans (see page 204).

Beans commonly eaten fresh include green (or French) beans, snake beans, yellow wax beans, broad beans, lima beans and purple climbing beans. The entire pod is eaten, except for older broad and lima beans, where the seeds are removed and the pod is considered inedible.

Broad beans originally grew in southwest Asia and the Mediterranean region. Green beans were first cultivated at least 7000 years ago in Central America and brought to Europe by the early Spanish and Portuguese traders. The lima bean is almost as old, and comes, along with its name, from Lima in Peru. Raw lima beans contain toxic substances called cyanogens which are destroyed by cooking.

There are also many beans whose seeds are eaten when dried. Among the richest vegetable sources of protein, dietary fibre and iron, dried beans come in many varieties, and are listed individually under legumes.

Nutritionally, beans are a good source of vitamin C and provide some iron, other minerals and vitamins as well as dietary fibre. The purple bean is a particularly good source of dietary fibre. Green beans have 90 kJ (21 Cals) per 100 g; the purple variety have 120 kJ (29 Cals) per 100 g.

Bean sprouts

Both beans and seeds can be sprouted by first soaking in water, draining and allowing to remain moist. Seeds are actually dormant embryos and once wet, they draw on their stored nutrients and begin to grow. The process of growth seems to excite the imagination and many people claim that sprouts have amazing nutritional virtues. In fact, sprouts use up some of the stored carbohydrates of the original bean or seed which reduces their kilojoules. They also produce vitamin C during the germinating process, although the quantities are quite modest when compared with many vegetables and fruits. The concentration of most other nutrients declines slightly due to an increasing content of water in the sprouts. The dietary fibre in sprouts may be valuable. Eaten raw in sandwiches or salads, or added to Asian-style foods, they provide a crunchy, nutritious food but they do not possess the 'wonder' properties sometimes attributed to them. They are a useful source of vitamin C for those who have no access to fresh foods.

Almost any bean can be sprouted but the term bean sprouts (or bean shoots) usually refers to the sprouts of the mung bean. Can be eaten raw or stir-fried. They are a source of dietary fibre and also contain some vitamin C. 50 g of bean sprouts have 40 kJ (10 Cals).

Beetroot

A root vegetable which contains about 8 per cent sugar — much more than most vegetables. The purple-coloured beetroot which we eat raw, cooked or canned, is a relative of sugar beet — a major source of sugar for much of the world's population. Beetroot is a good source of dietary fibre and contributes potassium as well as small quantities of other minerals and vitamins. 100 g beetroot contains 180 kJ (42 Cals).

Bok choy

Also known as baak choi, this Chinese vegetable is a type of cabbage. Both the leaf and the stalk are eaten. A dried form, known as 'choi gonn' is used in soups. Bok choy can be eaten raw or cooked in the same ways as cabbage or spinach. It is a good source of vitamin C, contributes small quantities of iron, calcium, various vitamins and dietary fibre. 100 g have 45 kJ (10 Cals).

Boletus

see Mushrooms.

Bracken

see Fiddlehead fern.

Brinjal

see Eggplant.

Broccoli

A green vegetable which is closely related to the cauliflower (both are members of the Brassica family and are descendants of wild cabbage). It can be eaten raw, steamed, stir-fried or made into soup.

Broccoli is one of the most nutritious vegetables available. It is an excellent source of vitamin C with 100 g providing more than 3 times the daily requirement. It is also a good source of dietary fibre and potassium and supplies useful quantities of iron, carotene (converted to vitamin A), vitamin E and several of the B complex vitamins. Broccoli also contains substances known as indoles which may have an anti-cancer action. 100 g broccoli have 100 kJ (24 Cals).

Brussels sprouts

First recorded as being grown in Brussels in Belgium in 1200, this vegetable is another nutritious member of the mustard or Brassica family. Brussels sprouts are an excellent source of vitamin C, containing a similar quantity to broccoli. They are also a good source of dietary fibre and potassium and contribute iron as well as a selection of other minerals, vitamins and indoles (see Broccoli). 100 g Brussels sprouts have 110 kJ (27 Cals).

Butternut pumpkin

see Pumpkin.

Cabbage

A member of the Brassica family, cabbage is one of the oldest cultivated vegetables, originally coming from the Mediterranean region. It also grows well in cold climates and, in its pickled form of sauerkraut, supplies much of the vitamin C during the winter months for people in very cold parts of Eastern Europe.

The longer cabbage is cooked, the stronger its flavour. Until recently, most people in countries such as the United Kingdom and Australia tended to boil vegetables until they were completely soft. The strong flavour (and the odour of hydrogen sulphide) of cabbage combined to make it a fairly unpopular vegetable. By eating cabbage raw or lightly cooked, this can be avoided. Chinese cabbage and various other types of cabbage generally have a milder flavour.

Red cabbage gets its colour from plant pigments known as anthocyanins.

Cabbages contain indoles (see Broccoli) and also substances known as goitrins which can interfere with the way the body uses iodine in the thyroid gland. Eating very large quantities of cabbage may aggravate an existing thyroid problem but will not usually cause the problem. Red cabbage also contains a substance which can destroy thiamin (vitamin B_1); this would only cause problems if very large quantities of red cabbage were eaten.

Nutritionally, cabbage is a most useful vegetable as it is an excellent source of vitamin C, a good source of dietary fibre (including some valuable soluble fibre) and potassium and supplies small quantities of other minerals and vitamins. Other varieties of cabbage have similar nutritional value. Chinese flowering cabbage and mustard cabbage have more carotene (converted to vitamin A in the body) and mustard cabbage is very rich in vitamin C. Red cabbage has almost twice the dietary fibre of regular cabbage.

100 g cabbage have 70 kJ (17 Cals). Chinese cabbage has even less with 100 g having just 35 kJ (8 Cals) while red cabbage has 95 kJ (23 Cals) per 100g.

Capsicum

In countries such as Australia, mild-flavoured red, green and yellow bell peppers are known as 'capsicums'. In the United States, the capsicum is an alternative name for the dried fruit of red peppers and is usually hot.

The capsicum (or bell pepper) is native to tropical America and is now grown all over the world, featuring in the cuisine of Mediterranean countries. The pimiento is a mild flavoured capsicum.

Nutritionally, capsicums are extremely high in vitamin C, with red capsicums having the most. One red capsicum has 11 times the average daily needs for this vitamin. Capsicums are also a source of dietary fibre and many vitamins and minerals. Red capsicums are rich in carotene (converted to vitamin A in the body). All varieties are low in kilojoules with 100 g having 65−105 kJ (15−25 Cals).

Cardoon

A thistle-like vegetable which grows in southern Europe and North Africa. Its inner leaves, stalk and thick root are boiled and eaten either hot or cold as a vegetable. It has almost a nutty flavour which is reminiscent of both artichoke and celery.

Nutritionally, the cardoon provides potassium, dietary fibre and small quantities of vitamins and minerals. 100 g have 85 kJ (20 Cals).

Carrot

A vegetable which is a native of Afghanistan. The early varieties were red, black or purple and the familiar orange type was not developed until the seventeenth century in Holland.

Nutritionally, the carrot is an excellent source of carotene (converted to vitamin A in the body), a good source of dietary fibre and provides small quantities of minerals and vitamins. 100 g carrots have 110 kJ (26 Cals).

Cassava

Also known as manioc, cassava is a large tuber which is grown throughout tropical regions for its roots which are eaten baked or boiled or made into flour for breads. Tapioca is also made from cassava. It is a good source of vitamin C, potassium and dietary fibre but has insufficient high quality protein to be used as a staple food. 100 g have 505 kJ (120 Cals).

See also Tapioca.

Cauliflower

A member of the Brassica family in which the partially developed flowering head is eaten.

Nutritionally, the cauliflower is an excellent source of vitamin C, a good source of dietary fibre and provides small but worthwhile quantities of various minerals and vitamins (including vitamin K). Cauliflower is also a good source of indoles (see Broccoli). 100 g have 80 kJ (19 Cals).

Celeriac

A distinctively flavoured root vegetable which is excellent served steamed or raw in salads. The flavour has a mild celery quality.

Nutritionally, celeriac is a good source of dietary fibre and provides small quantities of most vitamins and minerals. 100 g have 120 kJ (29 Cals).

Celery

A bunch of leaf stalks, celery is actually a member of the carrot family. Original versions of celery were bitter. These days, some celery is blanched by covering up the stalks with earth so that they are tender and sweet. Celery is most popular eaten raw.

Nutritionally, celery has not much to offer, providing small quantities only of minerals, vitamins and dietary fibre. The fact that celery appears stringy does not make it an especially good source of fibre. It is, however, a useful food for chewing to clean teeth. 100 g have 50 kJ (12 Cals).

Celtuce

A variety of lettuce with a celery flavour. Celtuce originated in China and is used in Chinese cooking. It is a good source of carotene, vitamin C and potassium. A 50 g serve has 45 kJ (11 Cals).

Chard

A vegetable rather like silverbeet. (Also called Swiss chard.) Both the green leaves and the reddish stalks can be eaten and are a rich source of vitamin C and carotene (converted to vitamin A in the body). Chard also contributes potassium and dietary fibre. 100 g have 85 kJ (20 Cals).

Chicory

A perennial plant with a blue flower, both the leaves and root of chicory are eaten as a vegetable, either raw or cooked. The chicory family includes Belgian endive, curly endive and escarole (or broad-leaf endive). The term 'chicory' is usually reserved for curly endive while Belgian endive is known as witloof (see page 373).

The leaves of chicory should be green, crisp and undamaged. They can be eaten raw in salads or steamed briefly to use as a hot vegetable. The roots can be steamed and eaten like any other root vegetable.

Nutritionally, chicory leaves are a good source of carotene (converted to vitamin A in the body), vitamin C and potassium. They also contribute dietary fibre and small quantities of many minerals and vitamins. 100 g of the leaves have 95 kJ (23 Cals). The root has only small quantities of minerals and vitamins but is a good source of dietary fibre. 100 g of the root have 305 kJ (73 Cals).

See also Endive.

Chinese spinach
see Amaranth.

Chive

A mildly flavoured miniature type of onion with a very small bulbous portion. Grows in clumps with small, white bulbs and green tubular leaves. Used to flavour omelettes and other egg dishes, salads (especially on tomatoes) and vegetables.

Chinese chives are long flat leaves, without a bulb. They have a stronger flavour than regular chives. If grown in the dark, this vegetable has a pale yellow appearance and is known as blanched Chinese chives. Flowering Chinese chives consist of a single tubular stem with a single conical bud at the top tip of each. If the bud has opened to a flower, the chive is considered too old to eat. The flavour is mild and the texture crisp but tender.

Nutritionally, chives are quite good sources of iron, dietary fibre and vitamins. In practice, however, the quantities eaten are too small to be significant.

Choko

A member of the gourd family. The fast-growing vine produces a smooth or prickly green fruit which can be used as a vegetable or added to cooked fruit dishes. Nutritionally, the fruit provides some vitamin C and dietary fibre and small quantities of other minerals and vitamins. 100 g have 75 kJ (18 Cals).

Courgette
see Zucchini.

Cress

A plant of the mustard family with small round leaves with a somewhat mustardy flavour. Usually grown to use in salads or sandwiches. Nutritionally, cress is rich in vitamins A and C but the quantity consumed is usually too small to make a significant contribution. See also Watercress.

Cucumber

Closely related to melons, cucumbers originated in India but many varieties are now cultivated throughout the world. Until 200 years ago, cucumbers were thought to be harmful and the skin was said to be poisonous.

Nutritionally, cucumbers contain small quantities of dietary fibre, minerals and vitamins. They are very low in kilojoules with 100 g having just 175 kJ (42 Cals).

Eggplant

Also known as aubergine or brinjal, this vegetable is a member of the nightshade family and is related to the potato. It is a native of India, and was introduced to Spain and North Africa in the middle ages. By the fifteenth century it was widely used in Italy and several hundred years later became popular in France. These days it features strongly in the cooking of Mediterranean countries.

The skin of the eggplant may be white or purple. The flesh has a spongy texture and will soak up vast quantities of oil if fried. Until recently it was advisable to sprinkle salt over eggplant slices, leave them for a while and then rinse and drain before cooking. This removed a slightly bitter flavour from the vegetable. Modern varieties of eggplant do not have this bitter taste and the salting step is no longer necessary.

Eggplant can be grilled, fried, used in casseroles, in moussaka, in vegetable dishes such as ratatouille or made into pickles. It can also be baked whole, cut open, the centre removed and mixed with various ingredients to produce stuffed eggplant halves. The cooked flesh can be pureed with a little olive oil and garlic to form the Lebanese dip known as baba ghannouj.

Nutritionally, eggplant provides small quantities of many vitamins and minerals as well as dietary fibre. It has no fat and is low in kilojoules with 100 g having only 70 kJ (17 Cals).

Endive

A member of the chicory family, native to India but widely cultivated in Mediterranean countries. Curly endive tastes like a bitter lettuce and can be eaten raw in a salad or cooked like spinach. Belgian endive is also known as witloof (see page 373). Escarole is a broad-leafed endive.

Nutritionally, endive is a good source of vitamin C and supplies carotene (converted to vitamin A in the body) as well as iron and dietary fibre and a selection of other minerals and vitamins. It is very low in kilojoules with 100 g providing just 40 kJ (10 Cals).

See also Chicory.

Escarole

see Endive.

Fennel

Also known as anise and finocchio, fennel is a white bulbous vegetable with feathery green leaves. The bulb looks a little like celery but has an aniseed flavour. It can be braised, steamed, eaten raw or blanched and used in salads. The leaves can be used to provide flavour to fish dishes, creamed soups or sauces or used in stuffings for lamb or fish.

Nutritionally, fennel provides some dietary fibre and small quantities of minerals and vitamins. 100 g of fennel have 80 kJ (19 Cals).

Fiddlehead fern

Commonly called bracken, the young shoots of the fiddlehead fern can be cooked or served raw in salads. Fiddlehead fern is a good source of vitamin C. A 50 g serve has 75 kJ (18 Cals).

Garland chrysanthemum

The green leaves of several varieties of chrysanthemum used in Japanese and Chinese cooking. As the leaves have a subtle but definite 'flower' flavour, they are used only in small quantities as part of a dish.

Chrysanthemum leaves are a good source of vitamin C, provide some calcium and other minerals and vitamins. A 30 g serve has 25 kJ (6 Cals).

Garlic

A member of the lily family and originally native to Asia, garlic has been used for 3000 years in China, and almost as long in Egypt. It also grows wild in Italy and southern France and is used in many of the dishes from these regions. In ancient Egypt, garlic was thought to contribute to the health and strength of the slaves who built the great pyramids. Since then, garlic has been used as an antibiotic, an antiseptic, and more recently, a method for lowering blood fats. A variety of other claims have also been made for garlic ranging from its alleged ability to cure warts, dandruff, worms and even prevent the greying of hair! Most of these claims cannot be substantiated.

Garlic does contain some sulphur components which have medicinal properties but whether it can live up to all the claims made for it is doubtful. The active principles in garlic include allicin (diallyl sulphide) which is also responsible for its characteristic odour and allyl propyl disulphide. They certainly function as antiseptics and the juice from garlic bulbs was used on wounds during World War I. There is also some evidence that the sulphur-containing substances in garlic can lower blood cholesterol levels. However, much greater effects can be achieved by eating less fat.

There is no real evidence that garlic cures the common cold — although it may well stop others from catching it!

See also Herbs.

Gourd

Vegetables/fruit of the melon family, edible when young but it is amazingly difficult to penetrate the tough skin of the older gourds. The gourds are probably native to Africa and China where they have been a staple part of the diet for thousands of years. The bottle gourd and the hairy gourd (a melon shaped rather like a baseball bat) are edible when young. The wax gourd is also known as 'winter melon' and is widely used in Asia. To prepare: remove the seeds and coarse fibres at the centre of the melon, slice or chop finely and stir-fry or use in soups. The shell can be dried and used as a bottle or bowl.

Nutritionally, gourds provide vitamin C, some varieties being rich sources. Others are good sources of carotene and provide some dietary fibre and small quantities of a range of vitamins and minerals. The kilojoule content varies from 55−125 kJ (13−30 Cals) per 100 g.

Green pepper

see Capsicum.

Jicama

Also known as the yam bean, the jicama is a tuber which grows in Mexico. Its white crunchy flesh is quite sweet and can be eaten raw or cooked. It is traditionally served with guacamole (see page 174). It can also be substituted for bamboo shoots in stir-fried or other Chinese dishes. It is a good source of vitamin C and dietary fibre and 100 g have 170 kJ (40 Cals).

Kale

A green leafy vegetable of the cabbage family (a Brassica). Very hardy and grows in cold climates when other greens are finished. Rarely seen in Australia.

A rich source of vitamin C, folacin and carotene, kale also has more calcium and iron than most other vegetables. It is also a good source of dietary fibre. 1 cup of raw kale (70 g) has 145 kJ (35 Cals).

Kohlrabi

A member of the cabbage family, kohlrabi looks like a small swollen turnip. However, it is not a root vegetable but is the swollen stem of a plant growing above the ground. Its purple skin hides a white interior with a flavour a little more delicate than that of a turnip. It can be eaten raw in a salad, steamed or stir-fried.

It is an excellent source of vitamin C, a good source of potassium and dietary fibre and provides some iron as well as other minerals and vitamins. 100 g have 140 kJ (33 Cals).

Kudzu

A root vegetable which can grow to about 50 cm in length. It looks a little like an irregular-shaped yam with tapered ends. Its white, slightly sweet flesh is a little like that of its relative the jicama. Unlike jicama, it is tough to chew and is used to produce a starch which can be used as a thickener. Although its name is from Japan, the kudzu has been cultivated throughout Asia for centuries.

To cook the kudzu, simmer its chopped flesh with chicken or beef bones for several hours. The resulting liquid will be quite sweet and you may even be able to chew the kudzu itself. If not, throw it out and drink the broth.

Lamb's lettuce

A soft-leafed lettuce used in Europe.

Leeks

First cultivated in the Mediterranean region, leeks are a member of the lily family and the national plant of Wales. This distinguished position was afforded to the leek as a result of a legend which said that during a battle between King Cadwallader and the Saxons, the Welsh wore leeks in their hats to distinguish themselves from the enemy.

The bulb of the leek and a variable part of its stem are eaten, either braised or cut into rings and added to soups, stews and casseroles. The famous soup, vichysoisse, is made from leeks and potatoes.

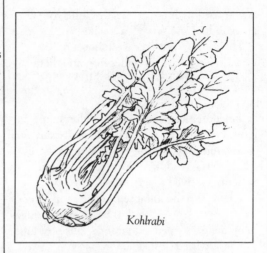

Kohlrabi

Leeks are a good source of vitamin C and provide dietary fibre and a number of minerals and vitamins. 100 g leek have 110 kJ (25 Cals).

Lettuce

Originally grown 5000 years ago in the Mediterranean region, lettuce now comes in many different forms. The best known lettuces are the iceberg with its round full head and crisp green leaves, cos with its long, firm green leaves, mignonette with its purple-tinged leaves and butter lettuce with its softer texture.

Lettuce is perhaps the most basic ingredient in salads but it can also be braised and served as a hot vegetable.

Nutritionally, lettuce provides some potassium, carotene (in the dark green outer leaves), dietary fibre and small quantities of minerals and vitamins. It has very few kilojoules; an average serving of 2 large or 4 small leaves has about 20 kJ (5 Cals).

Lotus root

The swollen brown bulbs of this Chinese vegetable look like a string of sausages. After washing, discard the neck, remove the skin, peel and cut up or slice to reveal the decorative pattern. The root can be steamed, baked, braised or fried. For special occasions in China, the whole lotus root is stuffed with mung beans and braised with pork. Slices of lotus root are also candied and served as snacks.

The lotus root is an excellent source of vitamin C and also provides iron and dietary fibre. 100 g of lotus root have 210 kJ (50 Cals).

Luffa

A dark green vegetable of the melon family, long and thin with a ridged skin and small 'warty' lumps. Only the young vegetables are edible as the seeds in older plants develop violent laxative properties.

To prepare the luffa, remove the top layer of skin, leaving the green skin between the ridges to produce a striped appearance. Slices of luffa can be stir-fried or steamed.

The luffa provides small quantities of minerals, vitamins and dietary fibre. 100 g have 70 kJ (17 Cals).

Mange tout

see Snow Peas.

Manioc

see Cassava.

Marrow

A vegetable of the cucumber or squash family, native to South America and the southwestern areas of the United States. Seeds of these vegetables dating back many thousands of years BC have been found in parts of South America.

Rather like a very large zucchini, the marrow generally has less flavour than its smaller counterparts. It can be steamed or microwaved and is probably at its best when seeded, stuffed and baked. Marrows have only small quantities of nutrients. 100 g have 30 kJ (7 Cals).

Melons

Most Westerners know melons as fruits, but the winter melon, the fuzzy melon and the bitter melon are used as vegetables in Asian cuisine. Their nutritional value is similar to that of the marrow.

The winter melon can weigh up to 45 kg and is a bland-tasting, white-fleshed cousin of the watermelon which has been bred from the cassaba melon. It can be stir-fried or steamed but needs only a short cooking time so that it keeps its texture.

The fuzzy melon looks like a large green cucumber with a few hairs. It is closely related to the winter melon and is eaten while quite young before its white flesh has become too bland in flavour. Can be used like zucchini.

The bitter melon has a ridged skin covered with 'warts'. The melon changes from a green colour to orange when ripe. It is best eaten somewhere in between the green and very bitter stage and the soft, ripe and slightly sweet orange stage. The bitter flavour is not usually liked by Westerners but is popular stir-fried, with beef or pork and black bean sauce in China. It is sometimes blanched, then salted for 15 mins before being rinsed and dried for use.

Mushroom

Although usually listed with vegetables, mushrooms are not vegetables but edible fungi. As such, their metabolism and nutritional value are different from other vegetables.

There are many varieties of mushrooms which grow wild, appearing in greatest numbers during autumn. They have been used as food since at least 3500 BC when the Sumerians put their wonderful flavour to good use.

Mushrooms are more closely related to moulds and yeasts and are unable to photosynthesise sugars. They usually live in symbiosis with the roots of trees, extracting sugars from the roots and providing minerals such as phosphorus in return. The cell walls of mushrooms are made of chitin, the same type of material which makes up the outer skeleton of insects.

Many varieties of mushrooms are quite toxic, so safe varieties are cultivated in most Western countries. Although these have less flavour than some of the wild mushrooms, the safety and convenience of cultivated mushrooms have made them a popular food worldwide.

Mushrooms grow from spores which appear just under the surface of the soil. The first flush produces many mushrooms, often growing close together. If these are picked a further flush will appear some days later.

The substrate on which the mushroom spawns influences the final nutritional value to some extent. For example, mushrooms grown on material which includes animal compost will contain vitamin B_{12} which migrates from the substrate into the mushroom. Since the diet of a complete vegetarian (a vegan) may be lacking in this vitamin, mushrooms are a useful way for vegans to replenish their supplies of B_{12}.

Nutritionally, mushrooms are a good source of niacin, containing as much of this vitamin as is found in meat. Mushrooms also contribute some dietary fibre and small quantities of many of the other B complex vitamins. They have no fat and are very low in kilojoules. 100 g of cultivated mushrooms have 95 kJ (22 Cals). Some varieties, such as straw mushrooms, have slightly higher values with 100 g having 140 kJ (34 Cals). These mushrooms are extremely high in niacin. For dried mushrooms, $\frac{1}{2}$ cup has 150 kJ (35 Cals).

Mushrooms should not be washed, but merely wiped immediately before use. They can be stored for a few days in a paper or cloth bag in the refrigerator. Do not keep them in a plastic bag or they will sweat and go bad. Some of the popular varieties of mushroom include:

- *Agaricus bisporus* — the cultivated mushroom. First cultivated in France in the seventeenth century, this variety is now grown throughout the world. It is grown in controlled conditions of temperature and humidity on a mixture of manure, straw and soil.
- *Agaricus campestris* — field mushroom. Found in meadows from late summer to autumn. Similar to the cultivated mushroom but may be larger and darker in colour. Its flavour is more intense and it is ideally suited for making soups and giving flavour to casseroles.

Cultivated mushrooms are commonly sold at three stages: buttons (or champignons), caps (beginning to open) and flats (fully opened, larger and with a more pronounced flavour).

- *Boletus cep* or yellow mushrooms. These excellent eating mushrooms have been favoured since the days of ancient Greece and Rome. They are found in conifer woods during late summer and autumn. They have stout fleshy stalks and delicately raised white veins running to the top. They have a superb flavour and may be used to prepare dried mushrooms. Known as porcini in Italy.
- *Chanterelles* — also known as egg mushrooms. These yellow-brown mushrooms grow in woods, especially beech woods. They have a funnel shape and a delicious flavour. During cooking, these yellow-brown mushrooms smell slightly of apricots. They take a little longer to cook than most other mushrooms.
- *Cultivated mushroom* — see *Agaricus bisporus* (above).
- *Field mushroom* — see *Agaricus campestris* (above).
- *Jew's ear mushrooms.* A European mushroom closely related to the wood mushroom of China. These mushrooms have a convoluted shape (a little like an ear) and grow on tree trunks. They are dried and used in Chinese cooking. Used raw, they have little flavour but contribute some texture and colour to a dish.
- *Morels.* A mushroom with a spongy cap and deep folds or hollows where the spores develop. They grow in spring and early summer and have a delicate flavour.
- *Puffball.* Edible when young, firm and white, the puffball appears during autumn. It has a mild flavour and traces of it have been

found in the remains of Stone Age settlements.

- *Shitake* — or winter mushrooms. These are widely used in Japanese cuisine and have been cultivated for more than 1000 years. They are grown on the wood of dead deciduous trees. In Japan they are cooked fresh; in China, they are dried and used in many soups, meat or fish dishes. The tough stems are removed from the fresh mushrooms and kept to give flavour to soups.
- *Straw mushrooms* — or grass mushrooms. These small conical-shaped, smooth brownish-grey mushrooms are widely used in Asia and are the only mushrooms which the Cantonese eat fresh. They are grown, as their name suggests, on straw and are eaten before their umbrella-like structure 'breaks out'. They are sliced or left whole and are often canned.

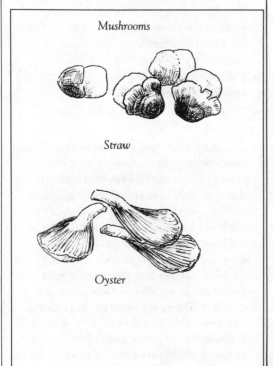

Mushrooms

Straw

Oyster

Mustard greens

The leaves of the white mustard plant can be eaten as a vegetable. This is the product usually grown with cress and sold as mustard and cress. Since the mustard is quite hot, very little is usually consumed. Nutritionally, mustard greens' high content of vitamins (especially vitamin C) is insignificant.

Nettle

In early spring, the young leaves at the tip of the common stinging nettle can be used as a vegetable, steamed or made into nettle soup. Nettles can also be fermented with sugar to produce alcoholic drinks. The 'sting' of the nettle comes from formic acid in the hairs on the leaves. By plucking just the end of the plant, the sting can be avoided. Like most green leaves, nettles have plenty of vitamins A, C and folacin (one of the B vitamins).

Okra

Also known as lady's finger or gumbo, okra is a vegetable which is native to tropical Africa and Asia. It has been cultivated in Egypt for about 800 years. It is related to the hibiscus and the edible portion is the immature pod. When cooked it becomes sticky and syrupy and is often used to thicken soups and stews. It can also be steamed and eaten as a vegetable. It is widely used in the southern states of America, mainly in rice and bean dishes. In India, okra is called bindi and in the Middle East it is known as bamia.

Nutritionally, the mucilages in okra make it an excellent source of soluble dietary fibre. It is also a good source of vitamin C and folic acid. 100 g of okra pods have only 70 kJ (17 Cals).

Onion

The onion is native to a wide region from the Middle East to India. It has been cultivated for about 5000 years and has been called 'king of the vegetables' because of its distinctive flavour and long and widespread use.

The onion is technically a stem and a leaf and each layer of onion is designed to provide food reserves for the new shoot which will grow from the centre of the onion.

The typical flavour and odour of the onion is noticed only when the onion is cut. With the disruption of the cells, an odourless sulphur-containing compound derived from the amino acid cysteine, is brought into contact with an enzyme. This immediately produces the substances which give onion its distinctive odour. Chives and garlic react in the same way but produce slightly different chemicals with their own distinctive odours.

The tears which we shed when cutting up onions are caused by another substance arising from cysteine. This volatile substance dissolves in the fluids in the eye and produces some mild sulphuric acid which stings and makes the eyes water.

When cooking, onions give off much of their odour compounds filling a kitchen with mouth-watering aromas. Some of these compounds are also turned into a sweet substance which accounts for part of the appeal of fried onions.

There are a number of different varieties of onions. Spanish onions (known as 'red onions' in the United Kingdom) are a purple colour and have a mild, slightly sweet flavour. Italian onions are smaller, also a reddish purple colour and have a mild flavour. White or brown onions (the latter is known as a 'yellow onion' in the United States and as a 'Spanish onion' in the United Kingdom) are available all year round. The brown skinned varieties have the best keeping qualities.

Nutritionally, onions contribute small quantities of many vitamins and minerals but are not rich sources of any. They do contribute some dietary fibre and their sulphur compounds may have some ability to lower cholesterol, if you could eat enough of them. A medium-sized onion (125 g) has 125 kJ (30 Cals).

Oyster plant
see Salsify.

Palm heart
Also known as 'hearts of palm', this vegetable is the pale coloured heart of the cabbage tree palm. At times, the terminal shoot of some varieties of palm is also sold as heart of palm. The products are usually only available canned. They are used in salads or as an appetiser.

Parsnip
A creamy coloured root vegetable of the carrot family. Native to the Eastern Mediterranean region, parsnips were used by early Greek and Roman civilisations. They have the best and sweetest flavour when grown in cold climates. They are suitable to steam, microwave (whole or in slices or chunks) or whole parsnips can be baked. They are also delicious mashed with a hint of finely grated orange rind.

Parsnips have a higher content of sugar than most vegetables (3 g per 100 g). They are a good source of dietary fibre and potassium and provide some vitamin C and other nutrients. Their kilojoule count is a little higher than some vegetables, but they can easily be included in any weight reduction diet. 100 g of parsnip have 210 kJ (50 Cals).

Peas, fresh
One of the oldest vegetables, peas were native to western Asia and were eaten dried until about the sixteenth century when fresh peas became a great delicacy, especially in France. A reverence for tiny new peas (petit pois), remains in that country. Recent developments in pea breeding have given us sugar or honey peas and snow peas (also known as mange tout). In these varieties, the pea pod has fibres going only in one direction rather than the criss-cross fibres in regular pea pods. The one-way fibre means they can be chewed easily and both pea and pod can be eaten.

In Western countries, most peas are removed from their pods and frozen. Nutritionally, this is an excellent move since most peas are frozen within about 20 mins of being picked and any losses of nutrients are halted. While frozen peas have a good flavour, peas which are freshly picked and eaten are even better.

Regular peas are high in protein (6 g per 100 g) and have more dietary fibre than most other vegetables. They are also a good source of vitamin C, iron and niacin (B_3) as well as providing zince and a good selection of other vitamins from the B complex. A typical serve of 50 g of peas has only 125 kJ (30 Cals). They do not deserve a reputation for being fattening. No vegetable does.

Snow peas have about half the dietary fibre and iron of regular peas but are still a worthwhile source. They also contain some protein and potassium and are an excellent source of vitamin C. A 50 g serve of snow peas has 70 kJ (17 Cals).

Peppers

see Capsicum.

Potato

Probably the most important vegetable in the world. Some populations have made this vegetable the staple part of their diet. Native to the Andes in South America and a staple food of the Incas, the potato is a tuber which belongs to the nightshade family. With its ability to grow in high and cold areas, it has proved invaluable in many areas.

The Spaniards took potatoes to Europe in the sixteenth century and they were eagerly grown in Ireland by the early part of the seventeenth century. The entire Irish economy became dependent on the potato and the crop failures of the mid nineteenth century caused widespread famine.

Potatoes have become especially popular in Germany, parts of Scandinavia and as the ubiquitous French fries throughout the world. They can be baked, roasted, steamed or boiled and mashed. Potato salads, pancakes, souffles and many dishes made from layers of sliced potatoes interspersed with other ingredients are all popular. Potato flour is also used in some German and Scandinavian breads.

In some countries, certain varieties of potato are marketed as being suitable for frying, baking or mashing. In other areas, they are merely designated as 'old' or 'new' potatoes, depending on how long they have remained in the ground. In general, new potatoes are immature and are most suitable for steaming or using in salads. Old potatoes can be stored for a longer time, have a dry mealy texture and are excellent for baking, mashing or making into chips.

Potatoes are a good source of complex carbohydrate, vitamin C and dietary fibre and supply small but significant amounts of minerals and vitamins. The fact that they are eaten so frequently makes them a significant source of many nutrients in the human diet. Their reputation as being 'fattening' is quite undeserved. An average-sized potato (125 g) has 345 kJ (82 Cals). It would be difficult to gain weight by eating potatoes — more than 90 would be required to increase weight by just 1 kg!

The major nutritional problem associated with potatoes comes from the oil or fat in which French fries or chips are cooked or from the sour cream or butter which is so frequently served with them. The potato itself is not to blame for excess weight.

The green colour which can develop on the skin of new potatoes may cause problems. Potato skins contain solanine and the level of this substance increases rapidly when the potatoes are exposed to light. Too much solanine can cause nausea, diarrhoea and vomiting. To guard against this, potatoes should be kept in a cool, well-ventilated, dark environment. Any green patches on the skin should be removed before cooking.

Pumpkin

A member of the cucumber family which originated in America, pumpkins are highly regarded as a food in some parts of the world but considered fit only for pig feed in others. There are many species of pumpkin and some have been cultivated for 9000 years. They range in size from 0.5 to 25 or 30 kg with the common varieties being 2–3 kg. Their growth rate can be fast with some pumpkins gaining 350 g per day!

In the United States, some varieties of pumpkin are known as 'winter squash'. The yellow fleshed vegetable with a pale orange-beige skin, known as a butternut pumpkin in some countries, is called a butternut squash in others. The butternut pumpkin is one of the most popular varieties. It has a rounded base containing seeds and a longish neck. Its pale brown skin is edible and the flesh has a sweeter flavour due to a higher content of sucrose.

Although some varieties have been valued for their nutritious seeds, the flesh of pumpkin is also a rich source of carotene which is converted to vitamin A in the body. They are also good sources of vitamin C and provide dietary fibre and potassium as well as some iron. 100 g of pumpkin has 65–190 kJ (15–45 Cals). They do not, therefore, deserve the reputation they have in some areas as being 'fattening'.

Pumpkins are used as a vegetable, a soup or in desserts. They can be baked, steamed, cooked in a fire (with skin on), made into soups, scones or steamed and used in a pie filling. They are also used for decoration at Halloween in the United States. The inside of the pumpkin is hollowed out, a face is carved in the shell and a candle or torch placed inside to shine out through the face.

Raddichio

A red, slightly bitter Italian lettuce. Available all year, its flavour complements that of other salad greens. Nutritionally similar to lettuce.

Radish

A root vegetable of the Brassica family. There are several major kinds of radish which probably originated in different parts of the world. They may be small and red, longer and white or even black skinned. In weight, radishes vary from a few grams for the tiny round red variety to a kilogram or so for the large white radishes used in oriental cookery. Their flavour varies from mild to quite pungent.

The large white radish probably originated in southern Asia and is finely sliced and stir-fried or used soups. The Japanese Daikon radish is mild in flavour and is usually served grated or pickled. The small red radish is eaten raw in salads.

Radishes are a good source of vitamin C and provide small quantities of other vitamins and minerals. They also contain dietary fibre, with the white radish having more than the red variety. The kilojoules are low, ranging from 35 kJ (9 Cals) for 50 g of the white radish to as low as 10 kJ (2 Cals) for each red radish. They will certainly never make you fat!

Rocket

see Arugula.

Rocket cress

Sometimes known as Italian cress, rocket is a spicy addition to salads.

Rutabaga

A root vegetable closely related to the turnip and first grown in Scandinavian countries in the eighteenth century. Its flesh is an orange-yellow colour and has a smooth dense texture and a strong flavour. Nutritionally, the rutabaga is a good source of dietary fibre, vitamin C and potassium. A 100 g serve has 145 kJ (35 Cals).

Salsify

Also called oyster plant, salsify is a root vegetable with a black or white skin, depending on the variety. Salsify is native to Europe and the Mediterranean regions and can be steamed, used for soups or casseroles or served in salads. After cooking, salsify looks shiny and slippery and this is presumably why it has been known as 'oyster plant'. It contains small quantities of minerals, vitamins and dietary fibre. 100 g of steamed salsify have 75 kJ (18 Cals).

Scallions

The vegetable known as a scallion in America is called a spring onion in Great Britain and a shallot in Australia. The Australian 'spring onion' differs from the shallot in having a more bulbous base. See also Shallot.

Shallots

A true shallot looks like a very small brown onion. It grows in small clumps and has a milder flavour than onions. Its name comes from the Greek word askalon which was the name of a small trading town in Israel where shallots were once sold.

The vegetable called a shallot in Australia is actually a spring onion. It is widely used in salads, for stir-frying or to give a fresh mild onion flavour to egg dishes, sauces, fish or other savoury dishes. The top part of the green shoot is not used.

Nutritionally, these shallots (or spring onions) are a good source of vitamin C and provide small quantities of other vitamins, minerals and dietary fibre. $\frac{1}{2}$ cup sliced shallots has 25 kJ (6 Cals).

Silverbeet

see Spinach.

Snow peas

see Peas.

Sorrel

Used as a vegetable and also as a herb, sorrel has an acidic, lemony flavour. French sorrel has a thicker, more succulent leaf and a milder flavour than the English variety (also known as wild or Russian sorrel). Both varieties have a high content of oxalic acid. Used in soups or sauces, sorrel finds a place in French cooking. Indian sorrel is used in curries and soups. Sorrel is high in vitamin C.

Spaghetti squash

Also known as vegetable spaghetti, this squash ranges in size from 800 g to several kilograms. It has a creamy coloured rind and is boiled or steamed whole for 20–40 mins, according to size. The squash is then cut open, the seeds removed and the flesh pulled out with a fork. It resembles long strands of spaghetti and can be served with any of the typical spaghetti sauces.

Nutritionally, it is a good source of dietary fibre and contains small quantities of minerals and vitamins. One cup of cooked spaghetti squash has 190 kJ (45 Cals).

Spinach

This green, leafy vegetable originated in Persia and some children wish it had stayed there! Because of its high iron content, spinach has been frequently given to children, some of whom do not like its rather strong flavour. Unfortunately for all the children who have reluctantly eaten their spinach, its iron is not very useful to humans as it is bound with oxalic acid. Many of the complaints of children regarding spinach should really be directed at the silverbeet which is grown in countries such as Australia and New Zealand and is commonly referred to as 'spinach'. Silverbeet has a much stronger flavour and a coarser texture than true English spinach. It is also likely that children's dislike of spinach is due to the common practice of boiling it until it is overcooked. Spinach needs just a few minutes of cooking or, if young, can be enjoyed raw.

Apart from the disappointment over its iron content, spinach remains an excellent source of vitamin C and also carotene which is converted into vitamin A in the body. It is also a good source of potassium and is, contrary to common belief, quite low in sodium. Silverbeet, by comparison, has much less carotene and does have a reasonably high level of sodium. 100 g of spinach have 65 kJ (15 Cals) while the same quantity of silverbeet has 55 kJ (13 Cals).

Spring greens

Sold in the United Kingdom, naturally enough in spring, spring greens are cabbages which are too young to have developed hearts. They are highly nutritious, being very good sources of vitamin C, carotene and dietary fibre and also supplying iron and other minerals and vitamins. 100 g of spring greens have only 45 kJ (10 Cals).

Spring onions

see Shallots.

Squash

Members of the cucumber family, squash come in all kinds of shapes and sizes and colours ranging from cream to yellow to light or dark green or variegated. Most squash are native to America and many were cultivated by American Indians 9000 years ago. In the United States, squash are divided into winter and summer squash. Winter squash fit a category called pumpkins by Australians (acorn, butternut and Hubbard squash). Summer squash include zucchini and smaller marrow-type vegetables which do not need to be peeled.

In Australia, squash include the small scallopini and button squash which are dark or light green or yellow on the skin and generally have pale green flesh. They are round or oblong and may have folded or smooth skin.

Nutritionally, the summer squash are good sources of vitamin C and provide some dietary fibre as well as a selection of minerals and vitamins. They are low in kilojoules, with 100 g providing approximately 85 kJ (20 Cals).

Swede

A fairly recent root vegetable first grown in the seventeenth century. Related to the turnip but has a stronger flavoured yellow flesh. Can be baked, boiled and mashed or stir-fried. The swede which is grown in Europe and Australia is very similar to the vegetable known as a rutabaga in the United States. Swedes are a good source of vitamin C and dietary fibre and provide some potassium and small quantities of other minerals and vitamins. 100 g of swede have 75 kJ (18 Cals).

Sweetcorn

Native to South America, sweetcorn is eaten as a vegetable when young (or in its immature state). For details about corn, see Grains and also page 83.

As a vegetable, sweetcorn is an excellent source of dietary fibre and complex carbohydrate. It is also a good source of iron and supplies small quantities of protein and many minerals and vitamins. An average cob (120 g edible portion) has 475 kJ (113 Cals).

Sweet potato

The root of a plant belonging to the morning glory family and native to tropical America. It is quite different from the yam or the ordinary potato. The colour of the flesh of the root of the sweet potato ranges from creamy white to orange. The skins are light brown, pink or even a purple colour. It is now grown in the United States, Europe, China and throughout the Pacific Islands.

Its 'sweetness' comes from its content of about 3 per cent sucrose. This increases during storage in warm climates and may reach 6 per cent. When cooked, enzymes also break down some of its starch to glucose. It is served baked in pieces, cooked and mashed, baked in slices with apples, made into pie fillings or served in a syrup with ham.

Nutritionally, the sweet potato is a good source of vitamin C and provides dietary fibre as well as a range of other minerals and vitamins. The yellow-fleshed variety is also rich in carotene. 100 g of sweet potato have 305 kJ (72 Cals) with the yellow variety having 280 kJ (67 Cals).

Taro

A vegetable grown for its tubers and leaves. Originally from southeastern Asia, it is now grown widely throughout the Pacific Islands. The tubers are steamed or boiled and made into a thick paste or a pudding. The large taro leaves are steamed. Both the leaves and the tubers of taro need to be cooked to destroy some of the calcium oxalate they contain. Taro is a good source of dietary fibre and provides vitamin C and potassium as well as small quantities of many minerals and vitamins. 100 g of taro have 455 kJ (108 Cals).

Tomato

A member of the nightshade family, the tomato is indigenous to the Andes region of South America. It was brought to Europe in 1523 and was regarded as an ornamental plant, known as 'love apple', in England. Only the Italians commonly ate tomatoes while the rest of Europe regarded it as being as poisonous as its relative, deadly nightshade. By the nineteenth century, its superb eating qualities were realised and consumption is now second only to the potato in most Western countries.

Tomatoes can be eaten fresh, grilled, stuffed and baked, made into soups, sauces or added to casseroles. They can also be used for jam. Canned tomatoes have similar nutritional value to fresh ones except for the added salt. However, tomatoes canned without salt are now widely available.

Nutritionally, tomatoes are a good source of vitamin C, carotene and dietary fibre. An average-sized tomato (125 g) has 295 kJ (70 Cals).

Turnip

This root vegetable has white flesh and can be either round or elongated. Baby turnips have the best flavour; older vegetables become rather strong.

Turnips can be steamed, roasted, mashed or used in casseroles or soups. Because of their strong flavour, only small quantities can be used in soups and casseroles.

Nutritionally, turnips are a good source of vitamin C, provide some dietary fibre and small quantities of minerals and vitamins. 100 g turnips have 80 kJ (19 Cals).

Water chestnuts

There are four major types of water chestnut — three of them are true water chestnuts.

The water chestnut most familiar to Western countries is usually the canned form of the Chinese water chestnut, a plant in the sedge family and not the true water chestnut. It is grown mainly in China and Japan and looks like a small ball covered in dirt. Once washed and peeled, the flesh is crunchy, succulent and sweet. These water chestnuts can be eaten raw as a snack, or steamed or added to soups or minced as a filling in wontons. Chinese people do not usually stir-fry water chestnuts. The canned water chestnuts are a good source of dietary fibre and supply small quantities of minerals and vitamins. 100 g have 210 kJ (50 Cals).

The true water chestnuts are *Tapa natans*, *Tapa bispinosa* and *Tapa bicornata*. They are native to Europe, Asia and parts of Africa. They have a tough outer shell which is removed and are then boiled or braised.

- *Tapa natans*, also known as the Jesuit's nut, was once commonly eaten in Europe. It has an edible seed (2–5 cm in diameter) which can be braised, steamed or minced and used in soups.
- *Tapa bispinosa*, also called the Singhara nut, is native to the Kashmir region of India. Its fruits are about 2 cm in diameter.
- *Tapa bicornata* was once an important food in China. It is also called the ling nut and has some resemblance to a potato in its texture.

Watercress

A member of the Brassica family, watercress is native to Europe. It has been used for centuries (it was previously called 'stime') and was once thought to have curative properties and an ability to repel evil! It has been cultivated throughout the northern hemisphere since the nineteenth century and is commonly grown in tanks or streams. Cultivated watercress has larger leaves than the wild variety.

The young leaves of watercress make a delightful addition to salads. The Chinese add watercress to soups and stir-fry it although it is generally recognised as being at its best when eaten raw.

Watercress is an excellent source of vitamin C and carotene. It is also a good source of dietary fibre, potassium and iron. An average serve of watercress has 20 kJ (5 Cals).

White radish

see Radish.

Winter squash

see Pumpkin.

Witloof

Also known as witlof, Belgian endive or Belgian chicory, this vegetable has been used in salads since ancient times. It is pale green with tightly folded leaves, unlike its relatives chicory and curly endive. Each head of witloof grows to a length of about 10−15 cm and is approximately 5−6 cm in diameter. The witloof can be steamed and served as a hot vegetable or the leaves can be separated and added to salads. A 50 g head has 32 kJ (8 Cals).

Wormwood

White wormwood is a variety of wormwood which is eaten in China. The vegetable has long purple leaf stalks and sparse leaves. It is a member of the chrysanthemum family and is served in small quantities stir-fried as a side dish.

Yam

Native to tropical regions of Africa, Asia and America, the yam is thought to have been cultivated since 800 BC. It is the tuber of a plant related to the lily. In parts of the United States, sweet potatoes are called yams; this is incorrect as they are quite distinct plants.

Some varieties of yam contain a bitter alkaloid which can be removed by peeling and cooking the vegetable. The yam contributes dietary fibre, potassium, some vitamin C and small quantities of other vitamins and minerals. It is low in protein. 100 g yam have 485 kJ (115 Cals).

Yam bean

see Jicama.

Zucchini

Known as the courgette in Britain, the zucchini is a small squash which is eaten without peeling. Usually steamed, stir-fried or fried in butter, zucchinis can also be eaten raw as long as the stem end is trimmed (it has a bitter flavour). Zucchinis are used in Italian cuisine and are an important ingredient in the French ratatouille.

Nutritionally, zucchinis are a good source of vitamin C, supply some dietary fibre and small quantities of many vitamins and minerals. 100 g of zucchini have 70 kJ (16 Cals).

VEGETABLE OILS
see Oils.

VEGETARIAN DIET

The majority of the world's population are vegetarian. Most of these people are not vegetarian by choice, but have found a diet of grains, legumes, seeds, nuts, fruits and vegetables is cheaper and more appropriate for living conditions without refrigeration. Most of these people have perfectly adequate diets which include ample quantities of protein, minerals and vitamins as well as plenty of complex carbohydrate and dietary fibre.

Within Western society, an increasing number of people are becoming vegetarian. Some believe such a diet is healthier, others do not like the thought of killing animals for food, some have religious reasons and many are just caught up in the fashion of it all. Some sportspeople also follow a vegetarian diet so that the percentage of energy coming from complex carbohydrate will increase.

Many people are concerned about the adequacy of a vegetarian diet, usually as regards protein. A meatless diet can be perfectly adequate, depending on the vegetarian foods chosen. Plants can provide every nutrient we need, including protein, as long as a variety of foods are eaten.

Lacto vegetarians avoid meat, fish and poultry, but are happy to include milk, cheese and yoghurt. Lacto-ovo vegetarians also include eggs. These animal products contribute vitamin B_{12} which can sometimes be low in a vegetarian diet. Dairy products also increase the calcium content of the diet.

A vegetarian diet is sometimes claimed to be healthier than one containing meat. There is no simple response to such a statement. There is ample evidence that vegetarians have less heart disease, less high blood pressure, fewer problems with their digestive tracts and a lower incidence of cancer than meat-eaters. However, most studies have compared vegetarians with populations who eat large quantities of animal protein foods. Comparisons with those who include more moderate quantities of meat or animal products may give different answers.

The traditional vegetarian diet included a wide range of grains, dried beans, peas and lentils, nuts, seeds, fruits and vegetables as well as milk and eggs. It was a totally adequate and healthy way of eating.

Some 'new style' converts to vegetarianism do not eat such a variety. Many women, for example, have cut out meat in an effort to reduce their weight. Since meats are often high in kilojoules, this tactic may work. However, many 'new style' vegetarians reject healthy products such as bread, grains, nuts, cereals and legumes. Cottage cheese, lettuce and other vegetables, salads and fruits dominate the diet. These foods are useful but cannot provide sufficient quantities of some nutrients. Foods such as grains, cereals, breads, seeds, nuts and legumes are needed in a vegetarian diet.

The protein in a vegetarian diet is almost always adequate (see page 241). Iron, zinc and calcium are more likely to be in doubt. They are found in plentiful supply in meat and milk. Women need more than twice as much iron as men (see page 192), so a vegetarian diet for a woman should be carefully selected to prevent iron deficiency occurring. Women are also more vulnerable to calcium losses.

The inclusion of dairy products (low-fat, if desired), eggs and legumes will add important nutrients, including calcium, protein, riboflavin, iron and other minerals and vitamins. Those who omit these animal foods should ensure they eat combinations such as those listed on page 282. For children, it is recommended that dairy products and eggs be included. If not, fortified soya milk should be a part of the diet.

Most vegetable foods are high in fibre, and therefore bulky. They take a long while to chew and the total quantity of food which needs to be eaten becomes large — especially for those requiring a high kilojoule intake.

Endurance athletes who train for many hours each week may need a diet with 16,000–21,000 kJ (4–5000 Cals) a day. Obtaining this quantity of food from purely low-fat vegetarian products can be difficult. It is easier if some fats from vegetable oils (preferably olive), nuts, peanuts and peanut butter are eaten along with grains, legumes, seeds, nuts and a variety of fruits and vegetables. If possible, add some more concentrated foods such as yoghurt, cheese, milk and eggs.

Rather than have some people who are vegetarian and others who loudly proclaim their meat-eating preferences, it would produce a better balanced diet if everyone ate the occasional vegetarian meal. Legumes and vegetables are excellent sources of particular types of dietary fibre, as well as being useful to supply a range of other nutrients.

A vegan diet is much more difficult for sportspeople and also children (see page 354).

VELOUTE
see Sauces, White Sauce.

VERBACOSE

A 5 unit sugar found in seeds.
See also Oligosaccharides.

VERBENA
see Herbs, Lemon Verbena.

VERMICELLI

A very fine noodle.
See also Pasta.

VERMOUTH
see Drinks, Alcoholic.

VICHYSOISSE

A cold soup made from potatoes and leeks, cooked in chicken stock and pureed to a smooth thick mixture with milk and cream. Vichysoisse was originally created by a French chef, Louis Diat, who named it after Vichy, the region in France near his childhood home. A serve of a typical vichysoisse (including cream) has 1150 kJ (275 Cals).

VIENNA COFFEE

Black coffee topped with whipped cream. An average cup of this type of coffee, without sugar, would have 335 kJ (80 Cals).

VILLI

Microscopic projections from the membranes of the small intestine. Under magnification, villi look rather like the pile on velvet. They serve to increase the surface area of the intestine, giving a much greater area for the absorption of nutrients.

VINAIGRETTE

A salad dressing made from oil, vinegar, lemon juice and seasonings. Each 30 mL of vinaigrette has 820 kJ (195 Cals).

VINEGAR

Vinegar is a by-product of fermentation, originally of wine. It is also made from various fruits. Vinegar undergoes two fermentations. The first occurs when natural yeasts turn the sugar in grapes or other fruits into alcohol. Vinegar yeasts, known as *acetobacters* are then added and form a vinegar plant which converts the alcohol into acetic acid. These vinegars obtain their flavour from chemicals called aromatic esters. These complexities of flavour are missing from vinegar which is simply manufactured acetic acid.

Some countries stipulate a minimum level of acetic acid in vinegars. In Britain and the United States, the level is 6 per cent for wine vinegars and 4 per cent for the rest.

• *White* vinegar is made from white grapes.

- *Malt* vinegar is made from malted barley, first made into a crude type of beer and then allowed to undergo its second fermentation with the vinegar yeast. The vinegar is then strained and coloured with caramel.
- *Herb* vinegars are made by steeping various herbs in white vinegar. They are used in salads, sauces and with fish.
- *Cider* vinegar is made from apples. It is cloudy but is often filtered to make it clear. It makes a good substitute for rice vinegars used in Asian cooking. Cider vinegar is also promoted for a wide range of ailments, including arthritis, heart disease and obesity. It has no special virtues for any of these.
- *Rice* vinegar is made in China and Japan and is added to soups and sweet-sour dishes. It can be red, white or very dark brown.
- *Wine* vinegars are sometimes left in oak vats to ferment slowly to produce a complex and full flavour. Red or white wines can be used.

VINE LEAVES

Originally from the Mediterranean region, vine leaves are also widely used in Middle Eastern cookery. They can be purchased fresh or canned in brine or oil and are usually stuffed with a mixture of rice, minced meat, nuts, garlic, herbs and vegetables.

VITAMINS

See following pages.

VITAMIN SUPPLEMENTS

An enormous industry supplying vitamin pills exists in Western countries. This is somewhat ironic when one considers that vitamin deficiencies are rare in these areas yet are common in some Third World countries. Even within countries such as Australia, studies have shown that those whose diets may be marginal in their vitamin content are not the ones taking the supplements.

The common nutritional problems in Western countries concern the high intake of fat, salt, sugar and alcohol and the lack of dietary fibre and complex carbohydrate. None of these problems is fixed by adding vitamins. If the diet is so poor that extra vitamins are required, it will be an unbalanced diet and, in most cases, its excessive amounts of fat, salt, sugar or alcohol will be damaging long before any signs of vitamin deficiency show up.

There are a few instances where vitamin supplementation can be useful. For example:

- Those who eat very little may need vitamin supplements until they can be persuaded to eat real foods
- Those taking particular drugs which affect vitamin metabolism may also need supplements
- Alcoholics will need vitamins

However, these instances do not mean that everyone who eats modestly, takes any drug, or has an alcoholic drink or two will need extra vitamins. Vitamin supplements cannot provide energy or undo the harmful effects of alcohol.

As can be seen from the individual entries for vitamins, a number of vitamins are toxic in excess doses. These include vitamins A, D, K, B_6, C and niacin. Gastrointestinal disturbances occur with some others such as vitamin E and pantothenic acid.

With the exception of toxicity of the high content of vitamin A in polar bear liver, it is difficult to take in too much of most vitamins from food sources. Supplements containing many times the recommended daily intake may cause overdoses all too easily.

Multivitamin supplements are commonly used. Many of these contain many times the RDI of some vitamins, yet for other vitamins, they have only a fraction of the body's needs. Vitamins which may be required to make up for the effect of drugs, such as biotin, are rarely found in multivitamin preparations. It is wise

VEGETABLES

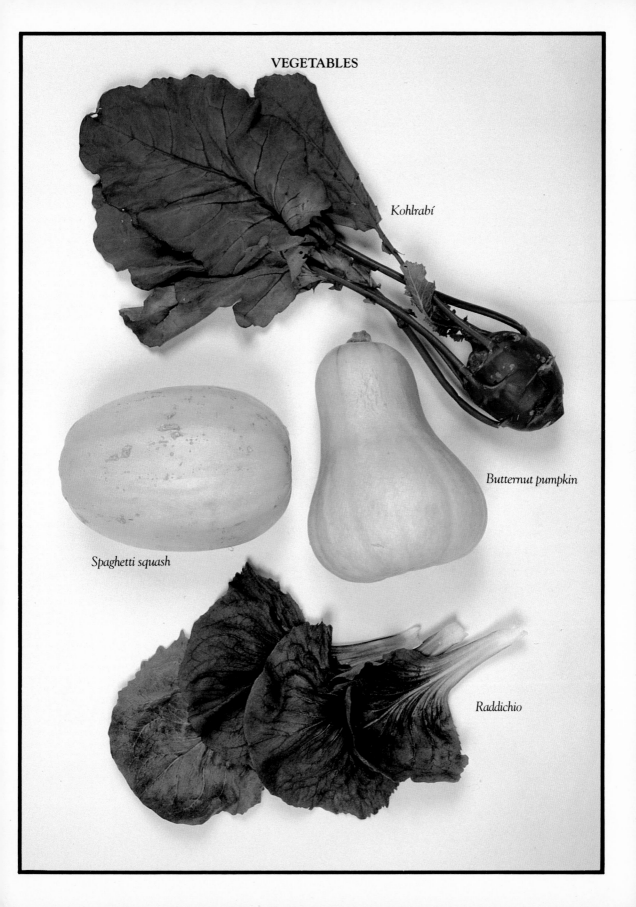

Kohlrabí

Butternut pumpkin

Spaghetti squash

Raddichio

VEGETABLES

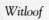

Witloof

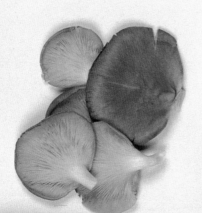

Oyster mushrooms

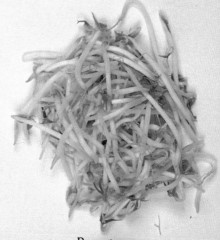

Bean sprouts

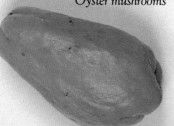

Choko

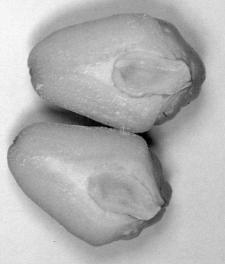

to check the quantities of vitamins against the RDI (see page 393).

Mega-dose vitamin supplements are those containing at least 10 times the RDI. In such doses, vitamins act as drugs rather than nutrients. Yet these high dose preparations are not subjected to the same rigorous testing that applies to drugs.

Claims made for high dose vitamin preparations — that they promote super health, increase resistance to infection, cure arthritis, cancer or heart disease — cannot be substantiated.

Similarly, the much-promoted idea that the current food supply does not contain adequate amounts of vitamins, also lacks evidence. In fact, tests of foods available show that most have more than adequate quantities of vitamins. Even fast foods, with their problems of high fat and salt content, still contain vitamins.

High doses of vitamins are only justifiable when there is evidence that the particular individual is suffering from a genuine vitamin deficiency. This requires proper medical testing. Simple tests of blood levels of some vitamins are not adequate since these do not always represent an accurate picture of the amount of the particular vitamin present in the body. Hair analysis, usually promoted for detecting mineral deficiencies, but sometimes used to 'diagnose' vitamin deficiencies, is considered to be fairly useless on both counts.

Vitamin supplementation is occasionally needed but should not be seen as a normal course of action for most people. Vitamins essentially come from foods.

VODKA

see Drinks, Alcoholic.

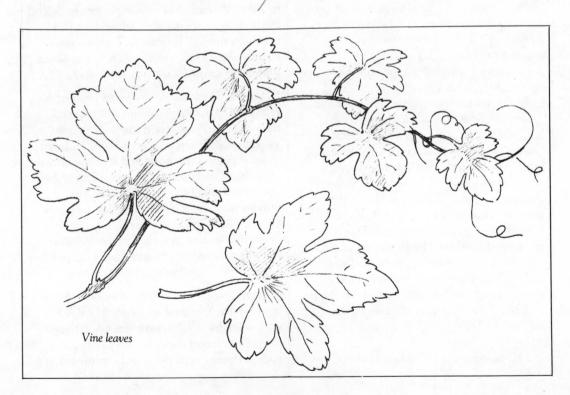

Vine leaves

VITAMINS

Vitamins are substances needed in very small quantities to act as catalysts in the many thousands of chemical reactions which occur in the body. They do not provide energy themselves but are essential for energy from proteins, fats and carbohydrates to be used by the body.

Vitamins fall into two major categories: water soluble and fat soluble. The 8 vitamins which make up the B complex and vitamin C are water soluble. This means they dissolve in cooking water and excessive quantities are excreted via the urine. Most are not stored in the body to any extent and need to be regularly supplied. Vitamins A, D, E and K are soluble in both the fats in foods and in the body's fat stores. A regular supply may be less crucial than is the case for the water soluble vitamins. Fat soluble vitamins are less easily lost in cooking.

Vitamin A

First discovered in 1913, vitamin A must be provided from foods as pre-formed vitamin A or as beta-carotene (also called provitamin A), which is converted into vitamin A in the wall of the small intestine and the liver. Other carotenoids can also be converted to vitamin A.

The correct name for vitamin A is *retinol* and the daily requirements are called retinol equivalents. The old terminology of international units (IU) was discarded in 1967, although some vitamin manufacturers have not yet caught up with this fact.

Beta-carotene is converted to retinol and one-sixth of the original carotene becomes retinol. Other carotenoids are less efficient sources of vitamin A and only one-twelfth of these becomes retinol. Thus the vitamin A content of a diet is calculated by dividing the carotene by 6 and adding this figure to the content of pre-formed vitamin A. If the content of other carotenoids is known, the figure for these should be divided by 12. In practice, usually only the pre-formed vitamin A and the beta-carotene are used. If the old international units are still used, these can be translated to micrograms of vitamin A as follows:

1 IU from retinol = 0.3 mcg of vitamin A

1 IU from beta-carotene = 0.1 mcg of vitamin A

Function: Vitamin A forms visual purple in the retina of the eye and is thus required for vision in dim light. This vitamin is also needed for growth and reproduction and to keep the epithelial tissue lining the mouth, respiratory tract and genito-urinary tracts moist and healthy. Vitamin A is thus important to defend the body against infections which try to find their way through this tissue. There is also some evidence that vitamin A may give some protection against some types of cancer.

Deficiency: Inadequate supplies of vitamin A take time to become apparent since several months supply is stored in the body. However, vitamin A deficiency occurs far too commonly in some parts of the world and is characterised by an inability to see in the dark, dry tear ducts and ulceration of the cornea, leading to blindness. Vitamin A deficiency is the major cause of blindness in the world. It is rare in Western societies. A lack of vitamin A also leads to stunted growth, increased susceptibility to infections, dry skin and hair.

Toxicity: Excessive amounts of vitamin A are stored in the liver and are toxic. The first signs are a dry red skin with eczema, fatigue, irritability, loss of appetite, loss of hair, haemorrhages, joint pains and vomiting. Later there is liver damage, leading to death. Excessive vitamin A intake is most likely to occur from overzealous use of vitamin supplements. However, there were deaths among early Arctic explorers who took in massive doses by eating polar bear liver — with 50,000 to 100,000 mcg/100 g, it is an extremely rich source of the vitamin. Toxicity is likely with a daily intake greater than 10,000 mcg per kg of body weight. However, adverse effects may occur with quantities as low as 200 mcg/kg body weight.

Excessive amounts of carotene come from habitual drinking of carrot juice. This causes carotenaemia, in which the skin and whites of the eyes turn yellow and the patient feels weak and nauseated. The body does not turn this excess carotene into vitamin A, but it still causes problems.

RDI: See table, page 393. Women taking oral contraceptives have higher levels of vitamin A in the blood and should not take supplements of this vitamin.

Major food sources (commonly consumed serves): Liver, dairy products and fatty fish are the best sources of retinol. Yellow, orange and green fruits and vegetables are the best sources of carotene (see page 57).

FOOD	RETINOL (mcg)	CAROTENE (mcg)
Breads, grains, cereals	0	0
Cream cheese, 30 g	115	65
Cheese, 30 g	105	135
Milk,		
regular, 1 cup, 250 mL	95	80
skim, 1 cup, 250 mL	0	0
Yoghurt, 200 g carton	70	95
Cottage cheese, 75 g	25	15
Butter, 20 g	180	130
Cream, 30 mL	140	75

* average figure taken. Dark leaves have much higher levels.

	RETINOL	CAROTENE
Margarine, 20 g	115	80
Oil, 1 tablespoon	0	0
Liver, cooked,		
lamb, 100 g	35 400	60
beef, 100 g	19 200	1920
calf, 100 g	18 100	670
Egg, 1	70	0
Meat, chicken	0	0
Fish	0	0
Eel, 100 g cooked	1 900	0
Salmon, canned, 100 g	100	0
Oysters, 1 dozen	90	0
Herring, 100 g	50	0
Cod liver oil, 20 mL	3 600	0
Carrots, 100 g		12 000
Kumera (orange sweet potato), 100 g		6780
Spinach, 75 g		4500
Spring greens, 100 g		4000
Pumpkin, 100 g		2780–3380
Broccoli, 100 g		2500
Capsicum, red, 100 g		1460
Endive, 50 g		1000
Tomato, 1, 150 g		900
canned, $\frac{1}{2}$ cup		630
Watercress, 25 g		500
Lettuce, 50 g		500 *
Asparagus, 100 g		500
Leek, 100 g		470
Brussels sprouts, 100 g		400
Beans, green, 100 g		400
Sweetcorn, 1 cob		360
Parsley, 5 g		350
Peas, 100 g		300
Cabbage, green, 100 g		300 *
Beans broad, 100 g		250
Mango, 1 medium		3800
Rockmelon, dark orange flesh, 150 g		3000
Apricots, dried, 50 g		1800
Apricots, 3 medium,		1500
Pawpaw, 150 g		1365
Jackfruit, 100 g		1130
Peach, dried, 50 g		1000
Tamarillo, 1 medium		930
Peach, yellow, 1 medium		600
Persimmon, medium		480

Guava, 100 g	440
Passionfruit, 50 g flesh	375
Avocado, $\frac{1}{2}$ medium	290
Orange, 1 medium	170

Cooking: There is little loss of vitamin A with normal cooking techniques. The carotene in foods such as carrots may even be a little more available after the heat of cooking has broken some cells so that carotene can be absorbed.

Vitamin B₁ (thiamin)

Also known as aneurine, this vitamin was first isolated in 1902 and its chemical structure was worked out in 1934. Thiamin created a milestone in nutritional research in 1901 when a doctor realised that there was some factor in rice polishings which could prevent the disease called beri beri, once common in countries where the diet consisted mainly of polished rice.

Function: Thiamin is important in the enzyme systems which work to release energy from carbohydrates. It is also important for growth and in the digestive and nervous systems and the heart.

Deficiency: Thiamin deficiency can occur in countries where the diet is poor. In Western societies, it also occurs in alcoholics. The early symptoms include muscle weakness and loss of limb function, memory and appetite. This progresses to affecting the brain more severely provoking symptoms such as vomiting, double vision, difficulty in walking and gross memory loss. The condition known as Wernicke's encephalopathy occurs when the brain is affected, usually in alcoholics. A progression to replacing memory with weird and wonderful tales is known as Korsakoff's psychosis.

Beri beri can be 'dry' with the symptoms listed above, or 'wet'. In this form, the heart is affected and the blood vessels do not constrict properly. The heart muscle fails and water accumulates.

Toxicity: It appears that large doses of thiamin are well tolerated. If given by injection, a large dose can cause shock.

Stability: Some thiamin is lost with cooking. Adding bicarbonate of soda hastens destruction of the vitamin. Sulphur-containing preservatives also cause a loss of thiamin. In general, about 25 per cent of the thiamin in foods is lost during cooking with greatest losses being from meats and vegetables. Baking losses in breads are less.

RDI: For adults, 0.7–1.1 mg (see table, page 393). Large doses are sometimes prescribed for alcoholics.

Major food sources (commonly consumed serves): Wholegrain products, pork, nuts and yeast extract are the best sources of thiamin. The thiamin in some vegetables is also useful.

FOOD	THIAMIN (mg)
Wholemeal pasta, raw weight, 100 g	0.99
Brown rice, raw weight, 100 g	0.59
Rolled oats, raw weight, 100 g	0.50
Pasta, raw weight, 100 g	0.22–0.49
Cracked wheat, raw weight, 100 g	0.48
Wholemeal flour, 100 g	0.47
Breakfast cereal, fortified, 30 g	0.28
Wheatgerm, 1 tablespoon	0.20
Wheat bran, 2 tablespoons	0.13
Wholemeal bread, 2 slices	0.12
Barley, raw weight, 100 g	0.12
White rice, raw weight, 100 g	0.08
White bread, 2 slices	0.06
Milk, 250 mL	0.10
Pork, leg steak, cooked, 100 g	0.59
Ham, cooked or canned, 100 g	0.38
Kidney, cooked, 100 g	0.38
Fish, cooked, 150 g	0.14
Meat or chicken, av. serve, 150 g	0.12
Oysters, 1 dozen	0.12
Sweet potato, white, 100 g	0.40
Peas, 100 g	0.31
Cassava, 100 g	0.23
Asparagus, 100 g	0.15

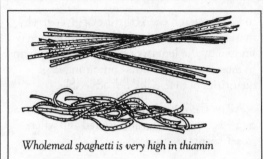

Wholemeal spaghetti is very high in thiamin

Rhubarb, 100 g	0.11
Brazil nuts, 50 g	0.50
Peanuts, 50 g	0.45
Hazelnuts, 50 g	0.20
Walnuts, 50 g	0.15
Almonds, 50 g	0.12
Dried yeast, 10 g	0.40
Yeast extract, 5 g	0.55

Vitamin B$_2$ (riboflavin)

A vitamin of the 1930s, riboflavin is associated with a flavoprotein, a yellow-fluorescent enzyme. If you have ever taken multivitamin preparations, you may have noticed your urine soon has a bright yellow-green colour. This is the excess riboflavin being excreted.

Function: Riboflavin is important for the way the body uses proteins. The growth and repair of tissues, including skin and eyes, need riboflavin.

Deficiency: A lack of riboflavin shows up with cracks at the corners of the mouth and on the lips, a shiny sore red tongue and a waxy type of dermatitis in the creases around the nose and the scrotum (in males). There may also be a lowered resistance to infection and a possibly increased risk of certain types of cancer.

Toxicity: No effects are apparent, probably because excess riboflavin is soon excreted in the urine.

Stability: Riboflavin is easily destroyed by light. Milk should not be left in sunlight, especially in glass bottles. Some riboflavin is also lost into cooking water.

RDI: For adults, 1.0–1.7 mg (see table, page 393).

Major food sources (commonly consumed serves): Liver, kidney, dairy products, fish, meat, almonds and yeast extract are the best sources of riboflavin.

FOOD	RIBOFLAVIN (mg)
Breakfast cereal, fortified, 30 g	0.40
Rolled oats, raw weight, 100 g	0.11
Cracked wheat, raw weight, 100 g	0.11
Wheatgerm, 1 tablespoon	0.07
Yoghurt, 200 g carton	0.55
Milk, 250 mL	0.40
Cheese, 30 g	0.13
Liver, cooked, 100 g	4.20
Kidney, cooked, 100 g	2.60
Pork steak, cooked, 100 g	0.32
Chicken legs, 2, cooked, 100 g	0.29
Beef, cooked, 150 g	0.24
Veal chops, 2, cooked	0.20
Lamb leg, cooked, 100 g	0.14
Ham, lean, 50 g	0.12
Egg, 1	0.23
Eel, cooked, 100 g	0.40
Mackerel, cooked, 100 g	0.38
Sardines, canned, 100 g	0.36
Fish, grilled, 150 g	0.24
Oysters, 1 dozen	0.24
Broccoli, 100 g	0.30
Peas, 100 g	0.15
Dried beans, 100 g	0.13
Spinach, 75 g	0.11
Avocado, $\frac{1}{2}$ medium	0.11
Prunes, 100 g	0.20
Almonds, 50 g	0.46
Milk chocolate, 100 g	0.23
Yeast extract, 5 g	0.85
Dried yeast, 10 g	0.40

Vitamin B$_3$ (niacin)

This vitamin was once called vitamin P-P. It includes nicotinic acid (no relationship to nicotine) and nicotinamide. It can either be obtained from the diet or it can be made from an amino acid called tryptophan. The body converts nicotinic acid into nicotinamide. The term niacin was adopted to avoid confusion with nicotine in tobacco.

Niacin was discovered in 1937 when it was found to cure a disease in dogs which resembled pellagra in humans. Subsequent study found that niacin also cured the pellagra which was widespread in the southern parts of the United States (see Corn).

Function: Niacin is needed by every body cell since it plays a vital role in the release of energy from foods. Without niacin, tissues begin to degenerate. It is also involved in the synthesis of some fatty acids and steroids. Large doses of niacin can lower cholesterol levels in the blood, although the side effects make this an unpopular and unwise treatment. The amino acid, tryptophan, can also be made into niacin in the body. This conversion requires vitamin B_6.

Those who promote megavitamin therapy also claim that large doses of niacin help schizophrenics. This has not been proved and general medical opinion is that niacin has no special value, and some potential problems, for schizophrenics.

Deficiency: Early symptoms include muscular weakness and fatigue, rough skin, anorexia and indigestion. A continued lack progresses to dermatitis, diarrhoea and dementia (often called the 'three Ds'). This condition, known as pellagra, was once common. It is not seen in countries such as Australia.

Toxicity: More than 1 g (1000 mg) of niacin a day will open up the blood vessels to the skin, causing flushing and rashes. These are usually so unpleasant that large doses are inadvisable. Such quantities of niacin can also cause gout and diabetes in susceptible people. Self medication with niacin is thus unwise.

It is unwise for endurance athletes to take niacin since it hastens the use of glycogen by muscles. Since these athletes' performance is limited by the length of time glycogen remains in muscles, supplements containing large quantities of niacin are not advisable.

Stability: Cooking losses of niacin are not great. Some is lost when meat is grilled and when frozen meats are thawed.

RDI: For adults, 10–20 mg (see table, page 393).

Major food sources (commonly consumed serves): Liver, kidney, tuna, chicken, peanuts and peanut butter, game meats, wholegrain products, fish, yeast extract and meat are good sources of niacin.

FOOD	NIACIN (mg)
Wholemeal pasta, raw weight, 100 g	6.2
Wholemeal flour, 100 g	5.7
Brown rice, raw weight, 100 g	5.3
Cracked wheat, raw weight, 100 g	4.5
Wheat bran, 2 tablespoons	4.4
Pasta, raw weight, 100 g	3.1
Buckwheat, raw weight, 100 g	2.8
Breakfast cereal, fortified, 30 g	2.7
Barley, 100 g, raw weight	2.5
Wholemeal bread, 2 slices	2.1
White rice, raw weight, 100 g	1.5
Rolled oats, raw weight, 100 g	1.0
Yoghurt, 200 g carton	1.1
Lamb liver, cooked, 100 g	14.5
Calf liver, cooked, 100 g	12.3
Veal kidneys, cooked, 100 g	9.2
Pigeon, cooked, 100 g	8.9
Chicken breast, cooked, 100 g	8.7
Rabbit, cooked, 100 g	8.5
Turkey, cooked, 100 g	8.5
Beef, cooked, 150 g	7.0
Pork steak, cooked, 100 g	6.9
Game meats, cooked, 100 g	6.0
Chicken legs, 2, cooked	4.8
Lamb kidneys, cooked, 100 g	4.4
Veal chops, 2, cooked	3.8
Lamb chops, 2, grilled	3.4
Ham, 50 g	2.0

Tuna, canned, 100 g	12.9
Mackerel, cooked, 100 g	8.7
Sardines, canned, 100 g	8.2
Salmon, fresh or canned, 100 g	7.0
Fish, grilled, 150 g	5.1
Prawns, 100 g	3.0
Mushrooms, 100 g	3.2
Potato, cooked, 1 medium	2.7
Peas, cooked, 100 g	2.3
Broad beans, cooked, 100 g	3.0
Dried beans, raw weight, 100 g	2.0
Avocado, $\frac{1}{2}$	1.7
Broccoli, 100 g	1.0
Dried peaches, 50 g	2.6
Passionfruit, flesh, 100 g	2.5
Dried apricots, 50 g	1.5
Prunes, 100 g	1.5
Peanuts, 50 g	8.0
Peanut butter, 30 g	4.5
Almonds, 50 g	1.0
Yeast extract, 5 g	6.0
Dried yeast, 10 g	3.6

Vitamin B$_5$ (pantothenic acid)

After its discovery in 1933, pantothenic acid did not receive a lot of attention because it was so rare to observe any deficiency of the vitamin in humans. During the 1950s and 1960s, work on pigs provided more information about the role of this vitamin. It has probably achieved more publicity because of its alleged ability to prevent hair going grey. Unfortunately, even though a deficiency of pantothenic acid will produce premature greying of hair in rats, humans with grey hair do not have a deficiency of pantothenic acid and adding more of the vitamin as a supplement will not prevent or reverse greying of human hair.

Function: Takes part in many reactions involving fats and carbohydrates. Involved in the formation of fatty acids and cholesterol, and also in a chemical substance which is subsequently used to produce haemoglobin. Also important in the transmission of impulses to nerves and muscles.

Deficiency: Symptoms induced in volunteers given a substance which antagonised pantothenic acid included abdominal pains, vomiting, fatigue, cramps in the legs, 'pins and needles' in the hands and feet and personality changes.

Toxicity: With very large doses (10,000 to 20,000 mg), diarrhoea has been reported.

Stability: There are no great losses of this vitamin during cooking. Very high temperatures may destroy some and there are some losses after freezing of foods.

RDI: For adults, 4−7 mg has been recommended. Up to 20 mg may be needed during pregnancy.

Major food sources (commonly consumed serves): Liver, kidney, beans, watermelon, mushrooms, salmon, peanuts, poultry, meat and wholegrain products are the best sources of pantothenic acid.

FOOD	PANTOTHENIC ACID (mg)
Rolled oats, 100 g	1.1
Bran cereal, 50 g	0.9
Wholemeal pasta, raw weight, 100 g	0.8
Muesli, 60 g	0.7
Rice, raw weight, 100 g	0.6
Rye crispbread, 20 g	0.6
Barley, raw weight, 100 g	0.5
Wholemeal bread, 2 slices	0.3
Milk, 250 mL	0.9
Camembert cheese, 30 g	0.5
Liver, cooked, 100 g	6.9
Kidney, cooked, 100 g	4.0
Duck, cooked, 100 g	1.6
Chicken, cooked, 100 g	1.2
Pork, cooked, 100 g	1.0
Beef, grilled, 150 g	1.0
Salmon, cooked, 100 g	1.8
Lobster, cooked, 100 g	1.6
Mackerel, cooked, 100 g	1.0
Herring, canned, 100 g	0.9
Oysters, 1 dozen	0.6
Crab, cooked	0.6

Broad beans, cooked, 100 g	3.8
Mushrooms, 100 g	2.0
Broccoli, 100 g	1.0
Sweet potato, 100 g	0.9
Peas, 100 g	0.8
Sweetcorn, 1 cob	0.8
Watermelon, 150 g	2.3
Avocado, $\frac{1}{2}$	1.1
Peanuts, 50 g	1.4
Peanut butter, 30 g	0.6
Hazelnuts, 50 g	0.6
Yeast extract, 5 g	0.4

Vitamin B_6

There are several forms of this vitamin including pyridoxine, pyridoxamine and pyridoxal. Vegetable foods usually have their B_6 present as pyridoxine while animal foods have more as pyridoxal. Vitamin B_6 was found to be essential for animals in 1933 and for humans in 1939.

Function: B_6 takes part in the reactions in which amino acids are incorporated into body tissues. It is also involved in the transmission of impulses in nerves and muscles and is important in making red blood cells. B_6 is also needed for the conversion of tryptophan to niacin.

B_6 is sometimes used in hormonal disturbances in women, although its usefulness is not really clear. Some women taking oral contraceptives seem to benefit from a B_6 supplement. The vitamin is also often given to pregnant women who are suffering from morning sickness. Whether it really helps is unclear at present. Vitamin B_6 is also prescribed for women with pre-menstrual syndrome. However, recent studies have shown that it is no more effective than a placebo pill.

Deficiency: From such widespread functions, a lack of B_6 leads to many problems. The skin, nerves, muscles and brain are affected. Mental depression, convulsions, skin rashes, irritability, weakness, anaemia, smooth sore tongue and weight loss occur.

Toxicity: It was once said that excess B_6 was excreted and would do no harm. Such assumptions have now been shown to be false. Large doses (200 mg/day) can cause impaired sensation in the hands and feet leading to polyneuritis.

Stability: There are some losses of B_6 during cooking. Some dissolves into cooking water and microwave cookery has a better retention than boiling foods. Overcooking of meats, especially grilling or roasting, also results in losses.

RDI: For adults, 0.8–1.9 mg (see table, page 393). Some people taking particular drugs may need more vitamin B_6 than the usual levels. Some anti-tuberculosis drugs increase requirements and penicillamine (a different drug from penicillin) also requires a B_6 supplement. Those with a rare condition known as homocystinuria also need extra B_6, as do people with excessive thyroid function or some children on particular anti-convulsants.

Major food sources (commonly consumed serves): Fish, lentils and beans, bananas, pork, poultry, meat, avocado and nuts are the best sources of B_6.

FOOD	VITAMIN B_6 (mg)
Processed bran cereal, 50 g	0.4
Wheatgerm, 1 tablespoon	0.3
Bran, 2 tablespoons	0.2
Rolled oats, raw weight, 100 g	0.1
Wheat breakfast biscuits, 2	0.1
Liver, cooked, 100 g	0.5
Pork, cooked, 100 g	0.5
Rabbit, cooked, 100 g	0.5
Beef, grilled, 150 g	0.5
Chicken or turkey, cooked, 100 g	0.4
Lamb or veal chops, 2, grilled	0.3
Kidney, cooked, 100 g	0.3
Mackerel, cooked, 100 g	0.8
Fish, cooked, 150 g	0.7
Salmon or tuna, canned, 100 g	0.5

Sardines, canned, 100 g	0.5
Crab, cooked, 100 g	0.4
Lentils or beans, raw weight, 100 g	0.6
Brussels sprouts, 100 g	0.3
Leeks, 100 g	0.3
Sweetcorn, 1 cob	0.3
Broccoli, 100 g	0.2
Cabbage, 100 g	0.2
Capsicum, 100 g	0.2
Carrot, 100 g	0.2
Cauliflower, 100 g	0.2
Peas, 100 g	0.2
Potato, 1 medium	0.2
Sweet potato, 100 g	0.2
Tomato, 1 medium	0.2
Mushrooms, 100 g	0.1
Spinach, 75 g	0.1
Banana, 1 medium	0.6
Avocado, $\frac{1}{2}$	0.4
Raisins, 50 g	0.2
Melon, 150 g	0.1
Walnuts, 50 g	0.4
Peanuts, 50 g	0.2
Peanut butter, 30 g	0.2
Yeast extract, 5 g	0.2
Dried yeast, 10 g	0.2

Vitamin B_{12}

Pernicious anaemia was recognised in 1824, but it was not until 1948 that vitamin B_{12}, more properly known as cyanocobalamin, was isolated. Before that time, the vitamin was known as 'extrinsic factor' or the anti-pernicious anaemia factor. It was a difficult vitamin to study, since in many cases, problems due to a lack of B_{12} were caused by an inability to absorb the vitamin. This vitamin is only absorbed in the presence of 'intrinsic factor', a substance secreted by the stomach. B_{12} itself is an unusual molecule because it contains cobalt. An explanation of its chemical structure gave a Nobel prize to Dr Dorothy Hodgkin in 1964.

Function: Vitamin B_{12} comes in several different forms and these have a number of roles in humans. It has a role in the chemical processes which go into making DNA, including the formation of the nucleus of red blood cells. It also helps to form the fatty material in nerve cells.

Deficiency: The functions of B_{12} are intimately connected with those of folic acid. Deficiency of either vitamin leads to megaloblastic anaemia. However, a lack of B_{12} also leads to nerve damage, affecting the spinal cord and sometimes causing paralysis. It is important that the true cause of the anaemia be diagnosed since giving folic acid may fix the anaemia but mask the damage being done to the nervous system.

A deficiency usually occurs because of a lack of intrinsic factor. This means that dietary B_{12} is not absorbed. In such cases, supplements of the vitamin are useless and it must be given by injection. A deficiency of B_{12} may also occur in vegans, since the vitamin occurs only in animal products, or from bacterial sources. The main group at risk are babies and children of vegan parents. In adult vegans, in practice, B_{12} deficiency rarely occurs. This is partly due to the fact that the body keeps about 5 years' store of B_{12}. It may also reflect some bacterial production of B_{12}, either in the mouth or in the intestine.

Toxicity: No toxic effects of this vitamin have been reported, even at very high doses.

Stability: B_{12} losses during cooking and food preparation are minimal.

RDI: For adults, 2.0 mcg (see table, page 393).

Major food sources (commonly consumed serves): Vitamin B_{12} is found mainly in foods of animal origin, with liver and kidney being extremely rich sources. Mushrooms absorb some B_{12} from the compost in which they grow and some fermented products may also contain B_{12}, made by the bacteria they contain.

FOOD	VITAMIN B_{12} (mcg)
Milk, 250 mL	0.75
Cheese, 50 g	0.50
Egg, 1	0.9
Liver, cooked, 100 g	82.0
Kidney, lamb, cooked, 100 g	80.0
ox	31.0
Rabbit, cooked, 100 g	12.0
Liverwurst, 50 g	4.0
Duck, cooked, 100 g	3.0
Pork, cooked, 100 g	3.0
Beef, grilled, 150 g	3.0
Lamb chops, 2 cooked, 100 g	2.0
Turkey, cooked, 100 g	2.0
Chicken, cooked, 100 g	1.0
Oysters, 1 dozen	18.0
Salmon or tuna, canned, 100 g	5.0
Fish cooked, 150 g	3.0
Mushrooms, 100 g	.26

Both comfrey and spirulina are thought to contain B_{12}. In fact, they contain B_{12} analogues, substances which mimic the action of B_{12} but cannot act as a substitute.

Folacin (folic acid)

The yeast extract, Marmite, was at least partially responsible for the discovery of folacin. It had been recognised in 1842 that a particular type of anaemia of pregnancy was related to a lack of leafy vegetables, but it was not until 1930 that Marmite was recognised as containing some factor which could also prevent this type of anaemia. In 1946, folacin was identified as a separate vitamin. Later it was found to represent a number of different substances including folic acid and folinic acid. Folacin is the name given to all substances with folic acid properties.

Some forms of folacin are more easily absorbed than others. The state of the intestine' is also important for its absorption and those with untreated conditions such as coeliac disease may not absorb folacin well. Many drugs, including alcohol, also affect its absorption.

Function: Folacin is important in the formation of new body cells and also takes part in the process whereby information about proteins is transmitted from the genes to the cells. It is therefore needed for passing on hereditary characteristics. It is also important in making blood cells (hence the anaemia) and plays a role in the way fats are used within the body. Its functions are highly integrated with those of vitamin B_{12}.

Deficiency: The anaemia which accompanies folacin deficiency is characterised by a low red blood cell count with the cells being larger than they should be. The white cells and platelets in the blood can also be affected. A lack of folacin is probably the most common vitamin deficiency on a world scale.

Toxicity: Folacin seems to be well tolerated in large doses. However, large doses (more than 400 mcg a day) may mask an associated deficiency of B_{12}. There have been some reports of high doses causing gastrointestinal disturbances.

Stability: Folacin is lost during cooking with re-heating causing high losses. Vitamin C in foods protects folacin to some extent. Some folacin is lost during canning and processing of foods.

RDI: For adults, 200 mcg (see table, page 393).

Major food sources (commonly consumed serves): The best sources of folacin are chicken livers, dried yeast, liver, green leafy vegetables and yeast extract.

FOOD	FOLACIN (mcg)
Oats, raw weight, 100 g	60
Processed bran cereal, 50 g	50
Unprocessed bran, 2 tablespoons	39
Wheatgerm, 1 tablespoon	33
Muesli, 50 g	26
Wheat breakfast biscuits, 2	25
Wholemeal bread, 2 slices	20

Chicken liver, cooked, 100 g	500
Lamb or calves' liver, 100 g	300
Kidney, cooked, 100 g	77
Crab, cooked, 100 g	20
Endive, 50 g	165
Kidney beans, raw, 100 g	130
Butter beans, 100 g	110
Broccoli, 100 g	110
Spring greens, 100 g	110
Spinach, 75 g	105
Okra, 100 g	100
Beetroot, 100 g	90
Brussels sprouts, 100 g	90
Cabbage, 100 g, raw	90
cooked	35
Peas, 100 g	78
Sweetcorn, 1 cob	75
Sweet potato, 100 g	72
Cauliflower, cooked, 100 g	50
Tomato, 1 medium	42
Chickpeas, cooked, 100 g	40
Lentils, cooked, 100 g	35
Mushrooms, 100 g	23
Avocado, $\frac{1}{2}$	66
Orange, 1 medium	52
Melon, 150 g	45
Strawberries, $\frac{1}{2}$ punnet, 125 g	25
Banana, 1 medium	24
Peanuts, 50 g	55
Almonds, 50 g	48
Hazelnuts, 50 g	36
Walnuts, 50 g	33
Dried yeast, 10 g	400
Yeast extract, 5 g	95

Biotin

Once known as vitamin H (or occasionally as coenzyme R), biotin was first isolated in 1942 and assigned status as a member of the B complex. It has received less attention from many nutritionists than some vitamins because it is made by bacteria in the intestine so that dietary sources become less important.

Biotin was first discovered as a factor by feeding diets containing raw egg whites. Avidin, a substance in raw egg white, binds biotin so that it cannot be used. Cooking eggs destroys avidin. Only those who eat a large number of raw eggs need be concerned about avidin. Some body builders, seeking the excellent combination of amino acids in eggs, do consume hazardous quantities of raw eggs.

Function: Biotin is important in making fatty acids in the body and also functions in the body's ability to maintain an adequate level of glucose in the blood when carbohydrate is not being consumed. Biotin deficiency can lead to low fasting blood sugar levels.

Deficiency: This is rare since the vitamin is made in the intestine. It is a possibility, however, when antibiotics are taken over several weeks. Biotin deficiency shows symptoms of dry skin with scaly dermatitis, smooth tongue, loss of appetite, nausea, 'pins and needles', depression, hair loss and high blood cholesterol level.

Toxicity: No adverse effects have been reported.

Stability: Cooking in water causes some losses. In general, since biotin is mostly made in the intestine, these losses are unimportant.

RDI: Since the vitamin is made by bacteria in the intestine, exact requirements are difficult to determine. General recommendation is for 50 mcg per 4200 kJ (1000 Cals) consumed.

Major food sources (commonly consumed serves): The best sources of biotin are chicken livers, liver, dried yeast, oysters, egg and oats. The bran from rice is also a good source, although it is not a commonly consumed food.

FOOD	BIOTIN (mcg)
Rolled oats, raw weight, 100 g	20
Most grains, av. serve	3
Milk, 250 mL	5
Camembert cheese, 30 g	3
Egg, 1	12
Chicken liver, cooked, 100 g	170
Liver, beef or calves', cooked, 100 g	48

Duck, cooked, 100 g	6
Meat, av. serve	2
Oysters, 1 dozen	12
Herring, 100 g	10
Fish, grilled, 150 g	7
Salmon or tuna, 100 g	4
Artichoke, 1 medium	6
Vegetables, av. serve	4
Avocado, $\frac{1}{2}$	3
Dried yeast, 10 g	20
Yeast extract, 5 g	7

B vitamins, other

A number of other substances have been listed with the B complex vitamins from time to time. These include carnitine (vitamin B-T), choline (see page 73), inositol (see page 189), myoinositol (see page 239), para-aminobenzoic acid (see page 257), lipoic acid (see page 210), orotic acid (B_{13}), pangamic acid (B_{15}) and amygdalin (B_{17}). See individual entries where indicated.

B_{13} (orotic acid)

A substance present in all living cells and isolated from cow's milk. Orotic acid is important in RNA and DNA and thus takes part in the synthesis of all body cells. However, it is not recognised as a vitamin and seems to be synthesised within the body. Milk is the only significant food source and since the substance occurs mainly in the whey, products such as ricotta cheese would be a high source.

Orotic acid has been used in experimental work to see if it can repair damage to heart muscle or reduce blood cholesterol. More research is needed to clarify these issues.

B_{15} (pangamic acid)

This substance was first isolated from apricot kernels in 1943 and made popular after a review of its uses in the USSR was published in the late 1970s. It soon came to be regarded as a panacea for almost every human ailment and was used by many sportspeople in the hope that it would increase oxygen uptake.

Two preliminary studies claimed that those taking large doses of pangamic acid were able to exercise for longer. Many other studies have shown no significant improvement. Most of the claims made for pangamic acid cannot be substantiated. Most are anecdotal. Someone buys pangamic acid at a very high price, takes the tablets and feels cured of some condition. This is not proof of the substance but only proof that a belief in a substance can produce desired results. Such placebo effects may be of little consequence. However, in the case of pangamic acid, the prices charged for the substance are exorbitant and represent a rip-off for the gullible.

Tests on many of the substances labelled as pangamic acid have shown they contain a wide variety of substances, mostly calcium gluconate and dimethylglycine. Some pills labelled as pangamic acid have been found to contain a substance called diisopropylamine dichloracetate. This substance dilates the blood vessels, drops blood pressure and produces a 'kick'. Some of the substances found in preparations labelled as pangamic acid are potentially dangerous; a few are known to be possible cancer-causing agents.

B_{17} (amygdalin)

This supposed vitamin consists of a group of cyanogenetic glycosides with no known value in human nutrition. First proposed as a cancer remedy in 1845, it has been subjected to many tests which have not shown it to have any value. It is not a vitamin.

It is the harmful effects of amygdalin which are of greatest concern. It contains cyanide, the original reason why it was thought that it might kill cancer cells. Unfortunately, cyanide is deadly to all cells.

Amygdalin is marketed under the name laetrile. It is not a vitamin and is likely to be harmful.

B-T (carnitine)

First discovered in 1947, carnitine is needed for fatty acids to be metabolised for fuel, especially in muscles. Carnitine helps fatty acids move into a special part of the cell where they can be used as fuel for muscle contraction. Carnitine is made in muscle from the amino acid lysine, a process which requires vitamin C. The body does not need to obtain it from the diet or supplements as it appears to be made as required.

Further research into the actions of carnitine is continuing, but there seems little justification for taking high-priced supplements of the material at present.

Vitamin C

As long ago as the early part of the eighteenth century, it was recognised that scurvy was related to the diet. It occurred commonly among sailors and explorers who had no source of fresh fruit or vegetables for long periods.

James Lind discovered that citrus fruits would prevent scurvy in 1747, although he did not know that vitamin C was the important factor. He published a treatise in 1754 on the subject but the British Admiralty did not put his recommendations into practice for more than 40 years. British sailors after this time had to eat limes and were called 'limeys'.

In his voyage to Australia in 1770, Captain James Cook recognised the need for fresh food and made his sailors sprout wheat and eat the shoots to prevent scurvy. Later, the early European settlers in Australia forgot the vital need for fresh foods and scurvy was common. Even as late as the early part of the twentieth century, explorers to the South Pole neglected to take any source of vitamin C. The frostbite which did not heal and brought about the death of Scott's party was probably due to vitamin C deficiency.

Vitamin C, more properly known as ascorbic acid, was finally isolated in 1928, and identified as the agent which prevented or cured scurvy in 1932.

Function: Vitamin C is needed in the synthesis of collagen, a protein found in connective tissue. It is important in forming a cement-like material in bones, capillaries, cartilage, gums and teeth. Vitamin C is also important in the production of some proteins and hormones, helps in the absorption of iron, prevents infection and may reduce blood cholesterol levels. Its antioxidant properties may also be important to the body's immune system. It certainly helps prevent nitrites being converted to nitrosamines (known to produce cancer). Vitamin C may also help the liver remove some unwanted substances from the body.

With such a range of functions, it is not surprising that so many people believe they should take extra vitamin C. However, large doses of vitamin C do not confer super health.

The commonly held theory that vitamin C gives protection against the common cold has not been substantiated in most double-blind studies. A few studies have suggested a slight reduction in the time a cold lasts when extra vitamin C is taken. Studies also show that if vitamin C does have any beneficial effects against the common cold, they are more likely to be confined to extra vitamin C intake at the time of the cold, rather than a continual high dose.

Taking vitamin C as protection against high blood cholesterol is sometimes recommended. At this stage, studies are giving conflicting results. Vitamin C influences the way the body uses zinc and copper and the protection against heart disease may be due to changes in these minerals.

It certainly makes sense to eat a food source of vitamin C at each meal. This is mainly to increase the absorption of iron from foods. It may also help prevent the formation of possible cancer-causing substances.

Deficiency: A lack of vitamin C causes scurvy. The first signs are weakness, bleeding gums, wounds which do not heal, joint pains, bruising and muscular weakness. Deficiency still occurs in some children in Western countries.

25

Toxicity: Excessive amounts of vitamin C from supplements is becoming a real danger as many people believe that 'if a little is good, more must be better'. The first symptom of an overload of vitamin C is diarrhoea. This may occur at intakes of 1000 mg a day or more. Those who take more than 4000 mg a day run an increased risk of kidney stones. If high levels of vitamin C are discontinued, there is also a risk of rebound scurvy. Babies born to mothers who have taken large doses of vitamin C during pregnancy have developed scurvy even when breast fed.

High doses of vitamin C also alter the effects of aspirin, anti-depressants and anti-coagulant drugs. They may also interfere with fertility and normal control of blood glucose levels.

Stability: Vitamin C is easily lost through exposure to heat, oxygen, water, alkali or copper. Damaged or wilted vegetables or fruits will have lost a considerable amount of their vitamin C. Microwave cookery, without water, causes the least loss of vitamin C. Steaming or quickly stir-frying foods is also better than boiling. Some raw fruits and/or vegetables should be included in each day's diet.

RDI: The normal requirement for adults is 30 mg/day (see chart, page 393). The body has enough vitamin C to last about 3 weeks. However, since some vitamin C is lost each day, regular replacement is advisable. The body's tissues will be saturated with vitamin C at a level of approximately 100 mg per day.

Smokers need more vitamin C than non-smokers and 100–130 mg/day may be required. Athletes do not benefit from massive doses of vitamin C.

Major food sources (commonly consumed serves): Vitamin C is found in breast milk, fruits, vegetables, liver and other offal meats and oysters.

FOOD	VITAMIN C (mg)
Guava, 100 g	243
Pawpaw, 150 g	90
Orange, 1 medium	76
Kiwi fruit, 1 medium	72
Rambutan, 4 medium	70
Strawberries, $\frac{1}{2}$ punnet, 125 g	56
Grapefruit, 1 medium	54
Rockmelon, 150 g	51
Mango, 1 medium	50
Loquat, 3 medium	49
Lemon, 1 medium	48
Custard apple, 100 g	43
Mandarin, 1 medium	41
Quince, 1 small	39
Carambola (star fruit), 1 medium	35
Pepino, 1 medium	31
Pineapple, 100 g	31
Honeydew, 150 g	24
Sugar banana, 1 medium	23
Babaco, 100 g	23
Persimmon, 1 medium	20
Prickly pear, 1 medium	18
Apricots, 3 medium	16
Tamarillo, 1 large	15
Capsicum, red, 100 g	172
Brussels sprouts, 100 g	110
Broccoli, 100 g	106
Capsicum, green, 100 g	92
Kohlrabi, 100 g	71
Cauliflower, 100 g	70
Cabbage, 100 g	46
Broad beans, 100 g	41
Cassava, 100 g	40
Okra, 100 g	34
Peas, 100 g	32
Kumera, 100 g	31
Leek, 100 g	30
Potato, 1 medium	27
Swede or turnip, 100 g	27
Tomato, 1 medium	27
Scallopini, 100 g	26
Watercress, 25 g	25
Pumpkin, 100 g	24
Sweet potato, 100 g	24
Artichoke, 1 medium	24
Snow peas, 50 g	23
Beans, green, 100 g	21

Spinach, 75 g	20
Chilli, 10 g	20
Taro, 100 g	16
Asparagus, 100 g	15
Spring onion, 3	15
Parsley, 10 g	11
Pacific oysters, 8	22
Sweetbreads, cooked, 100 g	18
Brains, cooked, 100 g	17
Liver, cooked, 100 g	13

See also Dehydroascorbic acid.

Vitamin D

A fat soluble vitamin which exists in several forms. It was isolated as an anti-rickets factor in the 1920s. The various forms of vitamin D include 7-dehydrocholesterol (found in the skin) and ergocalciferol. These substances are converted in the liver to 25-hydroxy cholecalciferol and then to the active form of vitamin D, 1,25-dihydroxy cholecalciferol, in the kidneys.

Function: The active form of vitamin D is important for calcium and phosphate to be absorbed from the intestine into bones.

Deficiency: A lack of vitamin D results in rickets in children or osteomalacia in adults. In both cases, bones fracture easily and are misshapen. Without vitamin D, calcium cannot be used. A lack of vitamin D usually only occurs in people who never expose their skin to sunlight. This is common in some Middle Eastern countries among women who are totally covered. Some babies are wrapped in clothing which also prevents sunlight getting to their skin. In extremely cold climates, there can also be a problem in exposing skin to sunlight.

Toxicity: Vitamin D is the most toxic of all the vitamins. Taking even 5 times the daily requirement can be harmful. With excessive vitamin D, too much calcium is absorbed and some is deposited in soft tissues such as the spleen and kidneys. This situation occurred in some countries a few years ago when baby foods were fortified with vitamin D. Some babies died.

Excessive amounts of vitamin D do not arise from sunlight. The tanning of the skin provides a natural barrier to excessive formation of the vitamin.

Large doses of cod liver oil can easily provide toxic levels of vitamin D.

Stability: Cooking losses are negligible.

RDI: It is generally recommended that 10 mcg of vitamin D is required each day. This is most likely to come from the action of sunlight on the skin. Smog, cloud and dust will interfere with the ultraviolet light required to supply vitamin D. Taking these factors into account, a few hours total exposure of some part of the skin to sunlight each week will ensure adequate supplies. Because of its toxicity, no more than 10 mcg of vitamin D per day should be taken as a supplement or from fish liver oils.

Major food sources (commonly consumed serves): Most vitamin D comes from the action of ultraviolet light from the sun. Some is found in fatty fish, dairy products and margarine.

FOOD	VITAMIN D (mcg)
Cod liver oil, 20 mL	42
Herring or kippers, 100 g	25
Mackerel, 100 g	18
Salmon, fresh or canned, 100 g	13
Sardines, 100 g	8
Tuna, 100 g	6
Liver, 100 g	1
Egg, 1	1
Margarine, 20 g	2
Cream, 30 mL	1
Cheese, 30 g	1
Butter, 20 g	0.2
Milk, 250 mL	0.1

Vitamin E

A fat soluble vitamin which occurs in a number of forms, known as tocopherols. These substances have been ranked in their order of biological activity as alpha-tocopherol, beta-tocopherol, etc. The most potent form is d-alpha tocopherol. Beta-tocopherol has about 50 per cent as much biological activity while the gamma form has only about one-tenth the level.

Vitamin E was discovered in 1922 and recognised as being essential for reproduction in rats. It was not isolated chemically until 1938. The vitamin is used commercially as an antioxidant to prevent rancidity in fats and membranes.

It is found mainly in plant foods.

Function: Vitamin E is an important antioxidant which means that it prevents damage to cells from oxygen. It is particularly important to prevent damage to polyunsaturated fatty acids from free radicals (see page 137) and functions in this role with the mineral selenium. Vitamin E also prolongs the life span of red blood cells and may be involved in the formation of haemoglobin. It also provides protection against toxic chemicals such as ozone or nitrous oxide.

Although claims are made that vitamin E will prevent ageing, heart disease, or encourage super sexual prowess, there is no substantial evidence that it has such functions.

Deficiency: The only sign of a deficiency of vitamin E is anaemia in newborn babies. There have been some reports of vitamin E-deficient people having greater break down of red blood cells, nerve and muscle fibres. Deficiency is rare as there are considerable stores in the body.

Toxicity: Vitamin E is not very toxic. At doses of 300 mg/day, there have been reports of nausea and gastrointestinal upsets. In animals, large doses interfere with the normal functioning of the thyroid gland, stop vitamin D fulfilling its usual role and prevent the normal clotting of blood. Whether these effects occur in humans is not yet known.

Stability: Some vitamin E is lost in food processing, but cooking causes little loss. Cold pressed oils may have a greater level of alpha tocopherol than those extracted with solvents.

RDI: Usual requirement for adults is 8–10 mg/day (see chart, page 393).

Major food sources (commonly consumed serves): Most vitamin E comes from plants, especially seeds, seed oils and nuts. Seafoods also provide some.

FOOD	VITAMIN E (mg)
Wheatgerm, 1 tablespoon	2.2
Muesli, 60 g	2.0
(higher if seeds included)	
Processed bran cereal, 50 g	1.0
Wheat cereals, 30 g	0.5
Wheatgerm oil, 20 mL	26.5
Sunflower oil, 20 mL	9.7
Cottonseed oil, 20 mL	7.8
Safflower oil, 20 mL	7.7
Palm kernel oil, 20 mL	5.1
Cod liver oil, 20 mL	4.0
Rapeseed oil, 20 mL	3.7
Corn oil, 20 mL	2.2
Soya bean oil, 20 mL	2.0
Olive oil, 20 mL	1.0

Vitamin F

see Linolenic acid.

Vitamin H

see Biotin.

Vitamin K

A fat soluble vitamin isolated in 1939. Vitamin K is made by bacteria living in the human intestine and includes a number of substances including K_1, phylloquinone (found in plants); K_2, menaquinone or multiprenylmeanquinone (made by bacteria and present in some animal tissue); and K_3, menadione (which can be produced synthetically). K_2 has only 75 per cent of the activity of K_1 while K_3 has twice the activity of K_1.

Function: Vitamin K is essential for the normal clotting of blood. It is involved in the manufacture of 4 blood clotting proteins, including prothrombin. Vitamin K is also needed to make particular proteins in bone and in the kidneys. These proteins may influence the way calcium is used.

Deficiency: Haemorrhages and bleeding accompany a lack of vitamin K. This can be a problem in newborn babies since they are born with very limited stores of the vitamin. The intestine of a newborn baby is also free of bacteria which could make the vitamin. Some antibiotics also destroy the bacteria which normally make vitamin K. Those with any form of malabsorption such as can occur in untreated coeliac disease, diseases of the pancreas or with a heavy intake of alcohol, may also lack vitamin K.

Some drugs act as vitamin K antagonists. These include warfarin and other drugs used to reduce blood clotting in cases of thrombosis. Anyone taking such drugs needs to keep their intake of vitamin K relatively constant so as to stay in balance with the prescribed dose of the drug.

Toxicity: Few toxic effects have been reported, but large doses may cause haemolytic anaemia.

Stability: There is little loss of vitamin K during cooking. Prolonged exposure to oxygen and light will cause some losses.

RDI: Approximately 2 mcg per kilogram of body weight.

Major food sources (commonly consumed serves): The best sources of vitamin K are leafy green vegetables. Apart from liver, most animal foods contain very little. Vitamin K is also made by bacteria within the intestine.

FOOD	VITAMIN K (mcg)
Soya beans, 100 g	190
Spinach, 75 g	180
Cauliflower, 100 g	150
Cabbage, 100 g	125
Lettuce, 50 g	100
Broccoli, 100 g	100
Liver, beef, 100g	100
pig, 100 g	17
chicken, 100 g	7

VITAMINS, RECOMMENDED DAILY INTAKE (RDI)

	Age (years)	Vit. A (mg)	Thiamin (mg) B1	Riboflavin (mg) B2	Niacin (mg) B3	B6 (mg)	Folacin (mg)	B12 (mg)	C (mg)	E (mg)
Men	19–64	750	1.1	1.7	18–20	1.3–1.9	200	2.0	40	10.0
	65+	750	0.9	1.3	14–17	1.0–1.5	200	2.0	40	10.0
Women	19–54	750	0.8	1.2	12–14	0.9–1.4	200	2.0	30	7.0
	65+	750	0.7	1.0	10–12	0.8–1.1	200	2.0	30	7.0
Pregnant		750	1.0	1.5	14–16	1.0–1.5	400	3.0	60	7.0
Lactating		1200	1.2	1.7	17–19	1.6–2.2	300	3.5	60	9.5
Infants	0–1/2	425	0.3	0.4	4	0.25	50	0.3	25	2.5–4.0
	1/2–1	300	0.4	0.6	7	0.45	75	0.6	30	4.0
Children	1–3	300	0.5	0.8	9–10	0.6–0.9	100	1.0	30	5.0
	4–7	350	0.7	1.1	11–13	0.8–1.3	100	1.5	30	6.0
Boys	8–11	500	0.9	1.4	14–16	1.1–1.6	150	1.5	30	8.0
	12–15	725	1.2	1.8	19–21	1.4–2.1	200	2.0	30	10.5
	16–18	750	1.2	1.9	20–22	1.5–2.2	200	2.0	40	11.0
Girls	8–11	500	0.8	1.3	14–16	1.0–1.5	150	1.5	30	8.0
	12–15	725	1.0	1.6	17–19	1.2–1.8	200	2.0	30	9.0
	16–18	750	0.9	1.4	15–17	1.1–1.6	200	2.0	30	8.0

W

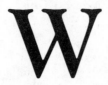

WAFFLES

A light, spongy batter made from flour, baking powder, eggs, milk and butter, cooked on a hot waffle iron which makes indentations in the finished product. Waffles are popular in Europe and North America. They are usually served as an afternoon tea treat or as a dessert with icecream and syrup. Commercially prepared frozen waffles may be heated in a home oven or toaster. Waffles have 1405 kJ/100 g (335 Cals) — approximately 360 kJ (85 Cals) for an average waffle or 1100 kJ (263 Cals) for a large waffle (75 g) — and contribute only small quantities of minerals and vitamins.

WAHOO
see Fish.

WAKAME
see Seaweed.

WALDORF SALAD
see Salads.

WALNUT
see Nuts.

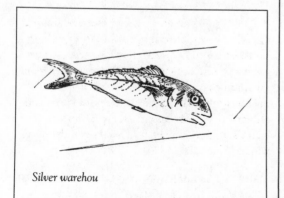

Silver warehou

WALNUT OIL
see Oils.

WAREHOU
see Fish.

WARFARIN

A drug used to prevent blood clotting. High doses of vitamins C or K can alter its action. A similar compound to warfarin is found in some types of clover and causes haemorrhages in cattle.

WASABI

The grated root of Japanese horse radish, a native plant that grows in the beds of mountain streams. Its hot flavour supposedly unlocks the subtle flavours of raw fish. Insufficient quantities are eaten for wasabi to make any nutritional contribution to the diet.

WATER

Water is more vital to life than food and the human body can survive only a few days without it. Around 50—60 per cent of the body's weight consists of water; leaner people having a higher percentage than those with greater levels of body fat.

Water exists both within the cells and around the cells in fluids, including the blood. Approximately two-thirds of the body's water is within cells and the remaining third is extracellular, or outside the cells. The body's water content can fluctuate to some extent but a drop of even 4 per cent can impair physical performance and lower the efficiency of the body. A lack of water leads to dehydration. A loss of 5—10 per cent of the body's water produces fatigue, mental confusion and apathy. If more than 20 per cent of the body's water is lost, death results.

Water is needed for the functioning of every cell and organ in the body. It is the solvent for all the body's chemical reactions. It transports nutrients, removes waste products, acts as a lubricant and maintains body temperature through sweating.

We obtain water from liquids and foods. Cooked meat is around 60 per cent water, fruits and vegetables contain 80−95 per cent water, cooked rice is over 70 per cent water and even bread is around 40 per cent water. The metabolism of proteins, fats and carbohydrates also produces water. Each day, most people take in more than a litre of water from food, about a litre and a half from fluids and obtain about 300 mL from the metabolism of food.

Water is lost from the body as sweat (at least 500 mL), expired air (about 350 mL), in faeces (about 150−200 mL) and in urine (more than 1500 mL per day). Heavy sweating during physical activity can lead to extra sweat losses of up to a litre an hour. Athletes therefore need to drink a great deal of extra water. Without it, performance falters.

Normally, we drink because we feel thirsty and thirst can be a good guide to water requirements. However, at times the thirst response takes too long to replace lost water. For example, after a heavy training session, an athlete who relies on thirst may take 48−72 hours to replace lost fluids. For athletes who train hard and regularly, more water is needed than thirst would dictate.

Heavy water losses can also occur with vomiting and diarrhoea and it is essential for recovery that victims of these conditions drink plenty of water. Severe burns can also lead to massive fluid losses.

Water retention can occur in the body but, contrary to popular belief, it is not usually the cause of excess body weight. Many women retain fluid just before menstruation and a few also have a temporary retention of fluid at the time of ovulation. This occurs because alterations in female hormones retain extra sodium in the body. Eating less salt and drinking more water to flush out the excess sodium give relief from the condition. Many women make the situation worse by trying not to drink anything, incorrectly believing that this will prevent greater fluid retention. When we feel thirsty and drink more water after a salty meal, the extra water 'flushes out' the salt. The same situation is necessary to remove the excess sodium which causes fluid retention.

How much water?
The exact quantity of water required depends on the individual. The body's surface area, the degree of physical activity and the sodium content of the diet will determine how much water is appropriate. For most people, 1.5−2.5 litres of water should be consumed each day. Both coffee and alcohol have a diuretic action in the body and at least some of the body's water requirements should come from other sources.

Hard or soft?
Hard water contains a high level of minerals such as calcium and magnesium and is more alkaline than soft water. Several studies reported less heart disease in areas where the water is hard. Whether this is due to the minerals in the water, or is simply a coincidence, is not yet resolved.

Hard water can affect the colour and texture of boiled vegetables. It does not lather well and for this reason, people in hard water areas may use water softeners which use an ion-exchange mechanism to replace the calcium and magnesium with sodium. If the hard water and reduction in heart disease theory is correct, water softeners may be undesirable for drinking water.

Mineral water
Water from springs in the ground or wells is

sold as mineral water. It may contain dissolved minerals including bicarbonate, sodium, chloride, sulphate, calcium, carbonate, magnesium, potassium, iron, fluoride and other minerals. In most products, the content of minerals reflects the natural mineral content of the water used. Some manufacturers may add small quantities of minerals, although this is now rare.

The actual quantity of minerals in most products is not much more than in most tap waters. Any alleged health properties are likely to be due to the placebo effect. Some mineral waters have a high sodium (salt) content; most of those on sale in countries such as Australia are now low in sodium. With 40–70 mg sodium/L, a glass of mineral water has only as much sodium as occurs naturally in a tablespoon of milk.

Most mineral waters are slightly alkaline. They may be still, naturally carbonated or they may be carbonated at the bottling plant. The addition of carbon dioxide has no harmful effects, but may cause burping.

Mineral waters are supposed to be good for health. In fact, their main advantage is in providing a socially acceptable non-kilojoule drink which acts as a useful alternative to sugary or alcoholic beverages. Bottled waters are certainly a healthier alternative in parts of the world where the local water supply is heavily contaminated.

Soda water

In the United States, soda water is referred to as 'club soda'. In the United Kingdom, Australia and New Zealand, soda water is a carbonated water. It has no added sugar and provides no kilojoules. The sodium content is usually low, although a few North American club sodas may have higher levels.

WATER CHESTNUTS
see Vegetables.

WATERCRESS
see Vegetables.

WATERMELON
see Fruit.

WATTLE
see Acacia.

WAX JAMBU
see Fruit.

WEANING FOODS

When an infant is about 6 months of age, small quantities of semi-solid foods are usually introduced. Over the ensuing 6 months, as the baby's teeth come through, the solid foods become more important and milk less so. Somewhere between 1 and 2 years of age, most babies are weaned from the breast or bottle onto solid foods. Milk, usually from cows, goats or soya beans, remains important as a source of protein, riboflavin and calcium (some of these nutrients are added to soya bean products for babies).

The order of introduction of foods into an infant's diet is relatively unimportant and should basically fit in with the usual family habits. Most babies begin having some cereal food; a few mothers prefer to begin with mashed fruits. Vegetables, pureed meats, fish and chicken follow until the child is eating a range of foods. The general family foods, chopped or mashed as appropriate, are quite suitable for weaning foods.

In some Third World countries, infants' diets deteriorate badly once the child is weaned. Foods of poor nutritional quality are given and gastrointestinal infections become common. In some areas, health workers have formulated special combinations of local foods in an effort to design a more complete weaning diet.

WEIGHT

Body weight represents the weight of the

bones, muscles, organs, fat and water present in the body. The most variable of these is the water which can be manipulated to give rises or falls of several kilograms in a day. There is no one exact weight which is correct for everyone of a certain height or frame size. The Body Mass Index (see page 40) gives an indication of the range of weights which are appropriate for people of different heights. There is no adjustment for age since there is no physiological reason for people to grow heavier as they become older. The fact that so many people in Western societies do is due to an overabundance of food and a lack of physical activity. See also the chart on page 7.

Excess fat can take up residence over most parts of the body. From the point of view of increased health risk, upper body fat creates the greatest hazard. Those who are fat in these areas have an increased risk of coronary heart disease, high blood pressure, diabetes, gallstones and certain types of cancer. Those whose excess fat is around the hips and thighs have fewer health risks associated with their weight.

Weight reduction is sensible for those with excess upper body fat. It will require:
- A reduction in the amount of fat eaten
- A reduction in the amount of sugar eaten
- A reduction in the amount of alcohol consumed
- An eating pattern not too far removed from current eating habits
- A possible increase in the quantity of foods containing dietary fibre and complex carbohydrate
- An acceptance that excess body fat can only be lost slowly
- Some type of exercise, such as walking, for at least 5 sessions of 20 minutes duration each week
- An acceptance of the fact that there is no fast, easy or magical way to remove body fat
- An acceptance of basic body shape
  Ideally there should be a balance between

the kilojoules from food and drinks entering the body on one side, and the kilojoules being used up in metabolism, physical activity and growth (in the case of children).

In Western society, many people have increased their intake of high kilojoule foods and drinks while decreasing their physical activity. The result is an increasing number of people with excess weight.

Effective weight reduction involves taking in less kilojoules than are being used by the body. The catch is that if you cut back very strictly and take in too few kilojoules, the body will simply burn less energy. Physical activity becomes more difficult and it therefore makes more sense for weight reduction to involve a moderate reduction in kilojoules with an increase in physical activity.

WEIGHT REDUCTION

There are considerable health risks associated with being overweight (see page 256). For this reason, the many people in Western societies who are overweight are usually advised to reduce their weight. Most are remarkably unsuccessful.

Weight reduction should involve a loss of fat from the body. Most weight reduction diets operate on the principle of weight loss from a loss of water. Loss of muscle accompanies this. Such diets may produce a quick weight loss but, in the longer term, they are worse than useless.

Weight reduction has become a search for a quick, easy, painless way to remove excess body fat. Even though the fat took many months, or perhaps years, to accumulate, most people want instant gratification and seek ways to lose weight in the minimum of time. Hence the succession of crazy weight reduction diets.

Most popular weight reduction diets work on a principle of reducing carbohydrate levels in the diet. With such a diet, the body is forced to use up its stores of glycogen (see page 165) in muscles. Since every gram of glycogen is stored with about 3 g of water, the loss of glycogen and its associated water shows up as a good weight loss on the scales. In reality, fat loss with such diets is minimal.

Many women also embark on weight reduction diets when they are not even overweight. Western society has placed such a high premium on women being thin that many perfectly normal and healthy-sized women have come to believe they are in need of weight reduction. Unfortunately, those who jump on the dieting merry-go-round may become fat in the future. This occurs because strict weight reduction diets cause a reduction in the muscle content of the body. Since muscle burns far more kilojoules than fat, a loss of muscle means a reduction in the body's kilojoule needs. After following many weight reduction diets, some women find they can no longer eat a normal amount of food without gaining weight.

WEIGHT WATCHERS

An organisation which has been involved in weight reduction for over 25 years. Begun by Jean Neiditch in New York, the Weight Watchers program is now followed in 25 countries and its meetings are attended by approximately half a million people each week. The program has 4 main elements:

- An eating plan which is nutritionally well-balanced, providing approximately 5000 kJ (1200 Cals) for women and 6300 kJ (1500 Cals) for men. An adolescent's program with slightly more than the men's program is also available.
- A graded exercise plan which gives members a choice of physical exercises at a range of levels. Members are encouraged to work their way up to the higher levels of the exercise plan.
- A behaviour modification plan which aims to help members become aware of the eating and exercise habits which made them fat in the first place. Leaders teach techniques to put changes in behaviour into practice.
- Group support. The success of Weight

Watchers is thought to be due to the members' understanding of each other's problems with excess weight. Each leader is a successful slimmer.

The Weight Watchers program does not offer a quick solution but is involved in teaching people how to buy, prepare and cook foods. Choices are designed so that members will lose weight and keep the weight off.

WEISSWURST
see Sausages.

WENSLEYDALE
see Cheese.

WERNICKE'S ENCEPHALOPATHY

Carl Wernicke was an eminent German neurologist who found that specific nerve disorders were related to particular areas of the brain. The condition which bears his name occurs when excessive alcohol intake leads to a deficiency of thiamin. Symptoms of the syndrome include gaps in memory. An associated disorder is Korsakoff's psychosis in which the memory gaps are filled with disturbing fantasies.

WEST INDIAN CHERRY
see Fruits, Acerola.

WHEAT
see Grains.

WHEATGERM

The germ or embryo of the wheat grain from which a new plant could be grown. Wheatgerm is rich in nutrients, as would be expected for the part of the grain which would initially support the life of the grain.

Wheatgerm is high in protein, dietary fibre (including both insoluble and soluble forms), iron, zinc, several other minerals, and vitamins E and the B complex. It also contains about 9 per cent fat, most of which is polyunsaturated.

Wheatgerm is removed from the wheat grain during the making of flour. Its removal is partly to produce a white flour and partly because its polyunsaturated fat content would quickly become rancid.

In making most wholemeal breads, the germ is returned to the flour.

Wheatgerm is used in biscuits, cakes, breads and other bakery products. It is also sprinkled over porridge or other breakfast cereals. 1 tablespoon of wheatgerm (10 g) has 125 kJ (30 Cals).

WHEATGERM OIL
see Oils.

WHELKS
see Seafood.

WHEY

The liquid left after milk has been coagulated to curds and whey and the curds have been removed. Whey has no special nutritional virtues, apart from the fact that it has almost no fat.

It contains a high quantity of lactose and products made from it can be a problem for those who have a lactase deficiency (see page 200). Ricotta cheese is made from whey.

WHISKY
see Drinks, Alcoholic.

WHISKY SOUR
see Drinks, Alcoholic.

WHITEBAIT
see Fish.

WHITENERS, COFFEE

A synthetic powdered product designed to replace milk in coffee. It is used by those wishing to avoid the fat in milk. However, most coffee whiteners will add more fat to coffee than regular milk. The products usually contain hydrogenated palm or coconut oil plus

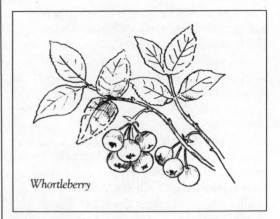

Whortleberry

corn or glucose syrup (a form of sugar), sodium caseinate (extracted from milk) and emulsifiers. They generally have as many kilojoules as the milk they are replacing — sometimes even more. One teaspoon of coffee whitener has 90 kJ (22 Cals).

WHITE RADISH
see Vegetables, Radish.

WHITING
see Fish.

WHOLEFOODS

Foods which are consumed with their edible parts intact. For example, products made from the whole of the wheat grain would be wholefoods; so would rolled oats or whole milk or sunflower seeds. In general, nutritionists recommend that more wholefoods are consumed. This usually provides a better balance of nutrients, especially more dietary fibre in the case of wholegrain cereal foods and fruits.

It is mainly by the process of refining foods that we create the possibility for imbalances in the diet. For example, it is difficult to chew enough sunflower seeds to take in an excess of fat but it becomes quite easy when the oil is removed from the seeds and converted into a concentrated margarine. Fruits also provide an example. Few people will overconsume apples when they have to crunch their way through the whole apple. When apples are processed to form apple juice, however, it becomes easy to consume 5 or 6 apples in a very short time. Wholefoods usually discourage overconsumption.

WHOLEGRAINS

Grains which are eaten along with their germ and bran. Wholegrain products have more dietary fibre as well as a higher level of minerals and vitamins. Some, such as wholewheat, also contain phytic acid which can form chemical complexes with minerals such as iron, zinc and calcium. However, since the wholewheat grain is rich in these minerals, the phytic acid only complexes with some of the minerals in the grain itself. Even taking this into account, the higher initial level of nutrients in the wholegrain product compared with refined grains means that the wholegrain contributes a higher level of nutrients.

See also Phytic acid.

WHOLEMEAL BREAD

Bread made from 90−100 per cent wholemeal flour. With its high content of dietary fibre and more complete array of minerals and vitamins, wholemeal bread is nutritionally superior to white bread.

See also Bread.

WHORTLEBERRY
see Fruit, Bilberry.

WINE

Wines have been made from fermented fruits, especially grapes, for thousands of years. Some grapes make better wines than others. The major reason for using grapes in preference to many other fruits is that they contain enough sugar to reach a fairly high level of alcohol but are acidic enough to prevent other bacteria spoiling the brew. Both the sugar and acidity influence the wine's keeping qualities as well as its final flavour. The balance of sugar and acid depends to a great extent on the climate in which the grapes are grown.

In making wine, the grapes are crushed, then fermented by yeasts which turn the sugar into alcohol. Red wines are made by fermenting the whole grape, including the skin. White wines can be made from green grapes or from red grapes without their skins. Once fermented, wines are then left to mature. This occurs either in stainless steel tanks, oak barrels or in the bottle.

Most table wines are fermented until all the sugar has been converted to alcohol. In making sweet wines, fermentation is stopped at a stage when some sugar still remains. To achieve the necessary sweetness, most dessert wines are made from grapes which have been left on the vine long enough to develop a high sugar content. Dessert wines include cream sherry (sweet, heavy and richly flavoured), Madeira (rather like a sweeter, darker sherry), marsala (used in Italian desserts), muscat (rich sweet wine made from muscatel grapes), port and tokay (a slightly nutty flavour).

Sparkling wines are made by natural fermentation (see Champagne) or, in the case of some very cheap products, are carbonated.

Most wines have about 10 per cent alcohol. An average 125 mL glass has about 460 kJ (110 Cals) and contains appoximately 13 g of alcohol. White wines generally have as much alcohol as red wines.

Some people have adverse reactions to wines. These may take the form of a sensitivity to the amines present, producing headaches or other symptoms (see page 21). Shiraz grapes are especially high in amines. White wines, on the other hand, may have a higher level of the preservative sodium metabisulphite and this can produce asthma or other reactions in sensitive people.

On the whole, however, there seem to be few nutritional problems in those who drink moderate quantities of wine. Heavy consumption (see Alcohol) causes considerable problems.

WINE, VARIETIES

Albillo
A grape variety used to produce sherry.

Blanquette
Also known as clairette, a grape used extensively in the South of France, blended with trebbiano to produce white wines with a fruity aroma. Grown in Australia.

Cabernet sauvignon
A variety of grape used for premium quality red wines, especially in Australia, the Bordeaux region of France, Chili and California. The wines have a fruity flavour and mature well.

Carignane
A variety of grape used for red wines and representing the most extensively grown variety in France. Also very commonly grown in California but not used to any extent in Australia.

Chablis
A dry, crisp, fruity white wine made from several varieties of grape.

Champagne
A sparkling wine made in the district of Champagne in France. Made from chardonnay, pinot and meunier grapes. It is allowed to undergo its first fermentation in the cask until it stops fermenting temporarily and is transferred to strong bottles. The second fermentation occurs in the bottles, producing a naturally sparkling wine. Vintage champagne is made from wines only of that particular year. Blended champagne is made from wines of different years, blended to produce the right flavour. For the first 3 months after bottling, champagne is gradually hand moved until the bottles are upside down and any impurities have collected on the cork. After some time standing in this position, the cork is released and the sediment removed. A small quantity of sugar may then be added before recorking. If no sugar is added, the champagne is labelled 'brut'. More sugar earns the word 'sec', followed by 'demi-sec' and finally 'doux' for the sweetest.

Champagne is absorbed more rapidly than most other alcoholic drinks. This is because the carbon dioxide relaxes the valve between the stomach and the upper part of the small intestine so the champagne quickly passes to this region and is rapidly absorbed into the blood. A 125 mL glass of champagne has 420 kJ (100 Cals).

Chardonnay
A grape grown extensively in northern France and used in the making of champagne as well as a dry white wine. Also grown extensively in California and Australia.

Chasselas
A grape variety used to make mild, fruity-flavoured white wines, especially in Alsace, parts of Germany and Switzerland (where it is called 'fendant'). In Australia it is used to make champagne-style wines.

Chenin blanc
A light-bodied, fragrant white wine which varies from being very dry to semi-sweet.

Chianti
An Italian wine, either red or white, with a dry, slightly tart flavour. Often presented in a raffia covered bottle.

Cinsaut
A grape grown for red wines, especially in South Africa (where it is incorrectly called 'hermitage'). Also used for port.

Doradillo
A grape variety used principally in making neutral flavoured wines to be distilled to produce brandy in Spain and Australia.

Frontignan

Red grapes from these vines are used in northern Victoria (Australia) to produce rich muscats. Green frontignan grapes can also be used to produce white table wines with a fruity flavour.

Grenache

A grape variety used to produce red wines, especially in parts of France and California. Also used for rose wine. Red wines made from grenache have a light fresh style but lack the character of some other red wines.

Malbec

A grape variety used for making red wines, especially in the Bordeaux region, Argentina and, to some extent, in Australia. The wines are rich in colour and tannin.

Mataro

A grape variety, also known as burgundy, and grown in small quantities in Australia, California and France. Used for red wines and ports.

Merlot

A grape variety used to make red wines, especially in France. Wines which include merlot grapes have a deep purple colour and a smoothness of taste.

Palomino

A grape variety used in making sherry, especially in Spain, California, South Africa and Australia. Not suitable for table wines.

Pinot noir

A grape variety which grows successfully in colder climates, especially in Germany, northern France and Switzerland. Used for red wines and also one of the main varieties grown for champagne (the pinot provides fullness to champagne while chardonnay gives a more delicate bouquet and elegance).

Rhine riesling

The premium grape variety of Germany, also

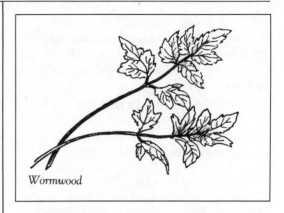

Wormwood

grown in Italy, Austria, Switzerland, Chile, California, South America and Australia. Wines made from this grape are fruity but crisp and have somewhat higher acidity levels than many white wines.

Sauterne

Sweet dessert wines from the Bordeaux district of France. These wines achieve their unique flavour partly from very late picking of the grapes, but also from the action of a mould which grows on the grapes in times of high humidity.

This mould damages the skin of the grapes, and when the weather becomes dry, some of the water in the grapes evaporates through the skin, leaving a grape with a very high sugar concentration. The mould also leaves the grape with a higher content of glycerol and less acid and this contributes to the smoothness of the finished product. 125 mL sauterne has 495 kJ (118 Cals).

Sauvignon blanc

A grape variety grown in France, California, and recently in Australia. Also grows well in hot climates and produces soft white wines.

Semillon

Used for making dry white wines, especially in the Bordeaux region of France (where it represents the major planting), other areas of France, California, Australia and South Africa.

Shiraz

Also known as 'hermitage', this grape is used in making red wines, especially those produced in Australia, and the Hermitage region of the Rhône valley. The colder the region in which shiraz grapes are grown, the greater the intensity of colour, tannin and acid, and consequently, the 'heavier' the wine. Shiraz grapes have a higher content of the types of amines which produce headaches in susceptible people. Many people who avoid all red wines need only avoid those made from shiraz grapes.

Sultana

A grape variety used for dry and sweet wines, sparkling wines and sherry. Very commonly used in California where the grape is known as 'Thompson seedless'.

Tokay

A grape variety which originated in Hungary and used to produce somewhat sweet wines with a higher alcohol content. Also used for fortified sweet dessert wines, sherry, or, occasionally, a rich full-flavoured table wine.

Tramminer

Also known as gewurztramminer, this grape variety is produced mainly in Alsace and other parts of France, with some plantings in Germany and Australia. The white wines produced are aromatic, spicy and strongly flavoured.

Trebbiano

Also known as white shiraz, this grape variety originated in Italy and is commonly grown in the south of France and Australia. In Italy, trebbiano is one of the wines used to make chianti. In other areas it is used alone or with other varieties to produce a dry white wine.

WINKLES
see Seafood.

WINTERGREEN

A small evergreen shrub which is a member of the heath family. Its leaves produce an oil which is used in linaments. Children with food sensitivity are often sensitive to this compound.

WINTER MELON
see Fruits.

WINTER SQUASH
see Vegetables, Pumpkin.

WITCHETTY GRUB

The true witchetty grub is the larvae of a large Australian moth of the genus *Xyleutes*. In some areas, any large white grubs are called witchetty grubs. The grubs can be eaten raw or roasted, but the heads are not usually eaten. The flavour is rich and almost nutty. Witchetty grubs are high in protein and rich in fat. 100 g (about 4 grubs) have 1150 kJ (275 Cals) and 19 g of fat.

WITLOOF
see Vegetables.

WONTONS

Small squares of pasta dough with a filling of meat (usually minced pork) and vegetables, either steamed or deep fried. Often served in soups as part of a Chinese meal.
  See also Short soup.

WORCESTERSHIRE SAUCE
see Sauces.

WORMWOOD

A bitter or aromatic herb whose leaves are used in making absinthe. White wormwood is eaten as a vegetable.
  See also Vegetables.

XANTHAN GUM

A gum produced by controlled fermentation of bacteria known as *Xanthomonas campestris* and containing glucose, mannose and glucuronic acid. Like other gums, xanthan is a form of soluble dietary fibre which forms a gel in the stomach (see Dietary fibre). It is fermented by bacteria in the large intestine. Used as a food additive in mayonnaise, dressings, desserts, icecream and drinks to provide 'body'. Food additive no. 415.

XANTHINES

Part of the group of substances known as purines. A related group of substances known as methyl xanthines include caffeine, theobromine and theophylline found in coffee, cocoa and tea respectively. These substances have a stimulating effect but do not accumulate in the body as they are rapidly excreted by the kidneys. Formerly used as diuretics to remove water from the body.

Uric acid is formed from the xanthines in purines found in some foods (see Purines). An enzyme, xanthine oxidase, catalyses the conversion of xanthines to uric acid. This can be a problem for those with gout (see page 168) and certain drugs can prevent the action of xanthine oxidase. The xanthines accumulate instead of uric acid and can be easily excreted by the kidneys.

XANTHOPHYLLS

Varieties of carotenoid or yellow pigments partly responsible for the colour of egg yolk, corn, pineapple, potatoes, onions and wheat flour. Flour for white bread (but not pasta) is bleached to remove xanthophylls. There is no nutritional reason for this process. If added to foods, listed as food additive no. 161.

XANTHURENIC ACID

One of the intermediate products in the metabolism of the amino acid tryptophan. Vitamin B_6 is required for the conversion of xanthurenic acid to other substances. A build up of xanthurenic acid indicates a deficiency of B_6. Measurement of xanthurenic acid after a known tryptophan load is used to determine B_6 deficiency.

XEROPHTHALMIA

A condition of the eye in which the conjunctiva of the eye becomes dry and hard. The cornea is then affected, becomes ulcerated and cloudy and eventually leads to blindness. Xerophthalmia is caused by a deficiency of vitamin A which normally keeps the lining of the cornea moist. Xerophthalmia due to vitamin A deficiency is the commonest cause of blindness in children and occurs all too often in poor areas of the world.

XYLITOL

A sweetener which occurs naturally in fruits and vegetables, especially in strawberries, raspberries and cauliflower. It is also produced commercially from wood. It is used as a sweetener in foods in some countries and is almost as sweet as sugar. Xylitol is classed as a 5-carbon sugar-alcohol. Its major advantage is that it does not cause dental caries and may even confer some protective effects on teeth. This occurs because xylitol blocks the uptake of glucose by the bacteria which cause tooth decay. Xylitol can also be heated or frozen without losing its sweet taste to any major extent. The major disadvantage of xylitol is that it causes diarrhoea if used in large quantities. The quantity will depend on the individual and xylitol is less of a problem in this regard than sorbitol. However, if diarrhoea develops after use, it should be discontinued.

XYLOSE

A 5-carbon sugar which is a form of dietary fibre. Found (in descending order of quantity) in guavas, spinach, pears, peas, blackberries, loganberries, raspberries, dried beans (such as haricot or kidney), swedes, cabbage, broccoli, green beans, okra and eggplant.

YABBIES

A freshwater crayfish. See Seafood.

YAM

see Vegetables.

YAM BEAN

see Vegetables, Jicama.

YEAST

Yeasts are living single-celled fungi which feed on sugar to produce alcohol and carbon dioxide. Some are a nuisance as they cause fruits and vegetables to rot or give rise to particular diseases (see Candida); other types are useful for making bread or beer. Yeasts make proteins and vitamins, especially the B complex vitamins, as they grow. This is why yeast extracts (Vegemite or Marmite) are such potent sources of these vitamins.

Baker's yeast is a strain of yeast which produces a lot of carbon dioxide but little alcohol. The yeasts used in making beer produce much more alcohol. In making sparkling wines and champagne, some of the carbon dioxide produced by the yeast is retained in the bottle.

Originally, raised breads were made using yeast taken from brewing (see Bread, page 43). Today, different types of yeast are produced for specific purposes.

Baker's yeast is made from molasses and water. Compressed yeast is partly dried and pressed into solid cakes. It should crumble easily, be a light cream colour and smell fresh and slightly alcoholic. If it has dried edges or smells stale, do not use it as it will be dead and will not cause dough to rise. Compressed yeast is activated by mixing it with a small quantity of warm water and leaving for 5 – 10 mins. It can be frozen.

Dried (or 'active') yeast has only about 8 per cent moisture. It must be kept perfectly dry until ready to be used. As soon as it is wet, it begins to 'work'. It can withstand much warmer water than compressed yeast and is most active at 41° to 43°C (105° to 110°F). During baking, all yeast is killed by the high temperatures.

Brewer's yeasts may be of two types. One falls to the bottom of the tank after fermentation, the other stays as a top-fermenting yeast (see Beer). In making beer, when the yeast cells die, their contents of B vitamins and protein are released into the brew. Unfortunately, since most people prefer clear beer, the dead yeast cells are filtered out. With them go most of the vitamins and protein.

Spent brewer's yeast is sometimes used as a food supplement. If does indeed have a high content of B vitamins and protein and also a high content of minerals such as chromium and selenium. Unfortunately, brewer's yeast also has a bitter taste. It is high in purines and is unsuitable for anyone with gout (see page 168).

Baker's yeast ('active' yeast) is not a suitable food as it destroys B complex vitamins in the intestine. It also causes digestive upsets as it continues to ferment in the intestine. Its own vitamins (present in much smaller quantities than in brewer's yeast) are not digested in the human intestine.

Torula yeast is made from wood cellulose or from sugar. The former is the more expensive. Torula yeasts are cultivated as a food supplement. They are high in protein and almost all of the B complex vitamins.

Special yeast products known as autolysed yeast extracts are also produced. These are used to intensify flavourings in foods such as soups and sauces. Their ability to 'boost' flavours comes from their high content of various nucleotides and monosodium glutamate.

See also Alcohol.

YIN AND YANG

In Eastern philosophy, yin and yang represent the two complementary forces of life. Yin is female, passive, receiving and conceived of earth and is represented in foods by fruit, dairy products, sugar, liquids and alcohol. Yang is male, light, active, penetrating and conceived of heaven. It is represented in foods by meat, animal foods and salt. Vegetables and grains are central and are considered neither yin nor yang. The macrobiotic diet (see page 214) is based on the principles of yin and yang. Western medicine does not recognise any scientific validity in the principles of yin and yang as they are applied to the diet.

YOGHURT

Milk which is soured by the use of bacteria, usually *lactobacillus bulgaricus* or *acidophilus* or *streptococcus thermophilus*. These bacteria break down some of the lactose in milk to form lactic

acid which thickens the milk and gives a slightly sour taste. The milk of cows, sheep, goats or buffalo can be used. In most Western countries, cow's milk is used whereas Middle Eastern countries use milk from goats or sheep. There is little nutritional superiority in any of these types.

The origins of yoghurt (or laban) remain a matter for argument. The Bulgarians and the Turks both claim it as their own but others maintain that it was discovered by accident by some nomads who carried milk in leather pouches made from sheep's stomachs. The bacteria present plus the warmth of the milk produced yoghurt which set in the cooler temperatures overnight. Whatever the real beginnings of yoghurt, it appears to be as old as recorded history.

Yoghurt has several reasons for being so popular. In areas without refrigeration, the bacteria in yoghurt prevent the growth of some other types of harmful microbes, thus making yoghurt a safer product than milk. The bacteria in yoghurt also change some of the lactose to lactic acid so that yoghurt can be eaten by those who are lactase deficient (see page 200). The tangy taste of yoghurt also contributes to its popularity.

Some of the claims made for yoghurt, however, cannot be substantiated. Its bacteria will not colonise the human intestine and wipe out harmful bacteria, as is often claimed. It will not, in itself, contribute to longevity.

Most yoghurts are made from milk (either regular or low-fat) with added milk solids. The milk is warmed and a small amount of a previous batch of yoghurt is added to introduce the bacteria. The mixture is kept warm for several hours until sufficient bacteria have built up to convert much of the lactose to lactic acid. This acid then curdles and thickens the mixture. Flavoured yoghurts have added sugar and fruit.

Sometimes yoghurt is drained by placing it in a cheesecloth-lined colander and allowing some of the water to drip out. This thickened product is also called yoghurt cheese.

Yoghurt can be eaten by itself, used as a topping for desserts or served on potatoes or with salads. It is also good to use in cooking Middle Eastern dishes, making cold soups, desserts, icecream or cakes and it can be added to sauces in place of sour cream. Since yoghurt will curdle when boiled, it should be brought to room temperature first, a small amount of the hot sauce mixed in with it, and then the yoghurt added to the bulk of the sauce. Heat gently without boiling. A small amount of

cream cheese added with yoghurt will prevent curdling.

Nutritionally, yoghurt is like a concentrated milk product. It is an excellent source of calcium, protein and riboflavin and contributes small quantities of other vitamins and minerals. A 200 g carton of natural yoghurt averages 670 kJ (160 Cals). The same quantity of low-fat yoghurt has 440 kJ (105 Cals) while the flavoured yoghurts average 795 kJ (190 Cals) and 695 kJ (165 Cals) for regular and low-fat varieties.

See also Milk.

Z

ZABAGLIONE

An Italian dessert made from egg yolks, marsala and sugar whisked in a double saucepan until thick. Usually served with sponge finger biscuits and/or fresh fruit. An average serve of zabaglione has 700 kJ (167 Cals).

ZEN DIET

see Macrobiotic diet.

ZEST

The fine outside part of the rind of citrus fruits (without the creamy white pith) is called the zest. It can be removed with a fine peeler and used to flavour custards, desserts, cakes or savoury dishes. The citrus oil in the zest provides a distinctive flavour and avoids the curdling effect which may come from using cirtrus juice to flavour some foods.

See also Rind.

ZINC

Zinc is an essential mineral for humans and approximately 2−3 g is found in bones, the skin, liver, pancreas, kidney, brain, red blood

cells, the eye and prostate gland.

Like many other minerals, zinc is part of many enzymes which catalyse various reactions in the body. It is important in wound healing, in the storage of insulin in the pancreas, in growth and reproduction, for the manufacture of some proteins and has a role in the structure of cell membranes. A zinc-containing protein in saliva is also involved in taste.

As is the case with iron, the more zinc you need, the greater the amount you absorb from foods. After breaking a fast, large amounts of zinc can be absorbed. Those who fast may need to be especially careful if they also take supplements. Phytic acid in grains and phosphates in soya beans and some cereal products can also interfere with the absorption of zinc. Those who use soya bean milk in preference to cow's milk will absorb less zinc. Very high doses of unprocessed bran can also reduce the absorption of zinc; 1−2 tablespoons a day will not cause problems. Some factor, as yet unidentified, in breast milk, also increases the absorption of zinc. Even though cow's milk has more zinc than breast milk,

ZINC

more is absorbed from the latter.

Deficiencies of zinc have occurred in parts of the world where the daily diet lacks zinc and intake of phytic acid from grains is high. Sexual maturation was absent under these conditions. A lack of zinc also occurs in heavy drinkers and in those whose diets consist mainly of vegetables and cereals. Symptoms include a lack of taste sensation, slow healing of sores and wounds, failure to grow and reduced sperm count. A lack of zinc cannot be reliably diagnosed by hair analysis.

Excessive amounts of zinc are dangerous. Even 10 times the recommended daily intake can present a health hazard. Symptoms of zinc toxicity include dehydration, diarrhoea, nausea, abdominal pains, dizziness and lethargy.

Daily requirement for zinc

Women	12–16 mg
during pregnancy	16–21 mg
during lactation	18–24 mg
Men	12–16 mg
Infants	1–3 mg
Children, 1–3 years	4.5–6 mg
4–7 years	6–9 mg
8–11 years	9–14 mg
12–18 years	12–18 mg

Food sources of zinc

FOOD	ZINC (mg)
Rolled oats, raw weight, 100 g	3.0
Unprocessed bran, 2 tablespoons	2.4
Rice, brown, raw weight, 100 g	1.8
Rice, white, raw weight, 100 g	1.3
Muesli, 60 g	1.3
Wholemeal bread, 2 slices	1.0
Puffed wheat, 30 g	0.8
White bread, 2 slices	0.4
Yoghurt, 200 g carton	1.3
Cheese, 30 g	1.2
Milk, regular or skim, 250 mL	0.9
Egg, 1	0.8

Oxtail, cooked, 100 g	8.8
Beef, cooked, 150 g	6.9
Liver, cooked, 100 g	6.0
Veal chops, cooked, 2	3.4
Kidney, cooked, 100 g	3.1
Pork steak, lean, cooked, 100 g	2.7
Lamb chops, grilled, 2	2.6
Chicken legs, cooked, 100 g	2.4
Ham, 50 g	1.1
Oysters, 1 dozen	54.0
Crab, cooked, 100 g	5.5
Prawns, cooked, 100 g	5.3
Sardines, 100 g	3.0
Tuna or salmon, canned, 100 g	0.8
Fish fillet, cooked, 150 g	0.6
Dried beans, raw weight, 100 g	2.8
Cassava, cooked, 100 g	2.4
Peas, 100 g	1.0
Av. serve of vegetable	0.2
Av. piece of fruit	0.2
Brazil nuts, 50 g	2.1
Almonds, 50 g	1.6
Peanuts, 50 g	1.5
Hazel nuts, 50 g	1.2
Walnuts, 50 g	1.0
Dried yeast, 10 g	0.8
Cocoa, 2 teaspoons	0.7

ZUCCHINI
see Vegetables.
ZUCCHINI FLOWERS

The flowers from zucchini plants, dipped into flour or a very light batter and fried, are considered a delicacy. They contain vitamin C, iron and calcium as well as small quantities of carotene and the B complex vitamins. 10 g of the actual flowers have only 10 kJ (2 Cals) — an insignificant quantity compared with the oil used for frying them.

ZWIEBACK

Literally meaning 'twice-baked', zwieback is a rusk of German origin. It is made from a sweet yeasted dough, baked as a loaf, cooled, sliced and the slices are then dried out in the oven until they are crisp and golden. Each slice has approximately 230 kJ (55 Cals).